Microsoft Word
for
Healthcare Documentation

A Guide for Transcriptionists, Editors, and Health Information Professionals

D1441675

Microsoft Word
for
Healthcare Documentation

A Guide for Transcriptionists, Editors, and Health Information Professionals

LAURA BRYAN, MT (ASCP), CMT, AHDI-F

Wolters Kluwer | Lippincott Williams & Wilkins
Health

Philadelphia · Baltimore · New York · London
Buenos Aires · Hong Kong · Sydney · Tokyo

Publisher: *Julie K. Stegman*
Acquisitions Editor: *Pete Sabatini*
Editorial Manager: *Eric Branger*
Managing Editor: *Amy Millholen*
Compositor: *Cadmus Communication*
Printer: *C&C Offset*

351 West Camden Street
Baltimore, Maryland 21201

530 Walnut Street
Philadelphia, Pennsylvania 19106

Printed in China

Library of Congress Cataloging-in-Publication Data

Bryan, Laura, 1963–
    Microsoft Word for healthcare documentation : a guide for transcriptionists, editors, and health information professionals / Laura Bryan. — 4th ed.
        p. cm.
    Rev. ed. of: The medical transcriptionist's guide to Microsoft Word / Laura Bryan. 3rd ed. c2005.
    Includes bibliographical references and index.
    ISBN 978-0-7817-9714-6 (alk. paper)
    1. Microsoft Word. 2. Medical transcription. I. Bryan, Laura, 1963- Medical transcriptionist's guide to Microsoft Word. II. Title.
    [DNLM: 1. Microsoft Word. 2. Word Processing—methods—Handbooks. 3. Forms and Records Control—methods—Handbooks. W 26.5 B915m 2011]
    Z52.5.M52B79 2011
    005.52—dc22

                                                                    2009033028

To purchase additional copies of this book, call our customer service department at **(800) 638-3030** or fax orders to **(301) 824-7390.** International customers should call **(301) 714-2324.**

Visit Lippincott Williams & Wilkins on the Internet: http://www.LWW.com. Lippincott Williams & Wilkins customer service representatives are available from 8:30 am to 6:00 pm, EST.

                            1 2 3 4 5 6 7 8 9 10

TO VICKI, WHO SHOWS ME EVERYDAY WHAT IT MEANS
TO HAVE A FRIEND AND BE A FRIEND.

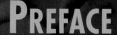

Starting with the first edition of *The Productivity Manual for Medical Transcriptionists* and continuing with this Fourth Edition of *Microsoft Word for Healthcare Documentation*, productivity with accuracy has been the hallmark of this book series. As financial pressures and time constraints continue to bear down on the healthcare industry as a whole, the need to work efficiently and accurately is more important than ever before. Microsoft Word is a veritable toolbox with many features designed to help you work more efficiently, so the challenge is not teasing functionality out of meager software, but knowing how to use the built-in tools to your utmost advantage. This text is uniquely designed to teach medical transcriptionists, editors, and health information specialists how to meet the challenges of the high-volume, time-constrained work of transforming dictation into an accurate and meaningful document.

After ten years of incremental changes, Word underwent a considerable facelift with the release of Office 2007. For new users, Microsoft is certain the revamped interface creates a friendlier environment for working with a very complicated, feature-rich application. For veteran users, however, the new interface is initially startling and very disorienting. "Where did that command go?" is a common refrain heard from long-time Word users. But veteran users will eventually realize that it is still very much the same Word underneath a new façade. Whereas previous editions of this text focused on facilitating the switch from DOS-based software to a Windows-based interface, this edition highlights the similarities between Word 2003 and Word 2007.

At first blush, one might wonder how a single text could cover two seemingly different versions of Word. One might also wonder why it is important to focus on what is the same, rather than focus on what is new to Word 2007—after all, Microsoft put a lot of effort into developing an easier-to-use interface. Even with all the cosmetic changes, Word 2007 has retained most of the "legacy" methods for completing tasks. Instead of describing every possible approach to completing a given task (of which there is always a minimum of three), this text emphasizes the methods that are most consistent between Word 2003 and Word 2007. Focusing on what is the same between these two versions of Word will help medical transcriptionists (MTs) be productive in a variety of educational and employment settings. It's not unreasonable to imagine a student or a practitioner (especially independent contractors) needing to quickly switch between the two versions of Word or even using both versions at the same time. Since speed and accuracy are gained by developing habits and muscle memory, maintaining consistent methods of working will maintain a consistent level of productivity regardless of the software version.

As with previous editions, this text focuses heavily on shortcut keys and keyboard commands as opposed to the mouse. Even with the extensive changes in Word 2007's user interface, the shortcut keys have remained largely the same, and key sequences for accessing commands on Word 2003's menus have been retained wherever possible. Learning shortcut keys works to the MT's advantage, since the goal is to keep the fingers on the keyboard while the foot is on the pedal. Transcriptionists using Word 2003 will be best served by memorizing as many shortcut keys as possible, so when the inevitable switch to Word 2007 occurs, the transition will be faster and easier.

The cosmetic changes in Word 2007 are symbolic of the changes happening throughout the healthcare industry—the underlying principles of healthcare documentation are still at work but there are tremendous external changes. The previous decade saw medical transcription move from analog tapes and paper-based documents to digital sound files and electronic delivery. The next era in transcription will be marked by the widespread adoption of speech recognition and the use of "smart" documents containing XML and other types of encoding. This edition supports both current and emerging healthcare documentation technologies. MTs moving into the role of Speech Recognition Editor (SRE) will need to hone their keyboard editing skills more than ever, as many platforms utilize keyboard commands to simultaneously control the audio playback and edit the speech-recognized drafts.

More and more, MTs are working with Word in conjunction with transcription platforms that control certain aspects of document management and patient demographics. Although this text does not describe any particular platform, it contributes to an understanding of these technologies by explaining the use of fields, document properties, template files, global templates, and other add-ins. This background information is also useful to health information professionals that process and edit documents before printing or exporting to an electronic record system. For these individuals, knowledge of fields and formatting will make editing easier and will avoid unintentional errors in the final report.

No doubt, technology will continue to have a tremendous impact on healthcare documentation, and the era of the "traditional transcriptionist" may give way to the "documentation specialist" whose role may include a mixture of transcribing, editing, and value-added tasks such as encoding and verifying data analyzed by natural language processing. The possibilities are exciting for individuals who enjoy learning and taking on new challenges. The traditional transcriptionist has always been characterized as a constant learner, and that same zest for learning a new medical term can and should be applied to learning technology. To secure a meaningful and profitable role in the future of health information, make a commitment to incorporate a new shortcut key, a new technique, or a new concept into your routine every few days. Incremental learning, as opposed to gorging and cramming, is more successful, more rewarding, and certainly less stressful.

While many perceive transcription as a manual job, MTs who hear "doctors' voices in their heads" on a daily basis know it is truly knowledge work. Critical listening and the ability to transform spoken English into comprehensible, written form are unique and valuable skills that still cannot be duplicated by computers. As technology inches its way into our lives and strives to replace us, it paradoxically proves the MT's true value. An underlying goal of this text is to demonstrate how the fusion of technology and the art of language are culminated in the extraordinary talents of the professional, knowledgeable, and dedicated healthcare documentation specialist.

Best wishes for a profitable and rewarding career,

Laura Bryan

July 2009

Microsoft Word for Healthcare Documentation: A Guide for Transcriptionists, Editors, and Health Information Professionals helps you work more efficiently by showing you how to use Microsoft Word's built-in tools to your utmost advantage.

This User's Guide introduces you to the helpful features that enable you to quickly master new concepts and put your new skills into practice.

CHAPTER 7

Formatting

OBJECTIVES

- Identify and use formatting marks.
- Recognize the role of styles in MS Word and manage the Normal style.
- Apply character formatting using the Font dialog box and shortcut keys.
- Use the Paragraph dialog box, Horizontal Ruler, and shortcut keys to format paragraphs.
- Format a typical SOAP note.
- Use headers and footers for letterhead and patient demographic information.
- Use section breaks to manage headers and footers and page margins.

Objectives help you concentrate on the most important information to glean from each chapter.

Formatting Basics

Understanding fundamental concepts and techniques related to formatting will increase your productivity and accuracy and create professional looking documents that are easy to edit. Word processors are designed to lay out text consistently and efficiently using standard paragraph formats and formatting commands. One of the most common mistakes a user can make is to treat their document creation software like an old manual typewriter! Software is *so much smarter* than typewriters. MS Word is a high-powered, world-class application with a tremendous set of features and functionality for efficiency, accuracy, and productivity. Using actual formatting commands (instead of repeatedly pressing Tab or Spacebar) can save hundreds of keystrokes over the course of a day of transcribing and make editing infinitely easier. Table 7-1 defines important formatting terms used in word processing.

The Insertion Point

The mouse pointer appears as an I-beam whenever it overlies an area that accepts text input. Clicking the I-beam in a given position sets the

KEYWORDS

default font
default tab stop
direct formatting
Font dialog box
formatting marks
hanging indent
header and footer
horizontal alignment
indent
line spacing
Normal style
Paragraph dialog box
paragraph mark
Reveal Formatting task pane
section break
set tab
style

Shortcut Keys
Shift+F1
CTRL+L
CTRL+R
CTRL+E
CTRL+J
CTRL+M
CTRL+Shift+M
CTRL+T
CTRL+Shift+T
CTRL+D

Keywords help you focus on the important terms that you should master.

Menu names and menu commands are typed in blue.

Galleries in Word 2007 are typed in blue.

Special formatting has been applied to the text to improve readability and comprehension. You will recognize common Windows elements by their font.

Button names and **tabs within dialog boxes** are bold with a box around them.

Tabs on the ribbon in Word 2007 are bold with a box around them.

Dialog box names and **folder names** are blue and bold.

Check boxes and *options listed within dialog boxes* are orange and italic.

Keystrokes are green.

<u>Toolbars</u> are blue and underlined.

<u>Groups within the ribbon</u> in Word 2007 are blue and underlined.

`Specific text to be typed` and `file extensions` are Courier font.

Tables summarize key information for at-a-glance reference.

Table 7-1	Formatting Terms Used in Document Creation Software.
Indent	The space between the margin and the edge of the text (to move text away from the right or left margin).
Hanging indent	A format in which the first line of a paragraph is closer to the left margin compared to the second and subsequent lines of the paragraph. This format is typically used in a numbered list where the number is at the left margin and the text is lined up ¼ to ½ inch from the number.
Center	A command that aligns text in the center of the margins.
Header and Footer	The space at the upper and lower edge of a document that typically contains the letterhead, page number, and patient demographic information. The header and footer space is separated from the body of the document so the text within the body of the report can be edited without affecting the placement of the text contained within the header and footer.
Hard page break	A forced page break inserted by the user (*cf* soft page break).
Soft page break	A page break which occurs automatically when the text reaches the lower margin of the page.
Justify	A command that aligns text even with both the right and left margins.
Template	A file that is used as the basis of a new document for a given document type or report type. A template contains formatted headings and other text that appears on all documents of that type.
Set Tab	A defined position on a line that determines where the insertion point will stop when the Tab key is pressed. Pressing Tab typically moves the cursor ½ inch, but a set tab stop will move the cursor to the exact position on the line defined by the tab stop.

Screen shots show you what you'll see on your computer screen as you perform each task.

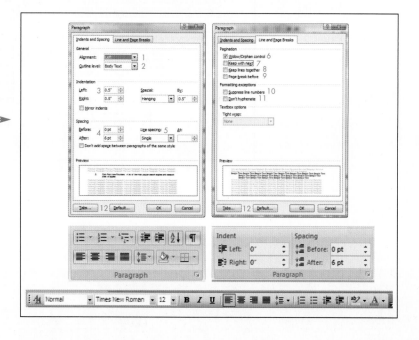

"Do It Quicker" boxes offer valuable timesavers, including shortcut keys and tips for maximizing efficiency.

 Since superscripts and subscripts are cumbersome to format, create Auto-Correct entries for items you use often (see Chapter 9).

"Caution" boxes alert you to common pitfalls and how to avoid them.

 Superscript and subscript characters are not compatible with all medical record systems, especially those that import text in plain-text format. Check with the provider or facility to determine which formatting characters are compatible with their document management system.

"Put It Together" boxes show you how various concepts discussed throughout the text work together.

 It's easy to demonstrate how a paragraph mark actually "carries" formatting information. Selecting and copying a paragraph mark (without any text) and pasting it in a new location will apply the formatting information stored in that mark to the text immediately preceding the paragraph mark.

"How I Do It" boxes are based on the author's first-hand experience, helping you apply what you've learned to be more productive and accurate in your work.

 Personally, I do not make extensive use of styles while transcribing (although they are indispensable when writing an article, a report, or a book). Instead, when starting a new account, I set up template files and apply as much formatting as possible to the template so there are very few formatting changes to make during routine transcription. Learn more about templates in Chapter 8.

Word logos are located in the margin for easily identifying keystrokes for opening dialog boxes.

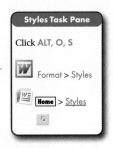

Clearly marked sections for Windows XP, Windows Vista, Word 2003, and Word 2007 direct you to the information specific to your operating system and version of Word.

5. With *Different First Page* selected, you will need to enter information into both the first-page footer and the second-page footer.

WORD 2003 XP

manage your file system. Use Windows Explorer to copy, delete, move, rename, and create files and folders. Windows Explorer should not be confused with Internet Explorer, which is used to browse web pages. Using Windows Explorer, you can also copy the contents of the first-page header to the second-page header. *This command will apply to the footer as well.*

WORD 2007 VISTA

Windows Explorer is used to see the hierarchy of folders on your computer and to manage your file system. Use Windows Explorer to copy, delete, move, rename, and create files and folders. Windows Explorer should not be confused with Internet Explorer, which is used to browse web pages. Using Windows Explorer, you can also view properties of disks, files, and folders, and perform maintenance tasks on disks (right-click a disk, file, or folder and choose Properties).

Access Windows Explorer by clicking the Computer icon on your Desktop or using the shortcut key Logo+E (see page XX for an explanation of the Logo key). **Computer** displays the disks and drives associated with your computer. From this

Content specific to Word 2003 is marked with Word 2003's icon.

Content specific to Word 2007 is marked with Word 2007's icon.

Shaded text and caution signs call special attention to critical information.

Blue background, white text: Changes screen to appear like Word Perfect 5.1 for DOS.

Provide feedback with sound: Associates sounds with certain events such as error warnings. Sounds may be disturbing or loud when wearing a transcription headset.

Provide feedback with animation: When turned on, Word will use special pointers to indicate certain automated procedures are in progress (eg, background saves).

Critical Thinking Questions at the end of each chapter promote a deeper understanding of fundamental concepts by encouraging analysis and practical application of information presented.

Critical Thinking Questions

1. Explain why an understanding of the paragraph mark is critical to understanding formatting and editing in MS Word. How does Word define a paragraph?

2. What are styles? How do they affect formatting in MS Word? In the context of transcription, what do you need to know about styles?

3. Define the default font and explain how to change it.

Glossary defines all the key terms used throughout the text.

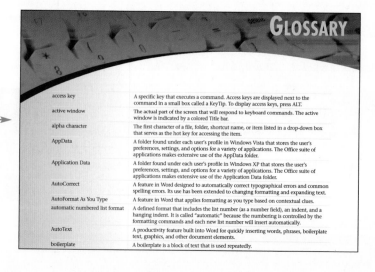

GLOSSARY

access key	A specific key that executes a command. Access keys are displayed next to the command in a small box called a KeyTip. To display access keys, press ALT.
active window	The actual part of the screen that will respond to keyboard commands. The active window is indicated by a colored Title bar.
alpha character	The first character of a file, folder, shortcut name, or item listed in a drop-down box that serves as the hot key for accessing the item.
AppData	A folder found under each user's profile in Windows Vista that stores the user's preferences, settings, and options for a variety of applications. The Office suite of applications makes extensive use of the AppData folder.
Application Data	A folder found under each user's profile in Windows XP that stores the user's preferences, settings, and options for a variety of applications. The Office suite of applications makes extensive use of the Application Data folder.
AutoCorrect	A feature in Word designed to automatically correct typographical errors and common spelling errors. Its use has been extended to changing formatting and expanding text.
AutoFormat As You Type	A feature in Word that applies formatting as you type based on contextual clues.
automatic numbered list format	A defined format that includes the list number (as a number field), an indent, and a hanging indent. It is called "automatic" because the numbering is controlled by the formatting commands and each new list number will insert automatically.
AutoText	A productivity feature built into Word for quickly inserting words, phrases, boilerplate text, graphics, and other document elements.
boilerplate	A boilerplate is a block of text that is used repeatedly.

Frequently Asked Questions Appendix lists the questions commonly asked by users of MS Word, especially those working within healthcare documentation.

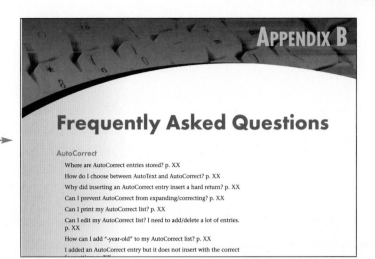

APPENDIX B

Frequently Asked Questions

AutoCorrect

Where are AutoCorrect entries stored? p. XX

How do I choose between AutoText and AutoCorrect? p. XX

Why did inserting an AutoCorrect entry insert a hard return? p. XX

Can I prevent AutoCorrect from expanding/correcting? p. XX

Can I print my AutoCorrect list? p. XX

Can I edit my AutoCorrect list? I need to add/delete a lot of entries. p. XX

How can I add "-year-old" to my AutoCorrect list? p. XX

I added an AutoCorrect entry but it does not insert with the correct formatting. p. XX

STUDENT RESOURCES

The student CD and online resource center reinforce what you learn in the text. Student resources include a question bank, templates, macros, and formatting exercises.

The Student Resource Center can be accessed at http://thePoint.lww.com/BryanWord4e.

INSTRUCTOR RESOURCES

The online instructor resources available for use with *Microsoft Word for Healthcare Documentation* include a test bank, an image bank, and PowerPoint slides for each chapter.

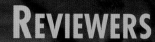

REVIEWERS

The publisher, author, and editors gratefully acknowledge the valuable contributions made by the following professionals who reviewed this text:

YVONNE ALLES, MBA
Department Coordinator
Allied Health
Davenport University
Grand Rapids, MI

DARLENE BOSCHERT, CPC, CPC-H, CPC-I, NCMA, CMT
Director
Medical Coding and Billing Program
Ultimate Medical Academy
Clearwater, FL

SUSAN D. DOOLEY, CMT, AHDI-F
Professor and Program Manager
Health Information/Medical Transcription
Seminole Community College
Altamonte Springs, FL

HOPE KREMER
Transcriptionist
Shelbyville, KY

BARBARA L. MARCHELLETTA, AS, BS, CMA (AAMA), CPC (AAPC)
Program Director
Allied Health
Beal College
Bangor, ME

B. JOY REYNO, CHIM
Faculty
School of Health and Human Services
Nova Scotia Community College
Halifax, Nova Scotia

CINDY THOMPSON, RN, RMA, MA, BS
Davenport University
Saginaw, MI

CONSTANCE WALLS, CMT
Associate Faculty, Health Information Technology
Health Sciences & Emergency Services
Collin College
McKinney, TX

ACKNOWLEDGEMENTS

Although a book displays the author's name on the cover, it is never a singular effort. I have come to realize that although books are commonplace, there is nothing common about the effort required to put one together. From the planning to the writing, editing, designing, typesetting, and publishing, many people contribute to the final product. So there are many people to thank.

First and foremost, I must thank my husband. I simply could not accomplish anything I do without Bob and his unwavering support of my seemingly endless projects and deadlines. Everybody needs a "Bob" in their life!

I would also like to extend my appreciation to the reviewers of the text who contributed valuable feedback throughout the writing and publication process. These reviewers contributed their time and offered their sincere and constructive opinions to create a more useful, relevant, and helpful text.

A special thank you to Susan Caldwell for so carefully and patiently preparing the screen shots for printing. And many thanks to the Medical Language & Reference group at Lippincott, Williams & Wilkins for continuing to support this book series. To Amy Millholen, the most patient, kind, and organized person I know, thank you so much for your expert management of this project and for working so hard to make my vision and expectations a reality. Every author needs an "Amy" in their life.

CONTENTS

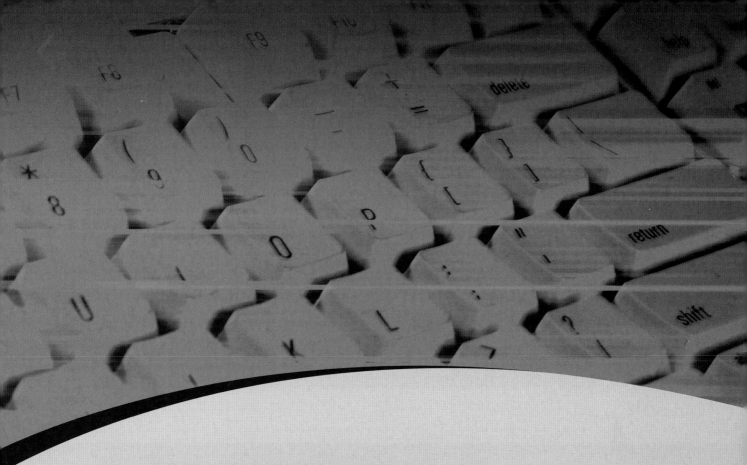

SECTION I

CHAPTER 1

Overview of Windows

OBJECTIVES

▸ Identify elements of the Windows graphical user interface and recognize how Windows uses various elements to give the user feedback.

▸ Identify the mode represented by each of the mouse pointers and use various mouse techniques.

▸ Manage windows using Minimize, Maximize, Exit, Close, and Restore.

▸ Describe fundamental Windows concepts: Select, View, Zoom, Default, Properties, and the Windows Clipboard.

To be truly efficient in your work as a transcriptionist, it is important to understand how MS Word interacts with Windows (the operating system). The operating system sets up the environment for all other applications on the computer, manages resources, provides security, and establishes network connections. Understanding the terminology and concepts described in this chapter will lay the foundation for learning MS Word as well as many other software applications, enabling you to work more efficiently.

KEYWORDS

active window
Clipboard
default
Desktop
dialog box
graphical user interface
menus
object
pointer
Properties
Quick Launch bar
Select
Start menu
task pane
Taskbar
View
Zoom

The Windows Interface

Windows uses a **graphical user interface** (GUI, pronounced goo-ey), which consists of a standardized set of graphical elements that create a consistent, predictable, and easy-to-use working environment. The advent of the GUI opened the world of computers to both novice users and professionals because a GUI does not require individuals to understand complex computer language. It is important to recognize the different elements that make up the Windows user interface and the terminology used to describe those elements.

Key elements of Windows include the Desktop, **Start** button, Start menu, icons, Taskbar, Title bar, menus, menu bars, toolbars, ribbons,

dialog boxes, and **task panes** as well as the various modes indicated by the mouse pointer. Figures 1-1 and 1-2 show the various elements in the Windows interface. The following pages describe these major elements.

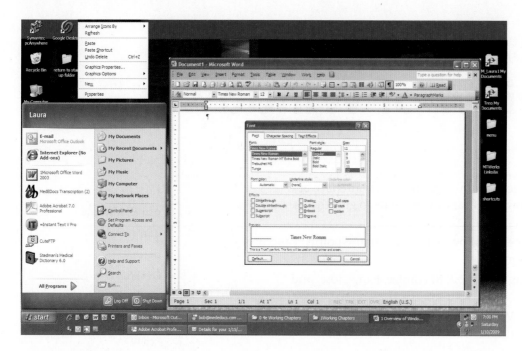

FIGURE 1-1 The major elements of the Windows XP user interface.

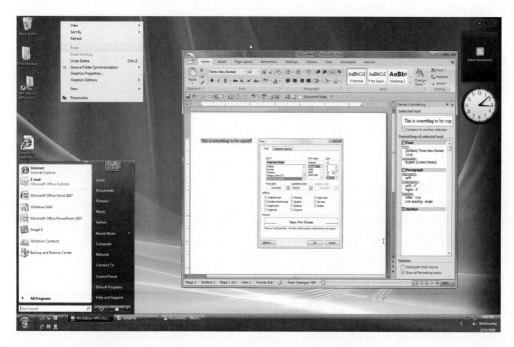

FIGURE 1-2 Elements of the Windows Vista user interface.

The Windows interface has so much detail and so many nuances that often escape the user's notice. Developing an eye for these details will make it much easier to operate your computer and will greatly decrease your confusion and frustration.

Object

Object refers to any distinct item on the display such as an icon, image (graphic), text, window, or part of a window. Almost any item displayed can be acted on in some way, and collectively these items are referred to as objects.

The Desktop

The **Desktop** is the main screen that appears after a full startup of your computer. The Desktop is meant to emulate the working surface of a traditional desk by providing convenient access to the items you use most. The Desktop can be customized with your favorite picture or background. A sample Desktop is shown in Figure 1-3.

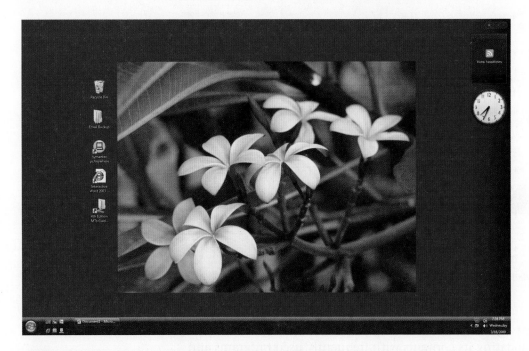

FIGURE 1-3 The Desktop showing icons to the left of the flowers and the Taskbar along the bottom edge.

Drag icons around on your Desktop to sort them into groupings that make it easier to locate icons when you need them. Right-click an empty area of the Desktop and choose Properties in Windows XP and Personalize in Windows Vista to change the picture displayed, background color, and other aspects of your Desktop.

The Start Menu

The **Start menu** (Figures 1-4 and 1-5) is the main menu in the Windows operating system and the gateway to the files and programs installed on your computer.

Access the Start menu by clicking / in the bottom left

corner of your screen or press the Logo key (see page 81).

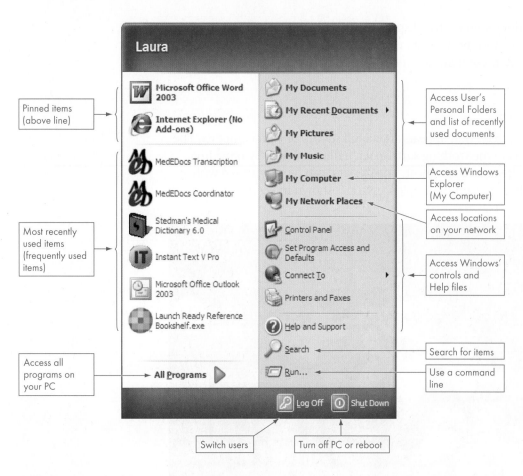

FIGURE 1-4 Details of the Windows XP Start menu.

The Start menu contains shortcuts to the items you will most likely use, and it adapts to your use by updating its contents with frequently used programs and files. Figure 1-4 and Figure 1-5 show typical Start menus in Windows XP and Windows Vista. Your Start menu may vary slightly depending on the programs you have installed. Generally speaking, items listed on the left side of the Start menu are shortcuts to programs, and items listed on the right side of the Start menu are shortcuts to "places" such as folders or networked drives. You will learn how to customize your Start menu in Chapter 3.

The All Programs menu displays a list of programs installed on your PC. Each software manufacturer determines how their program appears on your All Programs menu. Many create a program-group icon that includes the main program, help

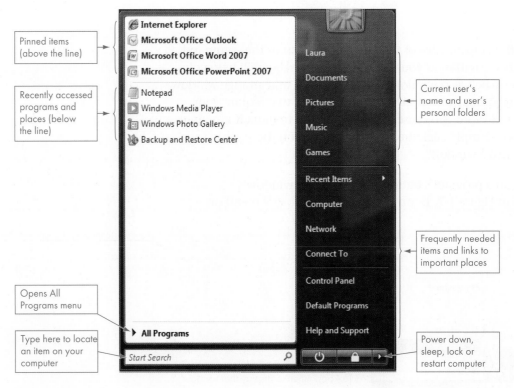

FIGURE 1-5 Details of the Windows Vista Start menu.

files, and utilities associated with that program. The name of the program group may be the name of the program or the name of the company that created the software. For example, all of the Office applications (Word, Excel, PowerPoint, etc) are located under the Microsoft Office program group, as shown in Figure 1-6.

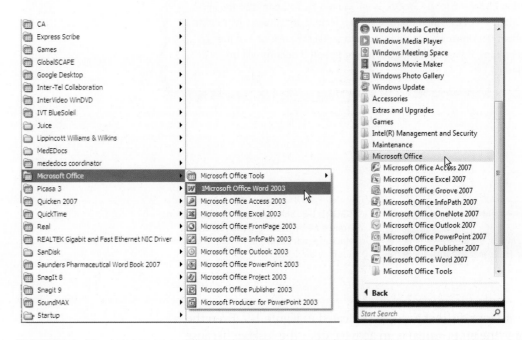

FIGURE 1-6 A program-group icon opens a submenu listing programs and utilities associated with a particular software program. The Microsoft Office group is shown in Windows XP on the left and Windows Vista on the right.

The Taskbar

The **Taskbar** sits along the bottom edge of the Desktop and acts as the command and control center for the activities on your computer. The Taskbar will help you track open windows, move between windows, close windows, and arrange windows on your display. The Taskbar may also notify you of programs that require your attention. For example, MS Word will cause its Taskbar button to blink if it requires a response to a message box. Simply click the window's button on the Taskbar to make that window the active window.

You can also right-click on a program's button to display that window's Control menu as shown in Figure 1-7. Learn more about the Control menu on page 22.

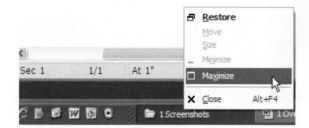

FIGURE 1-7 Right-click on a window's Taskbar button to display that window's Control menu.

 To close several windows at the same time, hold down **Ctrl** while clicking each corresponding window's button. Right-click over one of the selected buttons and choose Close Group as in Figure 1-8. You can also minimize several windows at one time using this same technique. Choose Minimize Group from the right-click menu. Be sure to right-click over one of the selected buttons; if you right-click anywhere else, the buttons will be deselected.

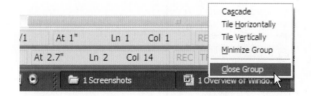

FIGURE 1-8 Select several Taskbar buttons at one time by holding down CTRL while selecting each button; right-click to close the group of windows.

The Taskbar is divided into four distinct areas, as indicated in Figure 1-9. Even the area without any buttons (the empty area) is an active part of the Taskbar because you can right-click this area to reveal a helpful shortcut menu.

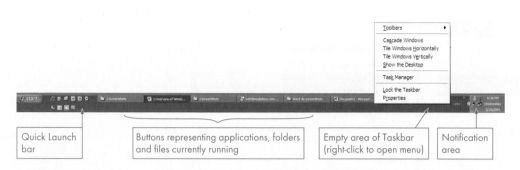

FIGURE 1-9 The Taskbar sits along the bottom edge of the Desktop. It is divided into four distinct areas and has its own right-click menu.

The Taskbar can also be used to minimize all windows (ie, show the Desktop). Right-click an empty area of the Taskbar and choose Show the Desktop. To return to the same window as before, click Undo Minimize All on the same right-click menu. You can also use the shortcut key **Logo+D** to show the Desktop (ie, minimize all). Toggle to switch back and forth between the Desktop and the most recent active window. Learn more about shortcut keys in Chapter 3.

Customizing the Taskbar

By default, the Taskbar is hidden along the bottom edge of the display and pops up when you move the mouse pointer toward the lower edge. You can also reveal the Taskbar by pressing the **Logo** key (see page 81 for a description of the Logo key).

The way the Taskbar behaves will determine how you use the Taskbar. There are several Taskbar behaviors that can be modified through the **Taskbar Properties** dialog box as shown in Figure 1-10. Right-click in an empty area of the Taskbar (away from any buttons) and choose Properties. Place or remove a check mark at any of the following options:

Lock the Taskbar: This command prevents the Taskbar from being changed. With the Taskbar unlocked, it is possible to resize the Taskbar by dragging the edges with the mouse or to move the Taskbar by dragging it to another edge of the Desktop. For example, the Taskbar displayed in Figure 1-9 has been resized to display two rows of buttons.

Auto-hide the Taskbar: Selecting this command causes the Taskbar to hide by sliding down below the edge of the display. To show the Taskbar, move the mouse toward the edge of the Desktop or press the **Logo** key. Remove the check mark if you would like to see the Taskbar at all times.

Keep the Taskbar on top of other windows: This command causes the Taskbar to always remain visible so that other program windows cannot overlap the Taskbar.

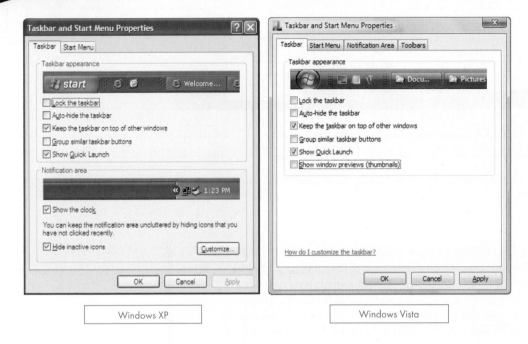

FIGURE 1-10 Change the way the Taskbar behaves in the Taskbar Properties dialog box.

Group similar Taskbar buttons: This option groups related windows together under a single button on the <u>Taskbar</u> as shown in Figure 1-11. It is intended to create space on the <u>Taskbar</u> when there are multiple windows running and the <u>Taskbar</u> is becoming too crowded. The number displayed in the program button indicates how many files are listed under that grouped button (eg, 7 in 1-11).

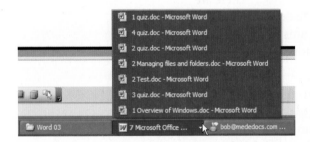

FIGURE 1-11 Windows can group Taskbar buttons that are associated with the same application under a single Taskbar button.

Show Quick Launch: This option displays the <u>Quick Launch</u> bar (see Figure 1-9).

Show window previews (Windows Vista only): This command is available to users running the Aero profile. With this option selected, a thumbnail view of the window appears when the mouse pointer hovers over a window's **Taskbar** button.

Since the Taskbar acts like a dashboard, I like to be able to see it at all times. I remove the check mark at *Auto-hide* and place the check mark at *Keep the Taskbar on top of other windows*. I also prefer to see a button for each window instead of grouping windows, as shown in Figure 1-11. If I am working on a project requiring many windows to be open at the same time, I resize the Taskbar so it accommodates two rows of buttons. This also allows each button to be wider and display more of the window name. To resize the Taskbar, first minimize all windows and then drag the upper edge of the Taskbar upward.

Be sure to minimize all windows before resizing or moving your Taskbar. If part of a window becomes hidden behind the Taskbar, close and reopen the program to reset the program's boundaries based on the new location of the Taskbar.

Quick Launch Bar

The **Quick Launch bar** sits between the `Start` button and the `Taskbar` buttons (see Figure 1-9) and provides an easy-access area for shortcuts to items that will open with a single click of the mouse. Simply drag and drop shortcut icons onto the Quick Launch bar for quick, one-click access to items you use often. (Learn how to create shortcut icons in Chapter 3.) Remove items from the Quick Launch bar by dragging them from the bar to the Desktop, or right-click the icon and choose Delete.

Notification Area

The Notification area sits at the far right of the Taskbar and shows the status of certain processes that are running in the background such as network connections and virus scanners. This area also displays the time and date. Bubbles with messages related to hardware and other peripheral devices often appear in the Notification area. Most importantly, security warnings generated by Windows and antivirus software appear in the Notification area.

Microsoft does not use pop-up boxes in the middle of the display to issue security warnings or to remind you to update your software, so be very cautious about acting on security messages that appear anywhere other than the Notification area. *Never click a link in an email, pop-up box, or web page to update security software!* Warnings in the form of pop-up boxes are most likely hoaxes.

Icons

Icons are small pictures that represent an action (a command), an application, a folder, a file, a file-storage disk, a printer, a camera, or a website. Icons are integral to the concept of a graphical user interface. You can gain a lot of information by looking carefully at an icon. The icon itself gives you information about the type of object it represents. Many applications have icons that are easily recognizable, such as Word's blue W and Excel's green X.

The following icons represent drives associated with your computer. The first icon represents a drive on your computer and the second icon represents a drive connected to your computer by a network.

Local and Network drives (XP)   Local and Network drives (Vista)

This next set of icons represents various folders. Icons from Windows XP are on the top row and the corresponding icons from Windows Vista are on the second row. The first icon might represent any folder. The second icon represents the **My Documents** folder (Windows XP) and **Documents** (Windows Vista) and is distinguished by a document popping out of the folder. Likewise, (**My**) **Music** is a folder icon with a music note. The fourth icon represents the **Recycle Bin**, a folder which contains files that have been "deleted" but can still be retrieved if needed.

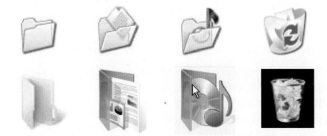

The following four icons represent specific applications: Internet Explorer, MS Word, MS Excel, and Windows Media Player. Icons on the top row are from Windows XP and icons on the bottom row are from Windows Vista.

The next four icons have a "page" with the application icon superimposed, indicating these are files with associated applications. The first icon represents a PDF file that will open with Adobe Reader; the second is a document that will open with MS Word. The third icon represents a spreadsheet that will open with Excel, and last is a media file that will open with Windows Media Player.

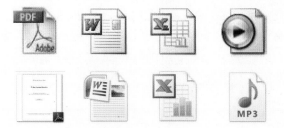

The following icons represent *shortcuts* to items, as indicated by the small curved arrow in the bottom left corner of the icon. Shortcuts are icons that will take you to a specific place or open a particular file but *are not the actual item they point to*. Shortcut icons can be copied, deleted, moved, and renamed without affecting the actual file (called the target). The first icon in each set is a shortcut to a folder, the second is a shortcut that will open Internet Explorer, and the third is a shortcut to a specific website that will be viewed using Internet Explorer. Learn more about shortcut icons in Chapter 3.

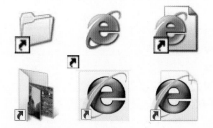

Folders

Windows (the operating system) uses electronic "folders" to sort and organize files. Just as a traditional office uses file folders to sort papers, Windows uses folders to organize computer files. Folders can have folders within them, called subfolders. Folders can contain a mixture of file types (documents, graphics, audio files) and are primarily used to sort and locate information in a way that is *meaningful to the user*. Most folders can be created, deleted, copied, renamed, or moved to a new location. Folders are managed using Windows Explorer. Figure 1-12 shows an Explorer window from Windows Vista with folders displayed.

Title Bar

One of the most overlooked, yet extremely useful elements of every window is the Title bar. The Title bar is the colored bar that creates the uppermost border of

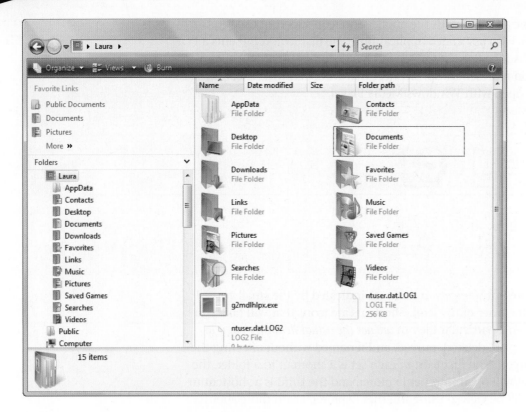

FIGURE 1-12 Folders are used to sort information on a computer.

windows and dialog boxes. The <u>Title</u> bar has many important functions, not the least of which is to identify the window. Always look at the name of the window as displayed within the <u>Title</u> bar. This will keep you oriented and often prevent confusion when working with new software or navigating the Internet. The <u>Title</u> bar, shown in Figure 1-13, also contains the window-control buttons (at the far right) for managing the window.

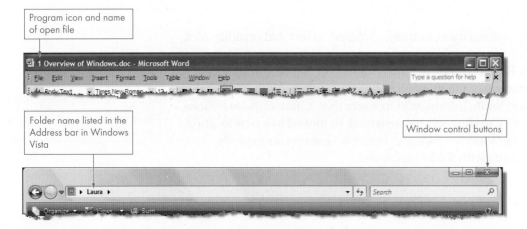

FIGURE 1-13 The Title bar displays the name of the window's contents and contains the window-control buttons.

Another important function of the <u>Title</u> bar is to indicate the **active window.** The active window is the actual part of the screen that will respond to commands from the keyboard. The active window can be a dialog box, a message box, an Explorer window, or the application window itself. The active window is always identified by a colored <u>Title</u> bar (ie, not grayed or dimmed) as shown in Figure 1-14. Learn more about the active window and keyboard commands in Chapter 3.

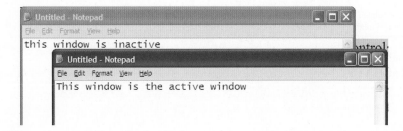

FIGURE 1-14 The Title bar indicates the active window. Notice the Close button (the red X) is also darker on the active window, especially in Windows Vista.

Status Bar

The <u>Status Bar</u> forms the lowermost border of most windows. As its name suggests, the <u>Status Bar</u> reports the status of a particular operation, gives feedback on certain commands, and gives statistical data about the program or the folder window (Figure 1-15). Develop a habit of glancing at the <u>Status Bar</u> for pertinent information while you are working.

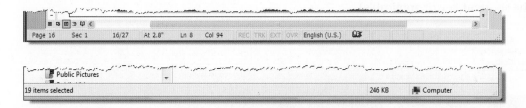

FIGURE 1-15 A Status Bar from a Word document (top) and a Status Bar from an Explorer window in Windows Vista (bottom).

Toolbars

Toolbars are collections of buttons that execute commands (Figure 1-16). Toolbars are also used to give the user feedback. Toolbar buttons change color to indicate the command is active, a feature is currently turned on, or the format is applied at the current location of the cursor. Depending on the color scheme you have selected for displaying windows, toolbar buttons may change color or they may appear clear or "pushed in." Study Figure 1-16 carefully and note the many features and functions of toolbars.

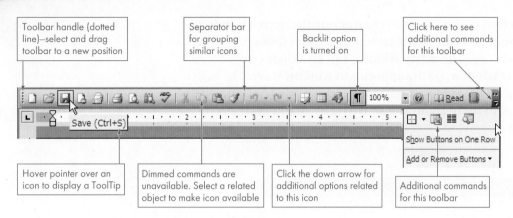

FIGURE 1-16 A toolbar from Microsoft Word 2003 showing typical toolbar elements.

Ribbons

Ribbons were introduced with the Office 2007 suite of applications and now other programs are incorporating this new approach to organizing commands. Ribbons replace the menu bars and toolbars that appear across the uppermost edge of the program's window (see Figure 1-17). Ribbons contain commands sorted by tabs. Within each tab, commands are further divided into groups. Commands located on the ribbon may have drop-down menus indicated by the downward arrow (▼) next to the command name. Some commands have a collection of preset formats called galleries that appear as drop-down menus. An icon, called a dialog box launcher, is located in the bottom right corner of some groups that have related dialog boxes. In addition to the static tabs that are always available, programs may also have contextual tabs that only appear when you are working with a related element. Like toolbars, the icons on ribbons change color to indicate the command is active or has been applied. Hover the mouse over any icon to display a ToolTip with the command name and the shortcut key (if applicable).

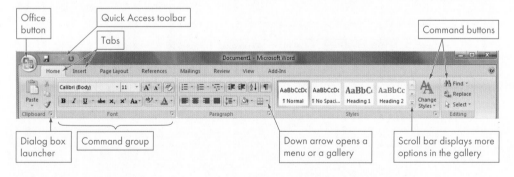

FIGURE 1-17 Ribbons were introduced with the Office 2007 suite of applications.

Ribbons only have one toolbar, called the Quick Access toolbar. By default, this toolbar sits above the ribbon at the far left. Commands traditionally located on the File menu are found on the program's main menu, accessible through the **Program** button in the upper left corner.

Menus

Menus contain a list of commands that are grouped by category or specific types of tasks. Menus are often listed horizontally, creating a menu bar. Most menu bars sit directly below the <u>Title</u> bar and typically contain 5-10 menus. Menus drop down from the menu bar or slide open to the right or left (submenus).

 The trend among Microsoft applications is to hide the menu bars so more work space is available on the screen. Hidden menu bars can be displayed (temporarily) by pressing the **Alt** key.

Menus are rich with information that may escape you at first glance. Study Figure 1-18 carefully, noting the underscored character, right arrow (▶), ellipsis (…), icons, and shortcut keys. Some menus include items with check marks to the left of the command to indicate features that can be turned on or off or items that can be displayed or hidden.

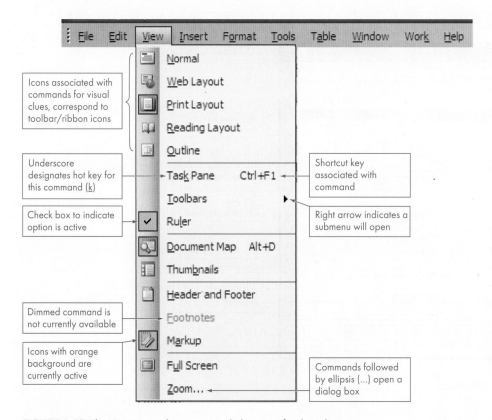

FIGURE 1-18 The View menu showing typical elements of a drop-down menu.

 Each menu command has a hot key, marked with an underscore character that is used to select that command with the keyboard. Menus also list keyboard shortcuts when available. Learn more about using hot keys and shortcut keys in Chapter 3.

Shortcut Menus

One of the best timesaving features in Windows is the **shortcut** menu. Shortcut menus appear when you right-click an object (files, folders, icons, toolbars, etc), and they contain the most common commands needed for that particular object. Almost every element displayed on the screen has a right-click menu associated with it. Learn more about right-click menus in Chapter 3.

Dialog Boxes

Dialog boxes are used throughout Windows and in all Windows-based programs. Dialog boxes use `tabs`, `buttons`, *check boxes*, *radio buttons*, *lists*, *slide bars*, `text input boxes`, and a variety of other methods for specifying options and settings. Commands that open dialog boxes are always listed on menus and buttons with an ellipsis (...) as in the `Default` button in Figure 1-19.

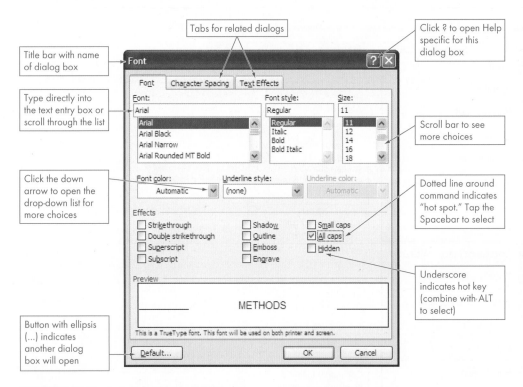

FIGURE 1-19 The Font dialog box in MS Word.

Dialog boxes always have a <u>Title</u> bar containing the name of the dialog box. Noting the name of the dialog box will help you stay oriented and will also help you describe the contents of your screen when working with technical support over the phone.

It can be very helpful to note the ellipsis listed after command names so you know you are about to open a dialog box versus executing a specific command. This can be very helpful when you are learning a new program and are not sure if clicking the command will take you to another window or to a "point of no return."

Task Panes

A **task pane** combines features of drop-down menus and dialog boxes. As their name implies, task panes assist the user in accomplishing specific tasks, and the options differ depending on the type of task to be completed. For example, MS Word includes task panes for creating a new document and revealing text formatting. Task panes run vertically along the left or right side of the window. Unlike dialog boxes, task panes remain open while you work. Figure 1-20 shows two typical task panes.

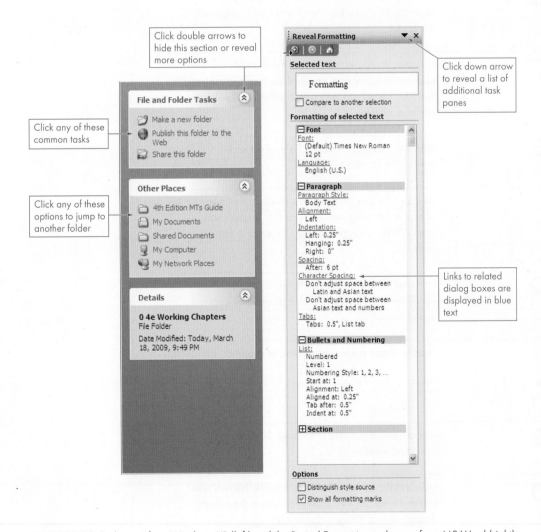

FIGURE 1-20 Task pane from Windows XP (left) and the Reveal Formatting task pane from MS Word (right).

Mouse Pointers and Techniques

The mouse and its on-screen **pointer** are integral to a graphical user interface. The pointer is used to select items anywhere on the display. The pointer not only points to objects on the screen, it also gives feedback to the user to indicate the computer's mode. The mode is indicated by the shape of the pointer or by another icon attached to the pointer as described in Table 1-1.

Table 1-1	**Mouse pointers and their corresponding modes.**	
Mode	**Pointer Shape**	**Description**
Normal select		Use to point and click on any object.
Help mode		Click an object or command for specific help related to that object.
Busy mode		Indicates Windows is working in the background. You may be able to continue working but the response time may be slower while the hourglass is displayed.
Wait mode		Indicates Windows is busy and the current application will ignore you until the task is completed. You may be able to switch to another window and continue working.
Precision select		Allows the user to more precisely select and manipulate graphics.
Text mode		Indicates the program is in text mode or that the pointer is hovering over an area that accepts text input. Often referred to as the I beam or insertion point.
Not allowed		Indicates the action you are trying to take is not allowed or the item you are pointing at is unavailable.
Resize mode		Used to resize a window, column or graphic.
Resize and Move mode		Use to move a graphic or to move or resize an individual window.
Link		Indicates the cursor is pointing to a link that will take you to a web page or a related topic in the current document or a different document.

Although a mouse may have only two buttons, there are many ways to use the mouse to give commands. Combining mouse techniques with modifier keys (Alt, Ctrl, Shift) further expands its capabilities. The following describes the most common mouse techniques used by Windows-based programs.

Left-click: Point to an object on the screen and click the left mouse button. This is by far the most common way to use the mouse, and unless noted otherwise, assume a "click" is a left click.

Right-click: Point to an object on the screen and click the right mouse button. This will open a shortcut menu with helpful commands.

Drag: Point to an object on the screen, press *and hold* the left mouse button while moving the object to a new location. Release the mouse button when the object is in the new location.

Drag-and-drop: Point to an object, hold down the left mouse button and drag the object toward another object. Continue holding the mouse button and hover the object over the target object (often a program button or folder icon). When the target object is selected, release the mouse button. Use this technique to move graphics, text, files, and folders.

Double-click: Point to an item and click the left mouse button twice in rapid succession without moving the mouse pointer. A double-click typically opens a file or folder without having to select the file first. If there is a delay between clicks, Windows will interpret two separate clicks and you will not get the desired result.

Ctrl+drag: Use the drag technique as described above while holding down the Ctrl key to copy selected item(s) such as files, folders, shortcut icons, text, or graphics.

Scroll: Scroll bars are used to move the contents of a window up, down, left and right. Scroll bars only appear if the window is too small to display the entire contents. Click the arrows located at either end of a scroll bar to move the screen in small increments, or drag the scroll button to move larger distances.

Scroll Wheel: Use the scroll wheel on the mouse to move up and down the window by spinning the wheel forward and back. Many scroll wheels also act as a third "mouse button" that puts the computer in "scroll mode." In this mode, you simply move the mouse forward and back to quickly scroll through a long document or web page. Click the scroll wheel again to turn off scroll mode. Scroll wheels may also act as a third button that can be pressed, not just rotated. Some software applications may include commands that are executed by clicking an object with the scroll wheel.

The various mouse techniques are possible because Windows' graphical user interface uses icons to represent both *files* and *commands*. Dragging items across the computer screen is the same as giving the computer a specific command such as move, copy, delete, and attach. You can drag objects from one open folder window to another open folder window, or you can drag and drop icons directly onto a folder icon to get the same results. Drag-and-drop can also be used to attach files to email or to open files with a specific program by dropping the file's icon onto an application's **Taskbar** button.

One of my favorite tricks is to drag icons from the <u>Address</u> bar of folders or websites onto the Desktop to instantly create shortcuts to that folder or website. Learn more in Chapter 3.

Window Controls

Commands for controlling windows are found on the right side of the <u>Title</u> bar and also on the Control menu that drops down from the <u>Title</u> bar. Figure 1-21 shows the window control buttons and the Control menu.

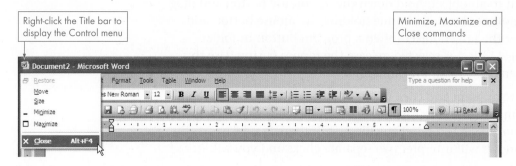

FIGURE 1-21 The commands on the Control menu correspond to the buttons on the right side of the Title bar.

The following commands are used to manage individual windows:

Close [×] : The **Close** button will close the current file. If there is only one open file associated with the application, the **Close** button will also quit (exit) the application. You may also encounter applications that display a **Close** icon for the file itself in addition to the **Close** button on the <u>Title</u> bar.

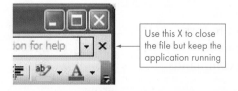

Use this X to close the file but keep the application running

Minimize [–] : This command causes the window to no longer be displayed, but the file or program will remain running and the program button will still appear on the <u>Taskbar</u>. Click the corresponding button on the <u>Taskbar</u> and it will become the active window again.

Maximize [□] : This command forces the window to occupy the maximum amount of space on the display, which may be either the full width and length of the display or the maximum size allowed by the application's programming.

Restore 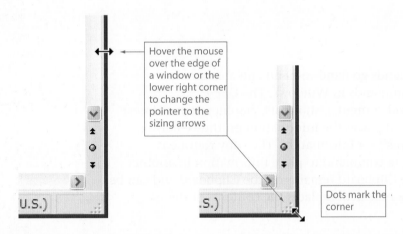 : This command resizes a window to its previous size before it was maximized. You will notice that the `Restore` and `Maximize` buttons are mutually exclusive. Only one or the other will be displayed on the Title bar.

These additional window-control commands are found on the Control menu:

Exit: This command quits a program.

Size: This command allows you to change the size of a window using keyboard controls, but it is almost always easier to size a window using the mouse. To resize a window using the mouse (not the Size command), hover the mouse pointer over the border of a window until it changes to a double-headed arrow as shown in Figure 1-22. Hold down the left mouse button and drag the border left or right. Windows can also be resized by dragging the bottom right corner (note the faint gray dots in the bottom right corner of many windows). With the exception of dialog boxes and message boxes, almost all windows can be resized.

Hover the mouse over the edge of a window or the lower right corner to change the pointer to the sizing arrows

Dots mark the corner

FIGURE 1-22 Hover the mouse over the edge of a window until the double arrow appears. Drag the edges left and right to resize the window.

 Maximized windows cannot be resized; click the `Restore` button first and then drag the edges to resize.

 Resize windows so you can see the contents of more than one window at a time. Drag the Title bar to rearrange windows on the screen. Double-click the Title bar to maximize a window or restore a window to its previous size.

Windows Concepts

Windows-based programs share fundamental concepts and conventions. Understanding these concepts will help tremendously in your overall understanding of your computer and decrease the learning curve for Windows and Windows-based programs. The following concepts are fundamental to a good working knowledge of Windows and will be referenced throughout the remainder of this text.

Select

Select means to distinguish the object on the screen from everything around it in order to perform an action on that particular item. Typically, the color behind the item changes when it has been selected. The selected object or the location of the cursor also determines what commands are available on menus, toolbars, and ribbons. For example, the cursor must be located within the boundaries of a table for certain commands on the Table menu/tab to be available.

Cut, Copy, and Paste

The Cut, Copy, and Paste commands go hand-in-hand and are among the most common and useful commands in Windows. The Copy command copies files, folders (and contents), shortcuts, graphics, text—almost any item that can be selected—and places the information on the Windows **Clipboard**, a temporary "container" for information. The copy routine is completed when you use the Paste command to place information in another location. Any item copied to the Clipboard remains on the Clipboard and can be pasted multiple times. Copying a new item replaces the contents of the Clipboard.

The Cut command is actually two commands combined: Copy and Delete. When you use the Cut command, the selected item is deleted from the original position and stored on the Clipboard in the same way as items that are copied. The item can then be pasted in a new location. The Cut, Copy, and Paste commands are located on the Edit menu of almost every window and often have icons on the toolbar/ **Home** tab (see Figure 1-23). If the window does not have an Edit menu, use the shortcut keys **Ctrl+X** (cut), **Ctrl+C** (copy), and **Ctrl+V** (paste). The right-click menu of most text input boxes (commonly found on dialog boxes) also contains Cut, Copy, and Paste.

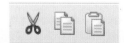

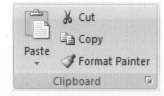

FIGURE 1-23 Cut, Copy, and Paste icons can be found throughout Windows and within applications.

If you accidentally use the Cut command instead of the Copy command, use the Paste command to place the item back in its original position or use the Undo command (see below).

There seems to be no limit to the ways you can use Copy and Paste. Develop a habit of using these commands for managing files and folders, editing documents, and gathering research information.

Using the Copy and Paste commands, you can

- copy a shortcut icon to one or several folders
- copy text from a website to a document
- copy graphics from a web page to a document
- copy files from one folder to another
- copy folders from a hard drive to a removable drive such as a USB flash drive
- copy text from one area of a document to another area or to an entirely different document
- copy text from a dialog box to a document
- copy text from a document into the text area of a dialog box
- copy Internet addresses from documents into the <u>Address</u> bar of your browser

The Print Screen key, typically located in the upper right corner of the keyboard, is a modification of the copy command. This key takes a snapshot of the current display and places an image of the display on the Clipboard. This image can then be pasted into a Word document or any other file type that accepts graphics. The key combination Alt+Print Screen will take a screen shot of the currently active window (window, dialog box, message box, etc).

Use Print Screen to document error messages or to help troubleshoot problems on your computer. Before clicking the message box to close an error message, hit Print Screen. Immediately paste the image into a Word document and make notes about the date and time and circumstances surrounding the error. When working with technical support, attach the document to email so that person can see the contents of your screen at the time the error occurred. You will find this to be an extremely helpful way of describing a problem and solving computer problems quickly.

Default

Default refers to something that happens if the user does not take an action or does not supply a preferred value. All programs, including the operating system, have default settings. These settings are typically based on the most common preferences, but there are many settings that you as an individual user will not like and some that are counterproductive for a medical transcriptionist. In Chapter 5, you will learn how to change default settings in Word so they are more amenable to your work as an MT.

View

One of the most important concepts to understand about computers is that you can change the way you see information without deleting or losing information. This concept is referred to as **View**. Since changing the way you see information is such an integral part of managing information effectively, almost every window includes view commands. The View menu/ View tab allows you to change the way information is displayed in order to filter information not needed or emphasize information that is needed. In folder windows, view commands change the way the folders and files are listed. When working in a Word document, various views change the amount and the type of information you see. Learn more about Word's views on page 123. The View menu/tab also typically includes commands for displaying or hiding toolbars, rulers, and the Status Bar.

Zoom

Another important concept related to view is **Zoom**, which allows the user to change the magnification of the text and objects on the display. A typical zoom setting is 90% to 100%; higher settings will make the text appear larger, and of course, lower settings cause the objects and text to appear smaller. Higher zoom settings are especially helpful for files with small font sizes (eg, Times New Roman 10 point). Like other view settings, *zoom does not affect the way the file will print.* Figure 1-24 shows the same document at a zoom setting of 90% and 200%.

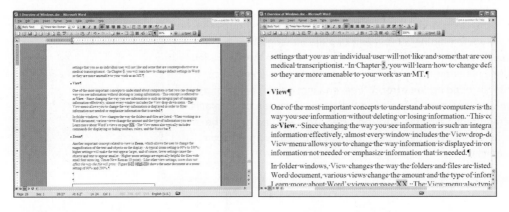

FIGURE 1-24 The same document displayed at a Zoom setting of 90% (left) and 200% (right).

I typically change the zoom setting to about 150% when proofreading a document. At this setting, the text is large and easy to read and greatly reduces eye strain. It also keeps me from leaning forward to focus on the monitor, lessening neck and shoulder pain. After proof-reading, I return the zoom setting to about 90% to make sure paragraph formatting, margins and other elements are properly placed on the page.

Quickly change the zoom by holding down **CTRL** while moving the mouse wheel forward or back. This works in Word, Internet Explorer, and many other applications.

Properties

In Windows, **Properties** refers to a file's attributes or the way an object appears or behaves. File properties include information about the file itself such as the size of the file, the date the file was created, the date the file was last modified, the author or creator of the file, etc. Properties associated with the Desktop, the Taskbar, and the Start menu change the way these items look and behave. Every object in Windows has its own properties and the information can be accessed by right-clicking the object/file and choosing Properties from the shortcut menu. Some shortcut menus may display Personalize or Customize in place of Properties. Whenever you want to change the way an object appears or behaves, right-click the object and modify the object's properties.

Critical Thinking Questions

1. Name at least three functions of the Title bar.

   _____

   _____

2. Why are the Maximize and Restore buttons never displayed at the same time?

   _____

   _____

3. Examine your Start menu. What can you say about the items listed in the left-hand column compared to items in the right-hand column?

   _____

   _____

4. Describe three ways to display the Control menu.

   _____

   _____

5. Describe at least five things you can determine just by examining icons (include all types of icons in your list).

   _____

   _____

6. Open a folder on your computer (preferably one with a lot of files). Change the view of the folder to each of the available views. Compare and contrast each view. Document these views using Print Screen and describe how each view can be used to locate specific information.

   _____

   _____

7. Open two or three windows at the same time. Right-click in an empty area of the Taskbar and use each of the available commands to tile the windows (cascade, horizontal/stacked and vertical/side-by-side). Describe how you might take advantage of each of the options. Document these views using Print Screen.

   _____

   _____

8. Right-click an empty area of the Taskbar and choose Properties. Select the Taskbar tab. Make a note of the settings (so you can return them to their original settings if you would like) and then change each of the options to see how each affects the Taskbar's behavior. Describe which options you prefer and why.

   _____

   _____

CHAPTER 2

Managing Files and Folders

OBJECTIVES

▸ Use Windows Explorer to manage files and folders.
▸ Identify key folders created by Windows and explain their purpose.
▸ Open and Save files.
▸ Use Search to find files and folders.
▸ Use the Task Manager to assess and manage the status of programs.
▸ Locate and describe the purpose of Word's program files.
▸ Back up critical data files.
▸ Recover files after a shutdown.

KEYWORDS

Application Data (Windows XP)
AppData (Windows Vista)
browsing
Documents (Windows Vista)
extension
My Documents (Windows XP)
path
RAM (random access memory)
read-only
Save
Save As
Search
Windows Explorer

Files and Folders

For a computer to be useful, the information needs to be organized. Just as we use manilla folders and file cabinets to sort and file information, Windows uses this familiar concept to organize electronic files. A disk is analogous to a filing cabinet which holds many folders. A file is analogous to a piece of paper or several pages stapled together. A computer file can be a small program or part of a program, instructions for running a program, a log that the computer creates, a graphic, or a document that you create.

Files

File names can be up to about 256 characters long, but it is not likely that you would ever use that many characters to actually name a file. File names can include letters, numbers, periods, commas, hyphens and underscore characters, but the following punctuation cannot be included in a file name: : \ / * ? < or >. A file name can contain several periods, but one last period is always used to separate the file name from the file extension. The **extension** is a three or four-letter suffix that is used by Windows to identify the file type and to associate the file with a particular program. For example, the `doc` extension is associated with Word, an `xls` extension identifies an Excel spreadsheet, and a `txt` extension is a plain text file that can be opened with most any word processing software.

It is important to become familiar with extensions and the applications associated with them. By default, Windows hides the file extensions. You will have better success managing your files if you display extensions, which will help you learn to associate extensions with their corresponding file icons (review icons on page 12). To display extensions, follow these steps:

1. Open Computer (**Logo+E**).

2. Press the **ALT** key to display the <u>Menu</u> bar in Windows Vista (it will already be displayed in Windows XP). Choose Tools > Folder Options.

3. In the **Folder Options** dialog box, select the ⏏ View ⏏ tab (Figure 2-1).

4. Under *Advanced Settings*, remove the check mark at *Hide extensions for known file types*.

5. You may also want to choose *Show hidden files and folders*.

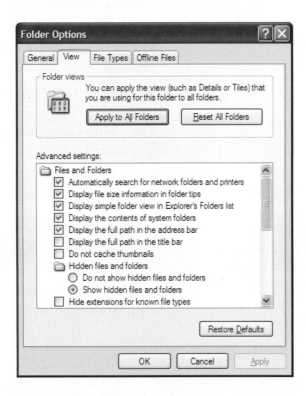

FIGURE 2-1 Use the Folder Options dialog box to display file extensions as well as hidden files and folders.

Files are stored on your hard disk (typically designated with the letter C) as electronic bits of information. Although you might think the information is stored in one "spot" on the disk, the contents of a single file might actually be scattered across the entire disk. Windows indexes the fragments so it can reassemble the file when needed. When you open a file, Windows retrieves all the fragments and moves a *copy* of the information to **RAM (random access memory)**. As long as you are working on the file (ie, the file is open), you are actually working on the data that has been copied to RAM. The original file (as it existed when you opened the file) remains on the disk. The information on the disk does not change until you use the Save command. This command takes any changes that have accumulated in RAM and transfers those changes to the disk where the original file is stored.

> *Any* file is subject to corruption while it is in RAM. Power surges or lulls (brown-outs) can affect files while they are open. Use the Save command often to protect your work by saving changes back to the hard disk. Although the hard disk is not fail proof, data is safer on the disk than in RAM.

Windows considers the copy of the file that is open to be a "temporary" file, often referred to as a "temp file," because this working copy is normally deleted from RAM when the file is closed. Files that are "open" are displayed in Windows Explorer with a tilde and a dollar sign (~$). If you view the contents of a folder (with hidden files displayed), you may see several temporary files, as in Figure 2-2. Ideally, they should only exist while a file is open, but it is not unusual for temp files to persist instead of being deleted. This happens most often when software shuts down abruptly, but there are many reasons why you may see an accumulation of temp files on your system. You can usually delete leftover temp files as you encounter them by simply selecting and deleting them (as long as the actual file is not currently open). Do not try to open a temp file; you will either receive an error message or open a file with nonsensical information.

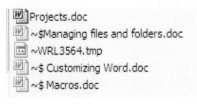

FIGURE 2-2 Currently open files begin with ~$ (tilde dollar sign) and temp files (.tmp) are marked with just a ~ (tilde).

Folders

A computer folder works just like a manilla folder to sort files. Within a folder, you can have files and/or more folders (called subfolders). Windows locates and identifies each file or folder by its unique address, called a **path** (or path name). The path lists the disk, folders, and subfolders that contain the file. Each folder in the path is separated by a backslash (\). A typical path would be C:\Documents and Setting\Laura\My Documents\Helpful inf.doc.

The path of the selected file or folder can be seen in the <u>Address</u> bar of an Explorer window. Two forward slashes (//) at the beginning of a path name (as in an Internet address) indicate the file is not located on the local hard drive (the computer you are currently using) but rather on another computer connected to your computer by a network.

Windows creates certain folders, called System folders, to locate information that it needs to run your computer. In addition to the System folders, Windows also establishes a set of user folders (also called personal folders) for each user account. Learn more about the user folders on page 32 (Windows XP) and page 49 (Windows Vista). System folders and user folders must remain in their exact location with folder names intact for Windows to operate correctly, but otherwise you are free to create as many folders as you like. Instructions for creating folders are given below for each version of Windows. Windows gives you almost unlimited options for creating folders and sorting information. Don't be afraid to use folders liberally. You can always combine the contents into other folders or delete the folder altogether. If you work with many documents on a daily basis, you can organize them into subfolders by month and day, or by category.

> All files on a computer must have a unique path name. Since Windows considers the folder and subfolder names (that contain a file) to be part of the actual file name, two or more files can have the same name as long as they are located in different folders.

Windows Explorer

Windows Explorer is used to see the hierarchy of folders on your computer and to manage your file system. Use Windows Explorer to copy, delete, move, rename, and create files and folders. Windows Explorer should not be confused with Internet Explorer, which is used to browse web pages. Using Windows Explorer, you can also view properties of disks, files, and folders, and perform maintenance tasks on disks (right-click a disk, file, or folder and choose Properties).

Access Windows Explorer by clicking the My Computer icon on your Desktop or using the shortcut key Logo+E (see page 81 for an explanation of the Logo key). **My Computer** displays the disks and drives associated with your computer. From this window, click any drive letter to access the folders and files stored on the disk. The Title bar will display the name of the folder that is currently displayed.

Figure 2-3 shows an Explorer window with the **Common Tasks** pane displayed on the left and the contents of the **My Documents** folder displayed in the file-list area. The **Common Tasks** pane, as you would expect, contains commands for the most common tasks performed on the contents of that particular folder. The commands on the **Common Tasks** pane change based on the contents of the folder itself.

Working with Folders

Windows creates a standard set of folders under each user's profile. Each person with their own login name has a profile. These folders are referred to as personal folders

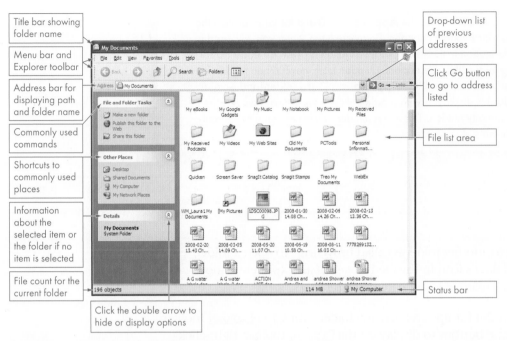

Title bar showing folder name

Menu bar and Explorer toolbar

Address bar for displaying path and folder name

Commonly used commands

Shortcuts to commonly used places

Information about the selected item or the folder if no item is selected

File count for the current folder

Drop-down list of previous addresses

Click Go button to go to address listed

File list area

Status bar

Click the double arrow to hide or display options

FIGURE 2-3 Details of an Explorer folder window.

and are the most commonly used folders. Important folders include **My Documents** and **Application Data**:

My Documents: This is the default working folder for the Microsoft Office suite of programs as well as many other applications. This means that when you save a file in Word, Excel, or other Office applications, **My Documents** will automatically appear in the **Save As** dialog box as the default folder for saving new files. The idea is that each user should save all their files within their own **My Documents** folder and its subfolders. Theoretically, this is not a bad idea, but after you have used your computer for a while, **My Documents** becomes crowded and difficult to manage. **My Documents** and its subfolders are a good place to store personal information, but most likely you will want to create other folders for specific projects or to sort your transcription work. See page 150 (Word 2003) or page 164 (Word 2007) for instructions on changing the default folder in Microsoft Office. Within **My Documents** you will find other folders such as **My Pictures**, **My Music**, and **My Videos**.

Favorites: This folder is used to store *shortcuts* to your favorite files, folders, and websites. **Favorites** is represented by a star icon ☆ that you will see on the toolbar in Windows Explorer and Internet Explorer. Learn more about shortcuts in Chapter 3.

Application Data: This folder contains user-specific information that is used by applications to store information about the way you use that application. For example, each user can customize MS Word with their own shortcut keys, toolbars, and macros, and this information is stored in the Normal.dot file within **Application Data**. Learn more about application files on page 71.

By default, Windows hides the **Application Data** folder to protect the folders from inadvertent changes. There are times when you will need to access information in this folder, so information is given on page 30 for displaying folders that are normally hidden from view. When hidden files and folders are displayed, the **Application Data** folder (and several other folders) is displayed with a pale yellow icon, which indicates the folder is normally hidden. This is a reminder to use caution when modifying the contents of this folder.

Browsing Folders

Moving from one folder to another folder is called **browsing**. To open a folder, simply double-click the folder's icon in the file-list area of an Explorer window. Folders with subfolders are referred to as "parent" folders.

Study the details of Figure 2-4 for tips on browsing folders using the Explorer toolbar. To choose which command buttons to display on the Explorer toolbar, right-click the toolbar and choose Customize.

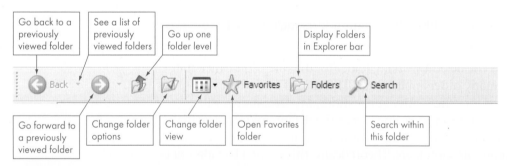

FIGURE 2-4 Use the Explorer toolbar to browse folders and manage folder options. The toolbar in this screen shot has been customized to display more icons.

Changing the View

To change the way the files and folders are displayed, select an option on the View menu (Figure 2-5). Folders and files are sorted separately, so a folder which contains both files and subfolders will sort the folders as a group and then files as a group.

Details view, as shown in Figure 2-6, displays detailed information in column form. Use this view to sort files alphabetically, chronologically or by type. Study the figure to learn ways to manipulate the file list so you can easily locate the information you need. Display or hide column headers by right-clicking any column header and choosing a heading from the menu.

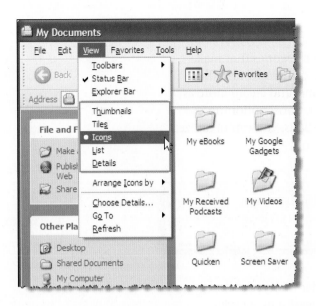

FIGURE 2-5 Use the View menu to display folder contents in various ways.

Click column headers to sort by name (alphabetically) or date (chronologically)

Drag columns left and right to change the order of the columns

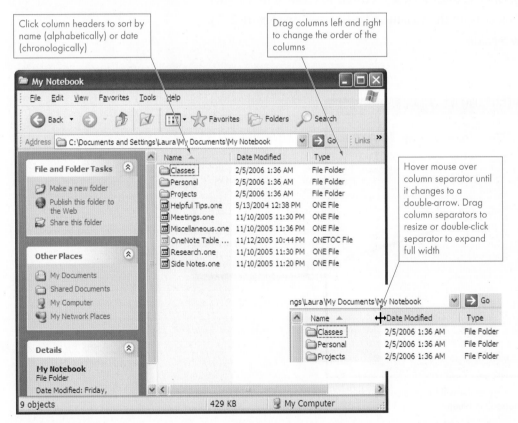

Hover mouse over column separator until it changes to a double-arrow. Drag column separators to resize or double-click separator to expand full width

FIGURE 2-6 Use Details view to display information about each file or folder and to sort by column headers.

When working with a folder containing a lot of documents, I like to use Details view. This allows me to sort by name or by date in order to locate files most recently changed. This can be especially helpful for locating files that you have worked on in the recent past.

Creating New Folders

Creating new folders will help you organize your work into categories that make sense to you. There is no limit to the number of folders you can create, and the decision is never permanent. Create, combine, delete, rename, and create more as needed to keep track of projects, tasks, research information, transcription notes, invoices, etc. If you work with many documents on a daily basis, you can organize them into subfolders by month and day or by client or doctor.

> Create shortcuts to your most commonly used folders so you can access them quickly (see page 103).

To create a new folder, display the parent folder (ie, the folder that you want to contain the new folder). Choose one of these methods to create a new folder:

- Click Make New Folder from the **Common Tasks** pane (see Figure 2-7).
- Choose File > New > Folder.

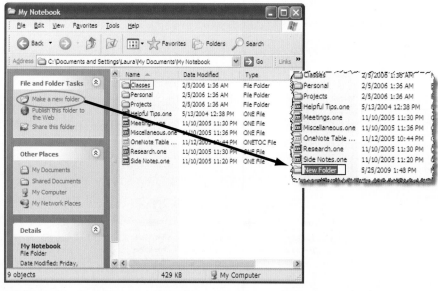

FIGURE 2-7 In this example, a new folder will be created as a subfolder in My Notebook. Type a new name to replace New Folder (backlit in blue).

A new folder will appear at the end of the list of files and folders. The folder name box will automatically open so you can type a new name for your folder. Press Enter to accept the new folder's name. If you do not name your folder, Windows will keep the name "New Folder."

Before creating a new subfolder, be sure the name of the parent folder is displayed in the <u>Title</u> bar. To create a new folder as a first-level folder under C, make sure the C drive is listed in the <u>Title</u> bar.

If you accidentally forget to name your new folder, select the folder, press **F2**, type a new name, and press **Enter**. You can name or rename a folder any time you like.

Working with Files

Most files are actually created within programs, so the easiest way to start a new file is to simply open the program that you normally use to work with the file. Most programs open with a new file already started. To create an additional new file, open the File menu/Program menu and choose New. In Word, you can use the shortcut key **CTRL+N** to start a new file. Always be sure you save a file (**CTRL+S**) as soon as you start the file. Although it is easy to get in a hurry and not pay attention to where you save a file, you will pay a larger cost in the long run when you waste time trying to locate files. In this section, you will learn how to manage your files using the **Save As** and **Open** dialog boxes.

Saving Files

The **Save As** dialog box is used to name a file and choose a location for storing the file. When a file is *first* created, the **Save** command opens the **Save As** dialog box, which allows you to name the file and designate a place to store the file.

There is not a **Save** dialog box in Windows. The first time you save a file, the program opens the **Save As** dialog box. Any subsequent saves simply write the changed information back to the hard drive (no dialog box needed). The Save As *command* is used to *change the name or location* of a file that has *already* been saved.

It is a good habit to name a file immediately after starting a new file. Don't hesitate to name a file because you are not sure what the file name should be—you can always rename the file. A file that has been named is much easier to recover in the case of a mishap. Immediately upon opening a new file, press **CTRL+S** or choose File > Save.

When saving files, you will encounter two types of **Save As** dialog boxes. Windows has a "native" **Save As** dialog box that is used by many different programs. Office has its own unique **Save As** dialog box that contains more features than Windows'. Each dialog box will be described below.

The Office Save As Dialog Box

The Office **Save As** dialog box is shown in Figure 2-8.

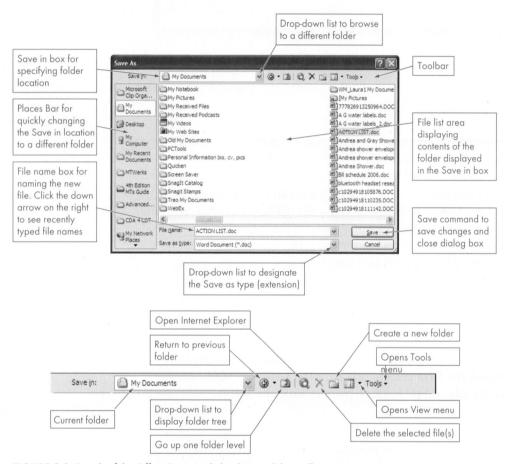

FIGURE 2-8 Details of the Office Save As dialog box and the toolbar.

To save a file from within an Office application, follow these steps:

1. From within the file to be saved, click File > Save (**CTRL+S**). The **Save As** dialog box will appear.

2. Click the down arrow next to the *Save in* drop-down list, as shown in Figure 2-9, and select a top-level folder or drive.

3. Choose a folder or subfolder from the file-list area. Continue to select folders in the file-list area until you drill down to the folder needed.

4. Make sure the *Save in* box displays the folder that you want to contain your new file.

5. If necessary, change *Save as type* to the desired file type (this is usually not necessary).

6. Type a name in the *File name* box.

7. Click **Save** or press **Enter**.

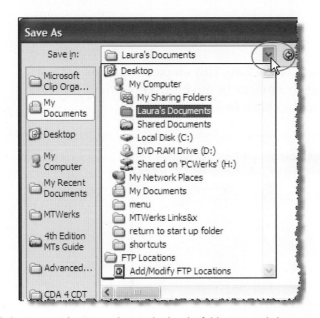

FIGURE 2-9 Click the arrow in the Save in box to display the folder tree and choose a top-level folder.

After a file is named, the **Save As** command allows you to save a copy of the file that is currently open using a different file name or a different file location. This can be helpful when you need to create "versions" of a file or when you need to create a new file that will look very similar to a file you have already created. With the original file open, choose File > Save As. Type a new name for the file and/or change the folder location by opening the *Save in* box and choosing another folder. Remember, you cannot have two files with the same name in the same folder, but you can have two files with the same name in *different* folders.

After completing Save As, the original file will be closed and the file with the new name or file location will be the currently active file. Be sure to save any changes to the original *before* using the Save As command.

The <u>Places</u> bar that runs down the left edge of the Office 2003 **Save As** dialog box can be modified to display shortcuts to the folders you use most. To add a shortcut to the <u>Places</u> bar, select a folder so that the folder name appears in the *Save in* box. Click Tools > Add to "My Places." Right-click the icons in the <u>Places</u> bar to remove, rename, or change the position of the icons. When saving a file, click an icon on the <u>Places</u> bar to quickly open that folder for saving the current file.

The Save As command results in two files-the original file and the copy of the original file with the new name. Compare this to renaming a file in Windows Explorer which results in one file—the original file with a new name.

Windows Save As Dialog Box

The Windows **Save As** dialog box is shown in Figure 2-10. This simpler dialog box has fewer tools on the toolbar, and the <u>Places</u> bar cannot be modified. Otherwise, this dialog box functions in the same way as the Office **Save As** dialog box.

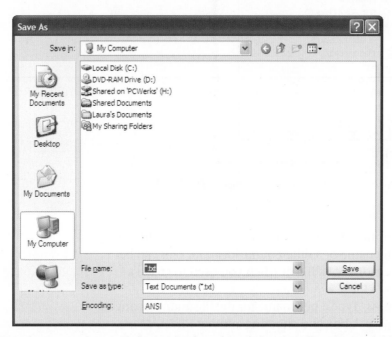

FIGURE 2-10 The common Save As dialog box has fewer features than the Office Save As dialog (compare to Figure 2-8).

Saving Files in a New Folder

You can create folders "on the fly" from within applications such as Word and Excel using the **Save As** dialog box.

1.   Click Save (**CTRL+S**) for a new file or Save As if the file has already been named.

2.   In the **Save As** dialog box, browse to the folder that will *contain* the new folder.

3.   Make sure that the folder name displayed in the *Save in* box is the correct parent folder.

4.   Click New Folder ▢ (see Figure 2-11).

5.   Type a name for the new folder and press **Enter**.

6.   Double-click the new folder (that you just created) to place the new folder in the *Save in* box.

7. Type a name for your file.
8. Click **Save** or Enter.

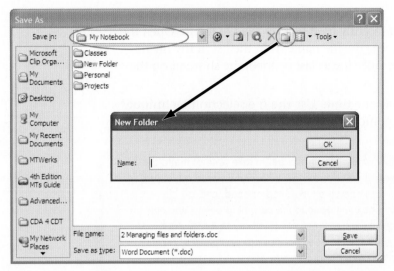

FIGURE 2-11 Click the New Folder icon to create a new folder "on the fly" while saving a file.

Opening Files

There are several approaches you can use to open files. Choose one of the following:

- Using Windows Explorer, locate the file by browsing to its folder and then double-click the file's icon (or select and press Enter). The file and its associated program will be displayed—you do not have to open the program first.

- If you have recently used the file, it will be listed on the Documents menu accessible from the Start menu. Simply open the Documents menu and select the file name.

- To open a file from within an application, choose File > Open. The **Open** dialog box, shown in Figure 2-12, looks and works very similar to the **Save**

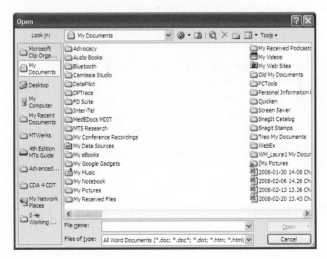

FIGURE 2-12 The Open dialog box is similar to the Save As dialog box and shares the same features. The Office 2003 Open dialog is shown here.

As dialog box. Locate the file by opening the *Look in* box and browsing to the folder containing the file you need. You can also click the folder name if available on the <u>Places</u> bar. Double-click the file's icon or select the file and press **Enter** to open.

- Word 2003 maintains a list of recently used files on the File menu. Open the File drop-down menu and choose the file name from the list. If the file has been moved to another folder since it was last opened, the shortcut on the File menu will not work.

- You can open multiple files at one time. Use the file selection techniques described on page 43 to select more than one file or folder.

It's easy to accidentally name a file and forget to take note of the folder where the file was saved. If you don't know where you saved a file, use the recent documents list to open the file. Once opened, choose File > Save As and the dialog box will open to the current folder so you can note the actual location of the file. Press **Esc** to close the **Save As** box without making changes. If the file does not appear on the list of recent documents, use Search, as described on page 45.

Read-Only Files

You may encounter files that are **read-only**, meaning the file can be opened, but it cannot be edited (ie, you can only read what's in the file but you cannot save any changes to that file). Often this happens when you try to open a file that is already open (in RAM). For example, if a program shuts down suddenly, it may fail to properly remove the file from RAM. The file may not appear open to the user, but as long as there are remnants of the file in RAM, Windows will not allow the same file to be opened again. Instead of opening the original file, Windows will present the user with another copy of the file that is marked read-only. Some files may be marked read-only on purpose, especially if the person who created the file selected that option when they saved the file (in order to prevent the file from being changed). See also information on ending programs using the Task Manager on page 68.

Using the Save As command is one way to get around a locked or read-only file. If you need to edit a file that is locked for editing, change the name using the Save As command. This will actually create a second document with a different file name. The original file will remain locked for editing, but you can edit the new file with the slightly modified name.

Organizing Files and Folders

In addition to creating, saving and opening files, you will also need to be able to move, copy, rename, and delete files and folders. Windows offers several methods

XP

for accomplishing these tasks. This section will describe commands on the **Common Tasks** pane; Chapter 3 will teach keyboard methods as well as how to use right-click menus.

Selecting Multiple Items

If you need to carry out the same command on more than one file or folder, it is more efficient to apply the command to all the files or folders at one time. Combining the mouse and the keyboard offers an efficient way of selecting several files and/or folders at once. Use these multi-select techniques for files and folders:

- To select several files or folders, hold down **CTRL** and click each file or folder icon.
- To select a range of files (a contiguous list), click the first file in the range, press and hold **Shift** while you click the last file in the range.
- To deselect any item, hold down **CTRL** while you click the item; the other selected items will remain selected.

 The easiest way to select all items listed in a folder window is to simply press **CTRL+A** (Edit > Select All).

Rename Files and Folders

Files and folders can be renamed at any time. Follow these steps:

1. Make sure the file to be renamed is closed and then locate the file in Windows Explorer.
2. Select the file (do not double-click as that will open the file).
3. Click *Rename this file/folder* from the **Common Tasks** pane.
4. Type a new name for your file and press **Enter**.

 If you have set file extensions to be displayed, as explained on page 30, then you must type the file extension when you type a new name for your file. If you do not type the extension, Windows will ask you if you are sure you want to change the file extension. Answer No and retype the new name including the extension.

Delete Files and Folders

Files can be deleted by dragging the file's icon to the Recycle Bin on the Desktop or simply selecting the file and pressing **Delete**. Deleted files go to the Recycle Bin where they can be retrieved if you later discover they have been deleted in error. If you are certain you want to permanently delete a file (and bypass the Recycle Bin), hold down **Shift** while deleting the file.

The **Save As** and **Open** dialog boxes are actually components of Windows Explorer. Notice the tools available on the toolbar—they are not limited to merely opening and saving files. Using commands on the toolbar and the right-click menu, you can actually perform many file and folder tasks, including renaming, deleting, moving, and copying files and folders—all within the **Save As** or **Open** dialog boxes. You are not limited to making changes to the file that is currently open within the application either. Once you are finished making changes to other files, press **Esc** to close the dialog without affecting the file that is currently open.

Moving and Copying with the Mouse

Dragging files in a graphical user interface is the same as giving the computer a specific command, so many file management tasks can be accomplished using drag-and-drop mouse techniques. To move files or folders using the mouse, open the destination folder (the folder where you want to move the files) as well as the folder containing the files to be moved. Select the files to be moved. Click the mouse pointer *directly over the selected items*. Drag the selected icons and drop them over the destination folder window.

You can also move items by dropping them on top of a folder's icon (ie, the folder window does not have to be open). Drag a selection toward another folder's icon (or shortcut icon) and hover over the icon until it too is selected. Once the destination icon is selected, release the mouse button.

When you drag files and folders between folders located on two different *drives*, for example, from drive C to drive D, Windows automatically assumes you want to *copy* the files, not move the files. Hold down the **Shift** key while dragging files between separate drives if you want to *move* the files.

To copy items between two folders, use the same technique as moving files but hold down **CTRL** while dragging with the mouse. You will know that you are copying the selected items when you see a plus sign attached to the mouse pointer as in Figure 2-13. The **CTRL** key instructs Windows to *copy* the files being dragged instead of moving the files.

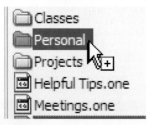

FIGURE 2-13 A plus sign attached to the pointer indicates the file is being copied.

Searching Your Computer

An extremely powerful tool in Windows is the **Search** feature. This utility searches your computer for files and folders based on whatever information you can provide. Windows allows you to search your entire computer or narrow your search to a folder and its subfolders.

Searching Your Computer

To begin a search, go to **Start** > Search > For Files and Folders (or press **Logo+F**). An Explorer window will open and the **Common Tasks** pane will be replaced with the **Search Companion**, as shown in Figure 2-14 .

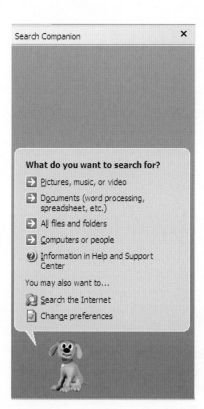

FIGURE 2-14 The Search Companion will step you through a series of questions to locate files on your computer.

By default, the **Search Companion** will present a series of questions to step you through the search routine, but this method can be rather time-consuming and even tedious once you are more experienced with searching. If you do not like the stepwise approach to entering search criteria, you may choose to go straight to the **Advanced Search** dialog instead. To forego the stepwise approach to searching, open the **Search Companion** as above and follow this sequence of commands:

Change Preferences > Change files and folders search behavior > Advanced

You do not have to make this change each time you perform a search; from this point on, each new search will begin with the **Advanced Search** task pane as shown in Figure 2-15.

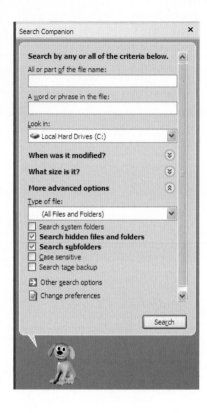

FIGURE 2-15 The Advanced Search task pane.

To perform a search, follow these steps:

1. Type part of the file name into the box labeled *All or part of the file name*. This information might include a word in the file name or even the file extension.

2. If you don't have information related to the file name, type information related to the file's contents into the second box labeled *A word or phrase in the file*. You can actually type information into either or both search boxes.

3. If necessary, narrow your search by expanding the advanced search options or clicking any of the options listed in the lower portion of the **Search Companion** task pane.

Type part of the patient's name into *A word or phrase in the file* box to locate a report on a specific patient. Type .doc in the *file name* box to speed up the search by narrowing the search to only Word documents.

Type your search criteria carefully. If you provide the wrong information, even a single character, you will exclude the file you are looking for. It is better to type *less* information that you know is correct rather than *more* information that is potentially wrong. For example, a search for a file name containing "johns" would find "Johns," "Johnson," "Johnston," or "Johnstone" and would be a better query if you were not sure of the exact spelling.

The search results will appear to the right of the **Search Companion** task pane in the file-list area. Notice that the Title bar and Taskbar button display "Search Results." The **Search Results** folder functions like any other Explorer window. You can perform any of the following:

- Select a file from the search results and double-click to open.
- Select the file icon and choose an option from the File menu such as Print, Delete, or Rename (as in Figure 2-16) or from the file's right-click menu (see page 96).
- To open the folder that actually contains the file, select the file and choose File > Open Containing Folder.

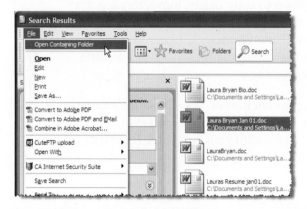

FIGURE 2-16 Open the actual folder containing the selected file using the command on the File menu.

 When the search routine returns a long list of files or folders, change the way the files are displayed in the search results pane to make it easier to locate the file(s) you need. See options for displaying folder contents on page 34.

 Examine the icons in the results pane carefully. Some files may be in the Recycle Bin; other icons may represent shortcuts. Most likely, you need to locate the actual *file* and not the *shortcut* for the file. Shortcuts will be displayed with a small curved arrow in the bottom left corner of the icon. Learn more about shortcuts on page 101.

Searching a Folder

You can also begin a search from a specific folder, which works really well if you know which folder or parent folder contains the file you need. To search within a specific folder, including its subfolders, follow these steps:

1. Locate the folder in Windows Explorer and open that folder.

2. Go to View > Explorer Bar > Search (or press **F3**). The **Search Companion** (as shown in Figure 2-15) will appear on the left with the folder's contents displayed on the right.

3. Type your search criteria. The folder name will already appear in the *Look in* box. The search routine will only search the open folder and its subfolders. The results will be displayed in a Search Results window as above.

For more on Windows XP, go to page 68.

Windows Explorer

Windows Explorer is used to see the hierarchy of folders on your computer and to manage your file system. Use Windows Explorer to copy, delete, move, rename, and create files and folders. Windows Explorer should not be confused with Internet Explorer, which is used to browse web pages. Using Windows Explorer, you can also view properties of disks, files, and folders, and perform maintenance tasks on disks (right-click a disk, file, or folder and choose Properties).

Access Windows Explorer by clicking the Computer icon on your Desktop or using the shortcut key **Logo+E** (see page 81 for an explanation of the **Logo** key). **Computer** displays the disks and drives associated with your computer. From this

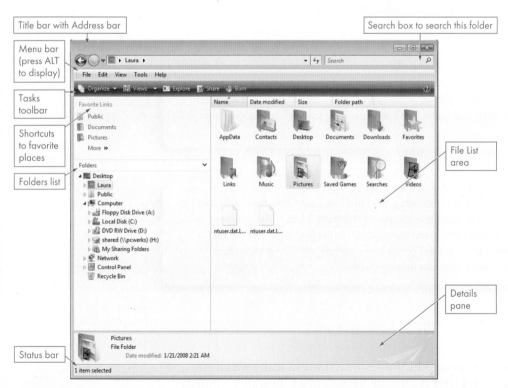

FIGURE 2-17 Details of an Explorer folder window. Click Organize and choose Layout to select panes to hide or display.

window, click any drive letter to access the folders and files stored on that disk. The Title bar will display the name of the folder that is currently displayed.

Figure 2-17 shows an Explorer window with Favorite Links and Folders displayed on the left and the contents of the **Laura** folder displayed in the file-list area. The Tasks toolbar, which runs below the Address bar, contains commands for the most common tasks you might want to perform on the contents of that particular folder. The commands on the Tasks toolbar change based on the contents of the folder itself.

Working with Folders

Windows creates a standard set of folders for each user called personal folders. You will notice that personal folders are displayed in a different color than other folders (compare the green and yellow folders in Figure 2-26). The folders you are likely to use on a daily basis are described below:

Users: This folder contains each user's profile information, so each user (an individual with a login name on this computer) has a folder within the **Users** folder. A user's profile includes their personal folders and their personal settings for the Desktop and Start menu as well as application settings and preferences.

Personal folder: This folder is the main folder for storing files created by the user. This folder always carries the user's name. This particular folder is easy to find because Windows places shortcuts to this folder in various places, namely the Start menu, **Save As** and **Open** dialog boxes as well as at the top of Favorite Links in the Explorer window. The path for the personal folder is C:\Users\Username.

Within the personal folder, you will find additional subfolders for storing various types of files. Figure 2-17 shows the subfolders in the personal folder. Notice the yellow folder named **AppData**. This folder contains user-specific information used by applications. For example, each user can customize MS Word with their own shortcut keys, toolbars and macros, and this information is stored in **AppData** (learn more at the end of this chapter).

The **Documents** folder within the personal folder (see Figure 2-17) is the default working folder for the Office suite of applications. This means that when you save a file in Word, Excel, or other Office applications, the **Save As** dialog box opens with **Documents** as the default location for saving new files. The idea is that each user saves all their documents, spreadsheets and slide presentations within their own **Documents** folder. Theoretically, this is not a bad idea, but after you have used your computer for a while, especially for transcribing, **Documents** may become crowded and unwieldy. The **Documents** folder is a good place to store personal information, but most likely you will want to create new folders for specific projects or to sort your transcription work. Learn more about creating new folders on page 52.

Favorites: This folder stores *shortcuts* to all your favorite items—files, folders, and websites. **Favorites** is represented by a folder with a star (see Figure 2-17).

VISTA

By default, Windows hides the **AppData** folder to protect users from making changes that might be harmful. There are times when you will need to access information in this folder, so information is given on page 30 for displaying folders that are normally hidden from view. Notice in Figure 2-17 that the **AppData** folder is displayed with a pale yellow icon to indicate the folder is normally hidden. This is a reminder to use caution when modifying the contents of this folder.

Browsing Folders

Moving from one folder to another folder is called **browsing**. To open a folder, simply double-click the folder's icon in the file-list area of an Explorer window. Folders with subfolders are referred to as "parent" folders. You can also browse folders using the Folders list on the left side of the Explorer window. Click the triangles next to folder names to display subfolders. The contents of the selected folder will be displayed in the file-list area.

Study the details of Figure 2-18 for tips on browsing folders using the Explorer Title bar.

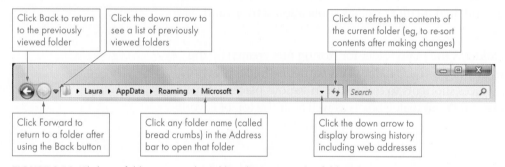

FIGURE 2-18 Click any folder name in the Address bar to open that folder.

One other way of browsing folders in the Explorer window is to use the arrows located between the folder names in the Address bar. Click the arrow to the right of the folder name, as shown in Figure 2-19, to display a drop-down list of that folder's contents. Choose any folder on the drop-down list to open that folder.

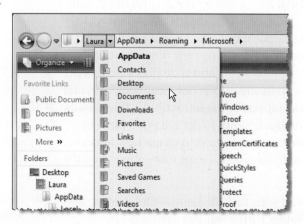

FIGURE 2-19 Click the arrow to the right of the folder name to select from a list of that folder's subfolders.

Changing the View

To change the way the files and folders are displayed, select an option on the View menu located on the <u>Tasks</u> toolbar (Figure 2-20) or move the slider button up and down. Folders and files are sorted separately, so a folder which contains files and subfolders will sort the folders as a group and then files as a group.

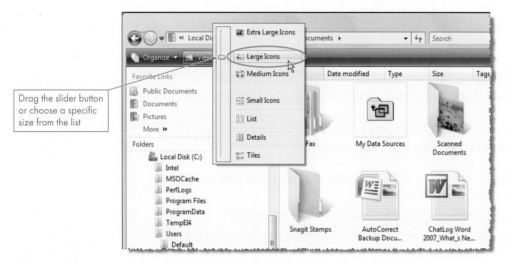

FIGURE 2-20   Use the View menu to change the way the folder contents are displayed. Select a specific view from the list or move the slider button.

 Click into the file-list area, hold down **CTRL** and move the scroll wheel on the mouse backward and forward to quickly change the size of the icons within the file-list area. The icons will "grow" and "shrink" as you move the wheel.

Details view displays detailed information about each file in column form. Use this view to sort files alphabetically, chronologically, or by type. Study Figure 2-21 to learn ways to manipulate the file list to easily locate the information you need.

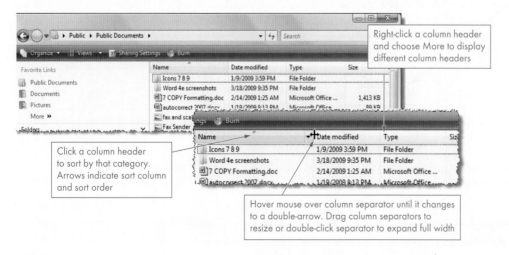

FIGURE 2-21   Use Details view to display information about each file/folder; click the column header to sort by that category.

VISTA

When working with a folder containing a lot of documents, I like to use Details view. This allows me to easily view dates in a column to locate files most recently changed. This can be especially helpful for locating files that you have worked on in the past few days or so.

Creating New Folders

Creating new folders will help you organize your work into categories that make sense to you. There is no limit to the number of folders you can create, and the decision is never permanent. Create, combine, delete, rename, and create more as needed to keep track of projects, tasks, research information, transcription notes, invoices, etc. If you work with many documents on a daily basis, you can organize them into subfolders by month and day, or by doctor/client.

To create a new folder, display the folder (that you want to *contain* the new folder) in the Address bar. Choose one of these methods:

- Using the Tasks toolbar, click Organize > New Folder (see Figure 2-22).
- Using the Menu bar, choose File > New > Folder (press the **ALT** key to reveal the Menu bar).

A new folder will appear as in Figure 2-22. The folder-name box will open so you can type a new name for your folder. Press **Enter** to accept the new folder's name. If you forget to name your folder, Windows will keep the name "New Folder."

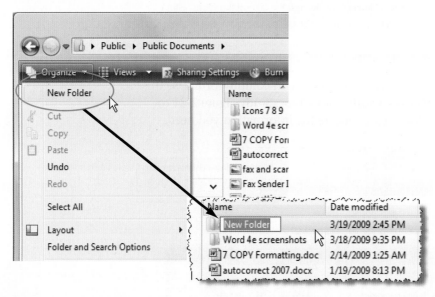

FIGURE 2-22 Click New Folder on the Organize menu. A new folder will be created as a subfolder in Public Documents. Type a new name in the folder name box to replace New Folder (backlit in blue).

If you accidentally forget to name your new folder, click the folder name (or select the folder and press **F2**) to open the folder-name box. Type a new name and press **Enter**. You can name or rename a folder at any time.

Before creating a new subfolder, be sure the name of the parent folder is displayed in the <u>Address</u> bar. To create a new folder as a first-level folder under C, make sure the C drive is listed in the <u>Address</u> bar.

Working with Files

Most files are actually created within programs, so the easiest way to start a new file is to simply open the program that you use to work with that type of file. Most programs open with a new file already started. To create an additional new file, click the **Program** button (or the File menu) and choose New. In Word, you can use the shortcut key **CTRL+N** to start a new file. Always be sure you name a file as soon as you start the file. Always pay close attention to where you save your files so you don't waste a lot of time trying to locate them. In this section, you will learn how to manage your files using the **Save As** and **Open** dialog boxes.

Saving Files

When saving files, you will encounter two types of **Save As** dialog boxes. Windows has a "native" **Save As** dialog box that is used by many different programs. Office has its own unique **Save As** dialog box that contains more features than Windows'. Each dialog box will be described below.

The **Save As** dialog box is used to name a file and choose a location for storing the file. When a file is *first* created, the **Save** command opens the **Save As** dialog box, which allows you to name the file and designate a place to store the file.

After a file has been named, the Save command will save changes to the file but will do so without opening a dialog box. The changes are saved to the hard disk so they are a permanent part of the file.

It is a good habit to name a file immediately after starting a new file. Don't hesitate to name a file because you are not sure what the file name should be—you can always rename the file. A file that has been named is much easier to recover in the case of a mishap. Immediately upon opening a new file, press **CTRL+S** or click **Program** > Save.

There is not a Save dialog box in Windows. The first time you save a file, Windows opens the **Save As** dialog box. Any subsequent saves simply write the changed information back to the hard disk (no dialog box needed). The Save As *command* can also be used to *change the name or location* of a file that has already been saved.

VISTA

Windows Vista Save As Dialog Box

The standard Windows Vista **Save As** dialog box is shown in Figure 2-23. The Office suite of applications uses a modified Windows **Save As** dialog box (described below).

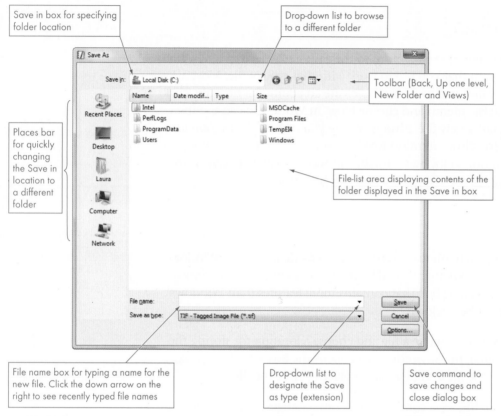

FIGURE 2-23 The standard Windows Vista Save As dialog box.

When presented with the standard Windows Vista **Save As** dialog box, follow these steps:

1. Begin by selecting a folder to store the new file. To do this, click the down arrow next to the *Save in* drop-down list, as shown in Figure 2-24, and select a top-level folder or drive. If available, you can also choose a folder from the Places bar on the left.

2. Choose a folder or subfolder from the file-list area. Continue to select folders in the file-list area until you drill down to the folder needed.

3. Make sure the *Save in* box displays the folder that you want to contain your new file.

4. If necessary, change the *Save as type* to the desired file type (this is usually not necessary).

5. Type a name in the *File name* box.

6. Click **Save** or press **Enter**.

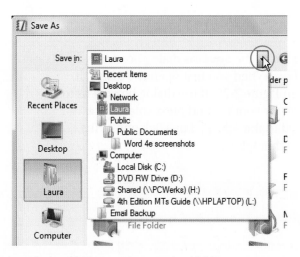

FIGURE 2-24 Drop down the list of folders to select a top-level folder.

After a file is named, the **Save As** command allows you to save a copy of the file that is currently open using a different file name or a different file location. This can be helpful when you need to create "versions" of a file or when you need to create a new file that will look very similar to a file you have already created. To rename a file, follow these steps:

1. With the original file open, choose File > Save As or Program > Save As (or **F12** in Word).

2. Type a new name for the file and/or change the folder location by opening the *Save in* box and choosing another folder.

Remember, you cannot have two files with the same name in the same folder, but you can have two files with the same name in *different* folders.

 After completing Save As, the original file will be closed and the file with the new name or file location will be the currently active file. Be sure to save any changes to the original *before* using the Save As command.

Notes

VISTA

Office 2007 Save As Dialog Box

When running Office 2007 under Windows Vista, the **Save As** dialog box looks more like Windows Explorer than a dialog box. When you first open the dialog, it will open in an abbreviated form as shown in Figure 2-25. If the dialog box opens to the folder you need, simply type a new name for your file and press **Enter**. If the folder you need appears in the path displayed in the <u>Address</u> bar, click one of the "bread crumbs" (a folder name) to change to that folder.

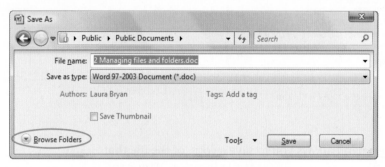

FIGURE 2-25 The abbreviated Office 2007 Save As dialog box.

To change to a completely different folder, click **Browse Folders** (**ALT+B**) in the bottom left corner. The **Save As** dialog box will expand to a full Explorer window as shown in Figure 2-26. Use the same techniques as discussed above for changing to a different folder. You can also select a folder from the Folders list or from the Favorite Links list.

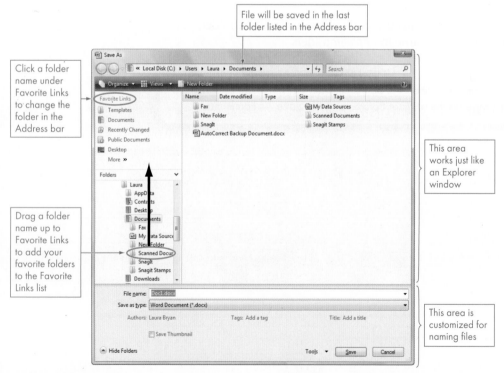

FIGURE 2-26 The Office Save As dialog box in Windows Vista looks and acts like an Explorer window with an additional area across the bottom for designating a file name and a file type.

VISTA

Drag folders from the Folders list upward into the Favorite Links area to create shortcuts to your most-used folders. To save an item in one of these folders, simply click the folder name in Favorite Links.

Saving Files in a New Folder

You can create new folders "on the fly" from within applications using the **Save As** dialog box. Follow these steps:

1. Click Save (**CTRL+S**) for a new file or Save As if the file has already been named.
2. In the **Save As** dialog box, browse to the folder that will contain the new folder.
3. Make sure that the folder name displayed in the *Save in* box or in the <u>Address</u> bar is the correct parent folder.
4. Click **New Folder** as shown in Figure 2-27.
5. Type a name for the new folder and press **Enter**.
6. Double-click the new folder (that you just created) to place that folder name in the *Save in* box.
7. Type a name for your file.
8. Click **Save** or **Enter**.

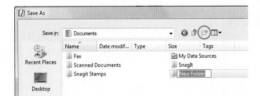 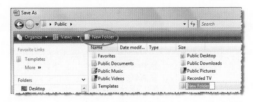

FIGURE 2-27 Click the New File icon to create a new folder "on the fly" while saving a file.

• •

Notes

Opening Files

There are several approaches you can take to opening a file. Choose one of the following:

- Using Windows Explorer, locate the file by browsing to its folder and then double-clicking the file's icon (or select the icon and press **Enter**). The file and its associated program will open—you do not have to open the program first.
- If you have recently used the file, it will be listed on the Recent Items menu accessible from the Start menu. Simply open Recent Items and select the file name.
- To open a file from within an application, choose File > Open or **Program** > Open. The **Open** dialog box, shown in Figure 2-28, looks and works very similar to the **Save As** dialog box.
- Many applications maintain a list of recently used files on the application's File menu/Program menu. Open the application used to edit the file and look on the menu for a list of recently used files. MS Word 2007 lists as few as 9 up to greater than 20 recent files on the right side of the Program menu. If the file has been moved to another folder since it was last opened, the shortcut on the File or Program menu will no longer work.

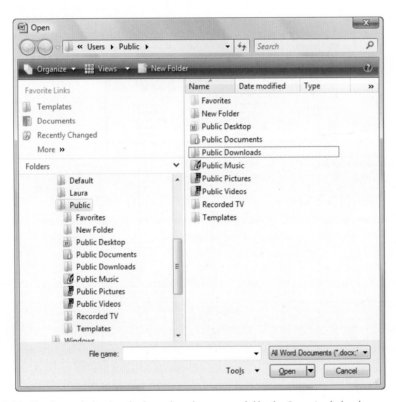

FIGURE 2-28 The Open dialog box looks and works very much like the Save As dialog box.

If you are opening a Word document from a previous version of Word, be sure that Word 2007's **Open** dialog box displays All Word Documents in the bottom right corner. The **Open** dialog box will display the contents of the currently selected folder based on the file type listed on the button. If the button displays Word Documents .docx, only Word 2007 documents will be listed in the file-list area.

The Office Program menu includes a list of recently used documents on the right side of the Program menu. To keep a document listed permanently, click the pushpin next to the document name. This will "pin" the document to the list so it remains on the Recent Documents list until you click the pushpin to "unpin" it.

Using Explorer or the **Open** dialog box, you can select multiple files to open at one time. Use the file selection techniques described on page 60.

It's easy to accidentally name a file and forget to take note of the folder where the file was saved. If you do not know where you saved a file, try using the recent documents list to open the file. Once opened, choose File > Save As or Program > Save As and the dialog box will open to the current folder so you can note the actual location of the file. Press **Esc** to close the **Save As** box without making changes.

Read-Only Files

You may encounter files that are **read-only**, meaning the file can be opened, but it cannot be edited (ie, you can only read what's in the file but you cannot save any changes to that file). Often this happens when you try to open a file that is already open (in RAM). For example, if a program shuts down suddenly, it may fail to properly remove the file from RAM. The file may not appear to be open, but as long as there are remnants of the file in RAM, Windows will not allow the same file to be opened again. Instead of opening the original file, Windows will present the user with another copy of the file that is marked read-only. Files may also be marked read-only on purpose if the person who created the file does not want that file to be changed. See also information on ending programs using the Task Manager on page 68.

VISTA

Using the Save As command is one way to get around a locked or read-only file. If you need to edit a file that is read-only, change the name using the Save As command. This will actually create a second document with a different file name. The original file will remain locked, but you can edit the file with the slightly modified name.

Organizing Files and Folders

In addition to creating, saving, and opening files, you will also need to be able to move, copy, rename, and delete files and folders. Windows offers several methods for accomplishing these tasks. This section will explain how to use the Tasks toolbar, and Chapter 3 will show you how to use right-click menus.

Selecting Multiple Items

If you need to carry out the same command on more than one file or folder, it is more efficient to apply the command to all the files or folders at one time. Combining the mouse and the keyboard offers an efficient way to select several files and folders at once. To select multiple files or folders, follow these steps:

- Hold down **CTRL** and click each file or folder icon.
- If you need to select a range of files (a contiguous list), click the first file in the range, then press and hold **Shift** while you click the last file in the range.
- To deselect any item, hold down **CTRL** while you click the item; the other selected items will remain selected.

The easiest way to select all items listed in a folder window is to simply press **CTRL+A** (Organize > Select All).

Windows Vista offers a new feature for selecting files using check boxes. This option allows the user to place check marks next to files instead of holding down **CTRL** or **Shift** while clicking with the mouse. To turn on this option, follow these steps:

1. Click **Organize** on the Tasks toolbar.
2. Choose Folder and Search Options.
3. Select **View**.
4. Scroll down the list of options and place a check mark at *Use check boxes to select items* as shown in Figure 2-29.
5. Click **OK** to close the dialog box.

Click each item in the file-list area to place a check mark. Click again to remove the check mark. Click in an empty area of the file-list area to remove all check marks.

VISTA

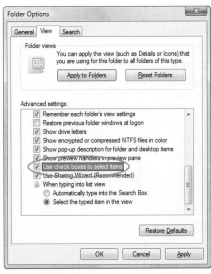

FIGURE 2-29 Turn on Windows Vista's check boxes to select files and folders.

Using the Tasks Toolbar and the Menu bar

The Tasks toolbar displays the most common actions performed on the selected item, and the commands change depending on the item selected. Typical file management commands include move, copy, delete, rename, and print. Select a file or folder from the file-list area then click a command from the Tasks toolbar. If the command you need is not displayed on the toolbar, click Organize as shown in Figure 2-30.

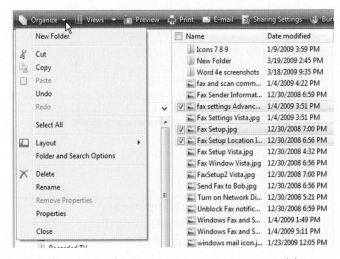

FIGURE 2-30 Use the Tasks toolbar or the Organize menu to print, cut, copy, delete, or rename files and folders.

VISTA

The Organize menu includes the command to rename files and folders. Typically, renaming is done one file/folder at a time. To rename several files, select the files and click Rename (or select the files and press F2). Type a new name for the first selected file and press Enter. The remainder of the selected files will be renamed using the same name as the first file and numbered sequentially (eg, NewName1; NewName2; NewName3, etc.).

If you have set file extensions to be displayed, as explained on page 30, then you must type the file extension when you type a new name for your file. If you do not type the extension, Windows will ask you if you are sure you want to change the file extension. Answer No and retype the new name including the extension.

Delete Files and Folders

Files can be deleted by dragging the file's icon to the Recycle Bin on the Desktop or simply selecting the file and pressing Delete. Deleted files go to the Recycle Bin where they can be retrieved if you later discover they have been deleted in error. If you are certain you want to permanently delete a file (and bypass the Recycle Bin), hold down Shift while deleting the file.

The **Save As** and **Open** dialog boxes are actually extensions of Windows Explorer. This is especially apparent with the new Office **Save As** and **Open** dialog boxes when running under Windows Vista. Notice the tools available on the **Open** and **Save As** dialog boxes—they are not limited to merely opening and saving files. Using commands on the toolbar and the right-click menu, you can actually perform many file and folder tasks, including renaming, deleting, moving, and copying files and folders within the **Save As** or **Open** dialog boxes. You are not limited to making changes to the file that is currently open within the application—you can perform tasks on any file while either dialog box is open. Once you are finished making changes to other files, press **Esc** to close the dialog without affecting the file that is currently open.

Moving and Copying with the Mouse

Dragging files in a graphical user interface is the same as giving the computer a specific command, so many file management tasks can be accomplished using drag-and-drop mouse techniques. To move files or folders using the mouse, follow these steps:

1. Open the destination folder (the folder where you want to move the files).
2. Select the files to be moved.
3. Click the mouse pointer *directly over the selected items*. Drag the selected icons and drop them over the destination folder window as shown in Figure 2-31.

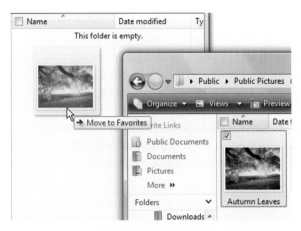

FIGURE 2-31 Windows Vista will display a ToolTip confirming that you want to move the selected file to the selected folder.

You can also move items by dropping them on top of an item's icon (ie, the folder window does not have to be open). Drag a selection toward another folder's icon (or shortcut icon) and hover over the icon until it too is selected. Once the destination icon is selected, release the mouse button.

When you drag files and folders between folders located on two different *drives*, for example, from drive C to drive D, Windows automatically assumes you want to *copy* the files, not move the files. Hold down the **Shift** key while dragging files between separate drives if you want to *move* the files.

To copy items between two folders, use the same technique as moving files but hold down **CTRL** while dragging with the mouse. You will know that you are copying the selected items when you see a plus sign attached to the mouse pointer as in Figure 2-32. The **CTRL** key instructs Windows to *copy* the files being dragged instead of moving the files. Remember, you can drop files onto any folder icon—regardless of where the icon is located.

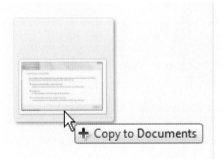

FIGURE 2-32 A plus sign attached to the pointer indicates the file is being copied.

Searching Your Computer

One of Windows Vista's notable improvements over previous versions of Windows is the **Search** feature. As hard drives have become enormous (in comparison to the drives of the 1990's), people have begun to accumulate more and more files. With the ability to store terabytes of information, "search" is now one of the most important features on a personal computer. Windows Vista indexes the information on your computer on an ongoing basis, so searching Vista is simple and amazingly fast. Search results are presented in real time—as you type your search criteria!

Searching from the Start menu

You can begin a search by opening the Start menu and typing into the Search text box located at the bottom of the Start menu. Simply press the **Logo** key and begin typing your search text, called a query. The Start menu will display up to 20 items based on your search, updating the results as you type. In the example shown in Figure 2-33, the search query was mede and Windows Vista immediately presented a list of results. Items that fit the search criteria are divided into categories and listed in the following order:

- Programs
- Favorites and History (includes links in Favorites and recent websites)
- Files
- Communications (includes email and chat transcripts)

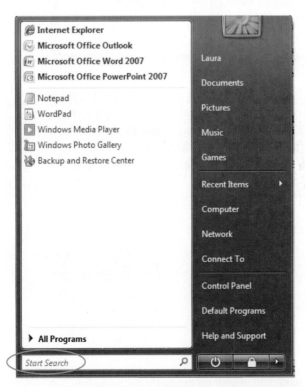

FIGURE 2-33 Type your search query into the Start menu text box to display the top 20 items that match your search.

If the item you are searching for is the first item on the list, simply hit **Enter**. If it is anywhere else on the list, click the item to open it or use the arrow keys to move up and down the list and press **Enter** to open the item. Hover over a search result to display a ToolTip with information about the item.

> Opening programs can be as simple as typing the program name and hitting **Enter**. For example, to open Word, simply click **Logo**, type word, and press **Enter**.

To cancel a search routine, press **Esc** to restore your normal *Start* menu contents.

If the *Start* menu does not display the file you need, click *See all results* at the bottom of the *Start* menu. An Explorer window will appear with *all of the results* of your search, which may be a surprisingly long list. Windows searches not just for the file name or words within the file, but also any information associated with a file, referred to as metadata (data that describes data). If the search results are unwieldy, click one of the *Show only* categories listed directly under the <u>Address</u> bar: *Email, Document, Picture, Music,* or *Other* (see Figure 2-34). In this context, *Document* refers to any file created by Office such as a Word document, an Excel spreadsheet, or a PowerPoint presentation.

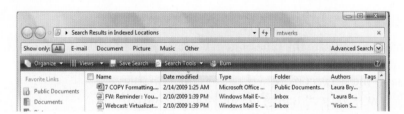

FIGURE 2-34 Choose a category from the Search pane to narrow your search results.

> When the search routine returns a long list of files or folders, change the way the files are displayed in the search results pane to make it easier to locate the file(s) you need. See options for displaying folder contents on page 51.

VISTA

If you still have not found the file you need or narrowed your choices sufficiently, click the Advanced Search button to expand the **Search** pane as shown in Figure 2-35.

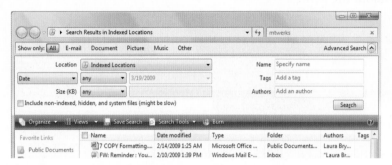

FIGURE 2-35 The Advanced Search pane drops open to display more search options.

Use the drop-down boxes to make selections as needed to narrow your search criteria and then click **Search**.

 You can search on partial words, but you must start at the beginning of a word. For example, `unger` would not find files with the word `hunger`.

A very efficient way to begin a search is to indicate the type of item you are searching for along with the search text. For example, to search for a file based on the file name, type `name: keywords` in the search box, where `name` is the Windows command to search file names only and `keywords` represents the word or words in your query (search). This technique works in any search box. Other search commands include `created:` (date the file was created), `modified:` (date the file was last changed), `type:` (file type such a .doc, .xls or .mp3) and `folder:`. The greater than (>) and less than (<) signs can also be used to indicate "since" and "before" respectively. Here are examples:

`Name:laura` (files with laura in the file name)

`Created:today` (any file created today)

`Created:>yesterday` (files created since yesterday)

`Created:<yesterday` (files created before yesterday)

`Modified:December 2007` (any files modified in the month of December)

`Modified:<January 2008` (any files modified before January 2008)

`first name:Bob` (people named Bob in your Contact list)

VISTA

The Search Results window behaves exactly like any other Explorer window. Sort and display the files as needed using the View menu. Once you locate the item, double-click the icon to open the file or right-click the icon to display a list of choices such as Print, Copy, Delete, or Rename. Open file location will open the actual folder that contains the selected file (see Figure 2-36).

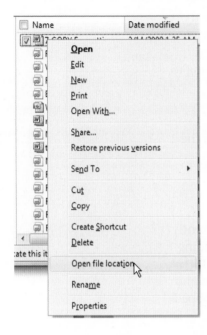

FIGURE 2-36 Right-click a result in the search pane to see a list of commands. Open file location will open the folder which contains the file you have selected.

 Examine the icons in the results pane carefully. Search results will include files in the Recycle Bin as well as shortcut icons (displayed with a curved arrow in the bottom left corner). Most likely, you need to locate the actual file and not a shortcut for the file.

Searching a Folder

You can also begin a search within a specific folder. This works very well when you know which folder contains the needed file but the folder has many files/subfolders within it. Using Windows Explorer, open the folder and press **F3** to open a search window using the current folder as the search location. In lieu of pressing **F3**, you can also type directly into the *Search* text box located in the upper right-hand corner of the folder window. If needed, display the **Search** pane with advanced search options by clicking Search Tools > Search pane (as in Figure 2-37).

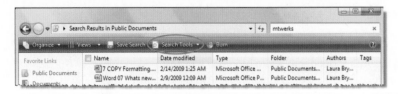

FIGURE 2-37 Display the Search pane to expand your search options.

Using the Task Manager

The Task Manager provides information about programs, processes and services running on your PC. It is helpful for assessing the status of programs, especially when a program has stopped responding (commonly referred to as "locked up"). Often users will restart (reboot) their PC when a program is no longer responding to the mouse or keyboard, but a much easier way to regain control of the PC is to use the Task Manager to end the individual program that is hung. Using the Task Manager is more efficient than shutting down your entire system because the Task Manager allows you to close the one program that is no longer responding without having to close all other open windows and running through an entire boot sequence.

Choose one of the following methods for opening the Task Manager:

- Right-click an empty area of the <u>Taskbar</u> and choose Task Manager from the shortcut menu.
- Press **CTRL+ALT+Del**. If given the option, click Task Manager.
- Press **CTRL+Shift+Esc**.

The **Applications** tab, as shown in Figure 2-38, displays programs that are currently running. If the program is hung, the *Status* column will display "Not responding." To end a program that has stopped responding, select the program and click **End Task** in the bottom right corner. Windows will ask you to confirm your decision and warn you that unsaved items will be lost. Of course, if the program has stopped responding, you do not have any choice.

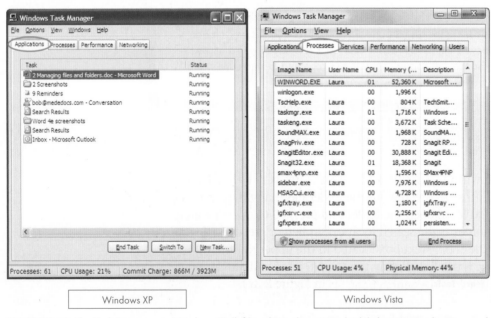

Windows XP	Windows Vista

FIGURE 2-38 The Task Manager in Windows XP (left) and Windows Vista (right) showing Applications and Processes.

 Be patient when using the Task Manager to end a program. It almost always works but it may take 30-60 seconds to complete. Avoid the temptation to click more buttons.

The Processes tab on the Task Manager displays all processes and services currently running. The number of processes running concurrently, as well as the CPU usage, is listed in the bottom left corner of the dialog box, as shown in Figure 2-39. Processes will include programs that are visibly running plus many that run in the background. Examples of background processes include mouse and keyboard controls, software controls for printers, faxes, and scanners, monitoring software such as virus scanners, and services such as Internet connections, software update services, as well as numerous processes and services required by the operating system. Items listed on the Processes tab are not always recognizable. For example, the *Image Name* for MS Word is WINWORD.EXE and the *Image Name* for Internet Explorer is iexplorer.exe. Click *Image Name* (column header) to sort the list alphabetically.

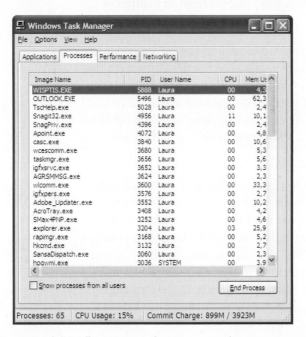

FIGURE 2-39 The Processes tab lists all programs and services currently running on your PC.

 When Word shuts down suddenly, it sometimes leaves "processes" still running. It will appear that Word is actually closed (ie, there are no buttons on the <u>Taskbar</u>), but there may still be remnants of the program left in RAM. When this happens, you may have problems reopening the file that was open when Word shut down. Windows may tell you the file is locked for editing or in use by another user. After a sudden shutdown, it is a good habit to make sure Word is completely closed. On the Processes tab, under *Image name*, look for WINWORD.EXE. Select this image name and click End Process. You will receive a warning that unsaved information will be lost, but if Word is supposedly closed, there is no additional information to be lost, so go ahead and answer Yes.

File Types in MS Word

Word uses several file types to store your actual work (documents) and to store information about how you prefer to work, including data files (see page 71) and document templates. File types are designated by the three- or four-letter extension that follows the file name. Documents are saved with the extension doc (for document) and templates (described in Chapter 8) are saved with the extension dot. These two file types are compatible with all versions of Word from Word 97 to Word 2007.

Word 2007 introduced a modification to the traditional file extensions. Documents originating in Word 2007 are (by default) saved as docx files. The 'x' indicates the file is encoded using XML (extensible markup language). There is no difference in the way the document appears, but docx files store information in a different format than doc files.

Word files created in previous versions of Word (ie, doc files) can be opened and edited in Word 2007. The Title bar will display the name of the file along with the phrase "Compatibility Mode" in parentheses. You can continue to work with the doc file in compatibility mode if you choose, or you can convert the file to Word 2007 docx format. To convert the file, open the file and choose **Office** > Save As (**F12**). In the **Save As** dialog box, open the *Save as type* drop-down box and choose *Word document (*.docx)*.

To open a Word 2007 file (docx) in previous versions of Word, you will need to download a file converter. The first time you attempt to open a docx file using another version of Word, a message will appear with the option to download the Microsoft Office Compatibility Pack. Once this file is downloaded to your computer, you will be able to open Word 2007 documents automatically. If you prefer to download the converter *before* attempting to open a docx file for the first time, locate the download page on the Microsoft website by performing an Internet search using the phrase Microsoft Office Compatibility Pack 2007.

Word 2007 files *may* contain functionality that will be lost when opened in previous versions of Word, but it is not likely that this will affect your medical reports. Features that may be affected include themes, mathematical equations, citations, art, and graphs. To learn more specific information about lost functionality, search the Internet using the search phrase Document element differences in previous versions.

> If you routinely exchange documents with others who do not use Word 2007, you can choose to automatically save all your documents in Word 97-2003 format (ie, as doc files). Follow the directions on page 164 for changing the default file format in Word 2007. Unless you are working with XML documents, it is not likely that any of the work you do as a transcriptionist/medical editor will be affected by this format change, and your coworkers and colleagues will appreciate receiving compatible documents.

Additional file types associated with Word 2007 include `docm` and `dotm`. These file types are equivalent to `docx` and `dotx` files except they contain macros. These file types will be explained in more detail in Chapters 8 and 12.

Safeguarding Your Data

If you use Word as your primary tool for transcription, you will have a large investment of time in your shortcuts, macros, and templates. Your speed and productivity will depend largely on how well you manage the tools provided to you in Word, and losing this data due to a hard drive failure or other mishap can cause a significant financial setback. *Backing up your program data is very important!* The following are the most important files to keep backed up:

- Template files including the Normal.dot and other document templates (see Chapter 8).
- The AutoCorrect list (see Chapter 9).
- The Custom dictionary (see Chapter 14).

You will learn more about these files in the remainder of this text. If you use a third-party counting program to track your line counts or a third-party text expander (eg, Instant Text or SpeedType), you will want to back up the glossary files associated with those programs, too.

Backing Up Data

The above-referenced files are located in various subfolders under each user's Microsoft folder. The exact folder locations depend on the version of Windows you are using. The paths for the various files are listed in Table 2-1 and Table 2-2 .

Table 2-1	Word's Program Data File Locations in Windows XP
Normal template (Normal.dot)	C:\Documents and Settings\Username\Application Data\Microsoft\Templates
User templates (dot files)	C:\Documents and Settings\Username\Application Data\Microsoft\Templates
AutoCorrect list (MSO1033.acl)	C:\Documents and Settings\Username\Application Data\Microsoft\Office
Custom Dictionary (Custom.dic)	2003: C:\Documents and Settings\Username\Application Data\Microsoft\Proof 2007: C:\Documents and Settings\Username\Application Data\Microsoft\UProof
Building Blocks (Building Blocks.dotx)	Word 2007 only: C:\Documents and Settings\Username\Application Data\Microsoft\Document Building Blocks\1033

Table 2-2   Word's Program Data File Locations in Windows Vista

Normal.dot	C:\Users\Username\AppData\Roaming\Microsoft\Templates
User templates (*.dot files)	C:\Users\Username\AppData\Roaming\Microsoft\Templates
AutoCorrect list (MSO1033.acl)	C:\Users\Username\AppData\Roaming\Microsoft\Office
Custom Dictionary (Custom.dic)	Word 2003 C:\Users\Username\AppData\Roaming\Microsoft\Proof Word 2007 C:\Users\Username\AppData\Roaming\Microsoft\UProof
Building Blocks Building (Blocks.dotx)	Word 2007 only: C:\Users\Username\AppData\Roaming\Microsoft\Document Building Blocks\1033

Figure 2-40 shows a folder with the Address bar displaying the path to the files in Word 2003 running under Windows XP. Figure 2-41 shows the folder with the Address bar and path for files in Word 2007 running under Windows Vista. The **Application Data** folder (renamed **AppData** in Vista) is normally hidden from view. *Before searching for these files, you will want to display hidden files and folders* (see instructions on page 30). You can locate the files using Windows Explorer to drill down through the folder path or you can use Windows Search (see page 45 for Windows XP or 64 for Windows Vista). If you use the Search feature in Windows, change the search results window to Details view so you can be sure to select the files that include *your username in the file path* (drag the column separator to the right so the entire file path is displayed). Also, look carefully at the icon to make sure you are not selecting a shortcut to the file (marked by a curved arrow in the bottom left corner of the file's icon).

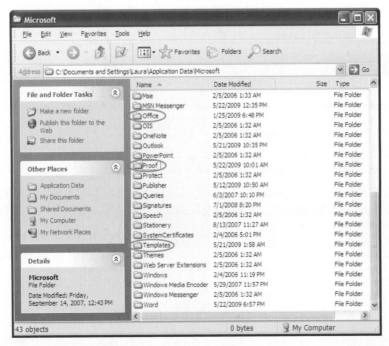

FIGURE 2-40 Folder locations for Word 2003 in Windows XP.

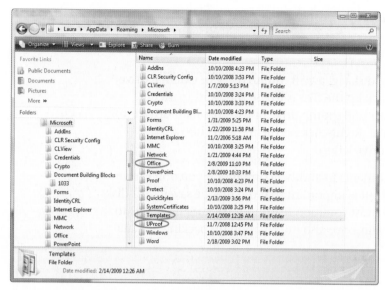

FIGURE 2-41 Folder locations for Word 2007 in Windows Vista.

Word must be closed in order to copy these files to a backup disk.

A quick way to locate the Word data files (on any version of Windows) is to type %AppData% (including the percent sign but no spaces) into the Address bar of any Explorer window and press **Enter**. Windows will open the **Application Data** or **AppData\Roaming** folder. From there, open the **Microsoft** folder that contains the data files for Word and other Office applications. (This method will open the **Application Data** folder even if it is hidden.)

The paths for the file locations are very specific and very literal. Word may store "native" copies of these files (with the same file name) in other folders, but only the folder paths under your profile that match the folder paths listed above will be the data files that contain *your user-specific information*. Be very careful that you are backing up the actual files that contain *your* information and not the native files. Word stores native copies of these files in order to reestablish the file in the event that the user's copy is moved or deleted.

If you have any doubt that you are selecting the correct data file to be backed up, use the file's modified date to confirm your file selection. Open Word and create a new AutoText entry, a new AutoCorrect entry, add a new term to your Custom dictionary, record a macro, or save a new custom shortcut key. These changes will modify the files that store the respective information. Close Word and search for the data files. The modified date should correspond to the current date and time.

To back up your data, follow these steps:

1. Close Word.

2. Locate the above files.

3. Copy the files to a removable disk (eg, a USB thumb drive or external drive) or a server. An easy way to back up the files is to use the Send To menu (described on page 98). Place a USB thumb drive or external hard drive into the USB slot on your computer. Right-click on the file and choose Send To > X (where X is the drive letter).

You can even email the files as attachments to another computer if you don't have an external drive or a server available. It is important that the files be saved on a disk other than your hard disk, since the most common reason for backing up files is to recover your data after a hard disk failure. See also information on backing up data in Appendix A on page 475.

Restore a Backup

To restore a backup copy, follow these steps:

1. Place the removable media containing the backup copies in the appropriate slot in your computer.

2. Open Windows Explorer (**Logo+E**) and select the removable media from the list.

3. Copy the file on the backup media using the Copy command (**CTRL+C**). *Do not try to open the file.*

4. On the destination computer, locate the corresponding folder and Paste (**CTRL+V**) the backup copy into its folder.

Most likely, there will already be a file with the same name in that folder, so you will want to answer Yes when asked to overwrite the existing file.

Move to a New Computer

The data files listed in tables 2-1 and 2-2 are compatible with all versions of Word. You can restore these files to any version of Word, regardless of which version was used to create the files (except the Building Blocks file which is only used by Word 2007). To move the files to a new computer, follow the steps above to restore a backup. Place the files in the corresponding folder based on the *version of Word and Windows that will be using the file*. For example, if the files originated in Word 2003 and you are moving to Word 2007, use the file locations for Word 2007.

To convert the Normal.dot file from Word 2003 format to the Word 2007 format, copy the Normal.dot file from the computer using Word 2003 and follow the steps below:

1. Close Word on the computer using Word 2007.

2. Following the directions above, open the Templates folder on the computer that is using Word 2007.

3. Locate the Normal.dotm file in the Templates folder and delete it.

4. Copy the Normal.dot file from the removable media and paste the file into the Template folder.

5. Double-click the Normal.dot file (in the Templates folder). This will open Word. Compatibility Mode will be displayed in the Title bar.

6. Immediately *close* Word. You will be asked if you want to save changes to the current document. Answer No. Next you will be asked to save changes to the Normal template. Answer Yes.

7. Reopen Word. Your Normal.dot will be converted to Normal.dotm.

8. Your favorite options and settings stored in Word 2003 will not transfer to Word 2007. Refer to Chapter 5 for guidance on setting options in Word.

Safeguarding Documents While You Work

Saving your files while you work is very important. Although Word has a file recovery feature to help prevent major losses, you still want to save your work often. Simply press **CTRL+S** every couple of minutes, especially after typing a very difficult section of a report. You will also want to develop a habit of pressing **CTRL+S** before you switch to another program, answer the phone, walk away from your desk, or as soon as you hear someone approaching your work area. If disaster strikes, you will lose very little work if you routinely use the Save command.

> If you keep several documents open at the same time, you can save or close all of your documents at the same time. Hold down Shift while opening the File menu and the menu choices will change from Save and Close to Save All and Close All.

AutoRecover

Word can automatically recover unsaved changes to documents if the program stops responding, shuts down unexpectedly, or there is a power failure. When AutoRecover is turned on, the changes you make are saved at set intervals (the default interval is 10 minutes) in a *temporary* recovery file. After a shutdown or failure, Word will automatically open the recovery file the next time Word is opened. The recovery file contains changes up until the last time AutoRecover took a "snapshot" of the document. For example, if you set AutoRecover to save every five minutes, you won't lose more than five minutes of work. See pages 141 (Word 2003) and 164 (Word 2007) for instructions on setting the AutoRecover feature.

> Always name new files immediately after creating. Unsaved documents may not always be recoverable. To recover work after a power failure or similar problem, you must have enabled the AutoRecover feature before the problem occurred.

After a shutdown, restart Word (see also caution on page 69). All documents that were open at the time of the incident will be listed in the **Document Recovery** task pane (Figure 2-42) that automatically appears on the left side of the Word window. Files that contain no changes since the last "hard" save (CTRL+S) will be marked [Original]. Files that contain information added between a hard save and an AutoRecover save will be listed as [Recovered] (Word 2003) or [Autosaved] (Word 2007). Theoretically, recovered files should contain more information than original files.

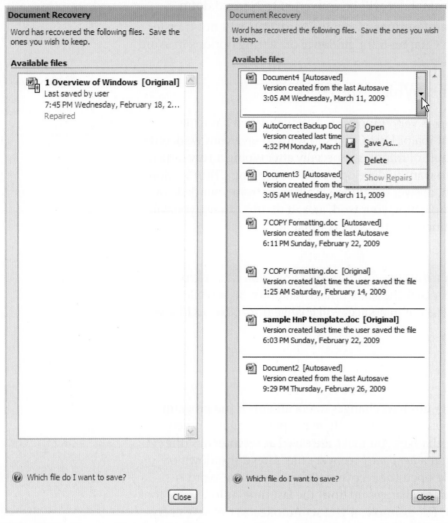

FIGURE 2-42 The Document Recovery pane will automatically appear when you reopen Word following an unexpected shutdown.

To open a recovered file, simply click the file name. Examine the file and see if everything appears to be OK. If so, save the file (CTRL+S). This will replace the original file as the "real" file on your hard drive and you can continue to work. You may have to retype or re-edit the file to replace the last few of minutes of lost information.

To discard a recovered file, click the down arrow associated with the file and choose Delete from the drop-down menu. If you are unsure which file you want to continue to use (original or recovered), right-click the recovered file name (in the task pane) and choose Save As. Give the recovered document a slightly different name than the original (eg, tack an 'R' at the beginning or end of the file name). Close the task pane. Compare the recovered and original versions of the file. After determining which file to keep, use Windows Explorer to delete any unneeded files. If you keep the recovered file, return the file name to the original file name (ie, remove the 'R' from the file name).

Critical Thinking Questions

1. Why is (My) Documents the most likely place to find a document?

_____

_____

2. Describe RAM and its relationship to open files.

_____

_____

3. Explain how Windows uses the file extension. List three examples of file extensions and their associations.

_____

_____

4. Describe at least three ways to select most (but not all) files in a folder (using mouse and/or keyboard techniques).

_____

_____

5. Name two ways to open a recently used document.

_____

_____

6. Follow these steps:

   a. Create a new folder as a subfolder on C (or the main disk on your PC). Name the folder Word4e Exercises.

   _____

   _____

   b. Move Exercise A, Exercise B, and Exercise B key provided on the accompanying CD to this folder (you will use these documents to complete exercises throughout the remainder of this text). Further details are provided on the CD.

   _____

   _____

7. Define the Application Data/AppData folder and explain its relationship to the program data files described on page 71.

_____

_____

8. Explain why it is important to back up program data files. Describe three reasons why you may need to restore these files.

_____

_____

9. On your computer, locate the program data files (described under Safe-guarding Your Data). Write down the modified date for each of these files.

_____

_____

10. If Word stops responding, what should you do?

_____

_____

CHAPTER 3

Using the Keyboard and Shortcut Icons

OBJECTIVES

▸ Navigate menus, dialog boxes, and Windows Explorer using the keyboard.

▸ Select text and objects using the keyboard.

▸ Minimize, maximize, and close individual windows using the keyboard.

▸ Use universal shortcut keys.

▸ Use right-click menus to carry out common file management tasks.

▸ Create and place shortcut icons in strategic places to access commonly used programs, files, and folders.

▸ Create and use shortcut icons to access websites and other resources.

KEYWORDS

access keys
alpha character
function keys
hot key
KeyTip
Logo key
modifier keys
navigation keys
Send To
shortcut icons
shortcut key
shortcut menus
toggle key
universal keys

Keyboarding refers to methods of controlling a computer using the keyboard instead of the mouse. In many instances, using the keyboard instead of the mouse to carry out commands is the most efficient way to accomplish a task. Once you learn the basic concepts for keyboarding in Windows, you can apply these concepts to any application designed for Windows. This standardization tremendously decreases the learning curve for any one application and increases your overall efficiency.

If you are accustomed to using the mouse, using the keyboard may be cumbersome at first—not because it is more difficult, but because you are changing a habit. Using the keyboard requires memorization of keystrokes, and it takes time to memorize a long list of key combinations. It may be mentally easier to click an icon to carry out a command, but it is much more time-consuming in the long run.

Make a gradual transition from mousing to keyboarding by learning a new technique or one or two new keyboard commands each day. Make a list of commands that you use often. Every few days, jot down two or three commands on a sticky note and place them on your monitor. Incorporate those shortcut keys into your routine and then repeat this for the next two or three commands on your list.

You will notice that many commands are universal (used by all applications), and many others follow a common pattern. Often a command that uses the CTRL key will use the first letter of the command name (eg, CTRL+P is often the shortcut key for Print and CTRL+S is typically the shortcut key for Save). If the initial-letter shortcut key combination is already assigned, then the second letter of the command name is used (eg, the shortcut key to center text in Word is CTRL+E because CTRL+C is globally assigned to Copy). Once you begin the process of going "mouse-less" you will become addicted to the ease and efficiency of keyboarding. After a few days, you will begin to see a difference, and after a few weeks you will be amazed at how much faster and more efficiently you can work.

Basic Keyboarding Concepts

A **shortcut key** is a key sequence that functions as if you clicked an icon or menu command using the mouse. Many shortcut keys act as toggles. A **toggle key** either alternates between "on" and "off" (think of a light switch), or cycles through a series of related commands or a collection of buttons. **Function keys** are the keys located across the top of the keyboard labeled F1 through F12. Many keyboards now come with function keys labeled with alternate commands such as Undo, Redo, Print, Save, etc. An F-Lock key located at one end of the F keys toggles the function of the F keys between the labeled command and the F key function (determined by the currently active program).

 If the F keys do not function as listed in this chapter or according to your software instructions, toggle the F-Lock key.

Modifier Keys

ALT, CTRL, Shift and Logo (see below) are called **modifier keys** because they are used to change the normal function of a key (eg, inserting the letter A versus the command Select all using CTRL+A). Modifier keys are either pressed simultaneously with the key they modify or they are pressed sequentially. If a keyboard shortcut is written with a plus sign in between the modifier key and the character key (eg, ALT+D), press the keys together. Be sure to press the modifier key slightly before the character key so that you do not press the character key alone—that will simply insert the character. Some commands use a combination of modifier keys and character keys (eg, CTRL+Shift+E). In this case, press the modifier keys at the same time, slightly before pressing the character key, so that all keys are pressed together.

If shortcut keys are written with commas in between (eg, ALT, D), press the two keys sequentially. Completely lift your finger off the modifier key before pressing the second key. You will also encounter commands that combine shortcut key techniques. For example, the command ALT+C, D means press ALT and C together, release both keys, then press the D.

A very helpful modifier key is the **Logo key**, also referred to as the Windows key. The Logo key, as shown in Figure 3-1, is marked with the Microsoft "waving" window logo (⊞) and is typically located on the left side of the Spacebar. Some keyboards may have a Logo key on each side of the Spacebar. Laptop keyboards are less standardized and the Logo key may be placed in the upper right corner. When pressed alone, the Logo key will open the Start menu; when pressed with another key, it executes a specific command. The Logo key is especially useful; no matter which window is active, you can *always* use the Logo key and its associated commands. See the list below under Universal Shortcut Keys for specific commands using the Logo key.

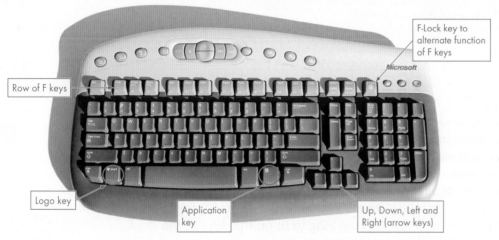

FIGURE 3-1 The Logo key is usually located to the left of the Spacebar and the Application key is located to the right of the Spacebar. (taken from *Technology for the Medical Transcriptionist*, reprinted courtesy of Sarah Bryan)

Application Key

An often overlooked key is the Application key, which is typically found to the

right of the Spacebar. This key is marked with a menu and a pointer. The Application key is the keyboard equivalent of the right mouse button. This particular key will open the shortcut menu associated with the selected item. You will learn more about shortcut menus later in this chapter.

Hot Keys

Virtually every command, whether listed on a menu bar, drop-down menu, submenu, shortcut menu, or dialog box, has a **hot key** which invokes that command when the menu or dialog box is active. The hot key is designated with an underscored letter within the command name. In Office 2007 and other applications that have adopted the ribbon (instead of a menu bar), hot keys are referred to as **access keys**. These keys are displayed next to the command in a small box called a **KeyTip**. To reveal hot keys, activate the menu bar or the ribbon by pressing ALT.

start You may prefer to display the underscore designations at all times—not just when a menu bar is active. To make this change in Windows XP, right-click an empty area of the Desktop and choose Properties > **Appearance** > **Effects**. Remove the check mark at *Hide underlined letters for keyboard navigation until I press the ALT key*.

You may prefer to display the underscore designations at all times—not just when a menu bar is active. In Windows Vista, go to **Start** > Control Panel > **Ease of Access** > *Ease of Access Center* > *Make the keyboard easier to use* > *Underline keyboard shortcuts and access keystrokes*. (Note: You can also press **Logo+U** to open the Ease of Access Center).

Alpha Characters

While commands on menu bars, drop-down menus, and dialog boxes always have designated hot keys (ie, underscored characters), items created by the user, such as files, folders, and shortcut icons, do not have underscored characters. For these items, the hot key is automatically the first letter of the item's name, called the **alpha character**. Also, items in a drop-down list within dialog boxes use the alpha character. *In all cases, when more than one item has the same alpha character, press the character repeatedly until the needed item is selected.* Once selected, press **Enter** to open/activate. Even if a list of items is too long to fit on the display, the alpha character will still select the item—an added plus for items located at the end of a long list.

Within any given folder, I often name files or subfolders using unique characters (including numbers and punctuation marks) as the alpha character. By doing so, I can always select a specific item with a single keystroke. This is infinitely faster than scrolling through the list, focusing on the file or folder name, and then clicking with the mouse.

Use numbers and letters to force a list of files and folders to appear in a certain order. For example, you may want your most important folders to always appear at the beginning of the list within their parent folder. Place a zero or a 1 at the beginning of the folder's name and sort the folder contents by *Name*. Your favorite folders will always be right at the top of the list.

Moving the Insertion Point/Cursor

The navigation keys are used to move the cursor/insertion point when working with both text and objects. **Navigation keys** include the four arrow keys and

Page up, **Page down**, **Home**, and **End**. When working with text, the arrow keys (**Up**, **Down**, **Left**, and **Right**) move either one character left/right or one line up/down. **Home** always moves the insertion point to the beginning of a line of text. Likewise, **End** moves the insertion point to the end of a line of text. **Page up** and **Page down** typically move the insertion point a distance equal to the height of the window (not the equivalent of a "page" as the name implies).

Adding **CTRL** to any navigation key moves the insertion point to the next "increment." For example, **CTRL+Left/Right** moves one word instead of one character. **CTRL+Home** moves to the top of the document or web page, and likewise, **CTRL+End** moves to the end of the document or web page.

When working with objects (eg, icons and graphics) **Left** and **Right** move one object left/right, and **Up** and **Down** move one line or object up/down. **Home** moves to the top of a window and **End** moves to the bottom of a window. **Tab** is used to move the cursor down through dialog boxes and through any window divided into panes (eg, Explorer windows and websites). **Shift+Tab** will reverse the direction of **Tab** key in almost every circumstance where the **Tab** key is used.

The location of the cursor is indicated by a dotted box around the item or by backlighting an item, as shown in Figure 3-2. Once an item is selected, hit **Enter** to open or **Spacebar** to place or remove a check mark.

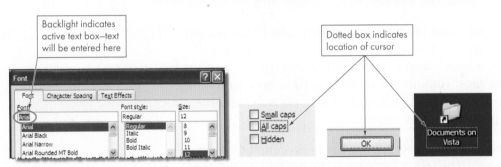

FIGURE 3-2 The location of the cursor is indicated by backlighting in a text box or by a dotted box around a command name, button, or icon.

Selecting Text

Selecting text within a document or in a text-input box is always accomplished the same way, using the **Shift** key combined with the navigation keys. Hold down **Shift** while pressing any **navigation** key or **CTRL+navigation** key combination.

The navigation keys are also used to "deselect" text (ie, remove the backlight) and move the insertion point to the beginning or end of the text. For example, when **Save As** opens, a suggested name for the file often appears in the *File name* box—already selected. Press **Right**, **Left**, **Home**, or **End** to deselect the text and place the insertion point at the beginning or end of the suggested file name. Remember, these keys work *anywhere* text is selected.

Navigating Menus

To access commands on menus, press the **ALT** key to activate the <u>Menu</u> bar. Once activated, the <u>Menu</u> bar is staged to "grab" keystrokes. File (always the first item on a menu bar) will be backlit or appear "pushed in" to indicate that the <u>Menu</u> bar is active (see Figure 3-3). For applications that have hidden menu bars, press the **ALT** key to both display the <u>Menu</u> bar and activate it at the same time.

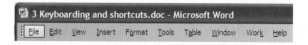

FIGURE 3-3 The File menu will be backlit or will appear "pushed in" when the Menu bar has been activated.

 Sometimes it appears that the program has stopped responding to the keyboard. If this happens, look at the <u>Menu</u> bar to see if you accidentally hit the **ALT** key by itself and activated the <u>Menu</u> bar. When the <u>Menu</u> bar is active, only the "hot keys" are active, so it may appear that the keyboard is not responding. Resist the temptation to pound the keyboard and simply press **Esc** to deactivate the <u>Menu</u> bar.

After activating the <u>Menu</u> bar, press the hot key corresponding to the needed drop-down menu. Using Figure 3-3 as an example, **ALT, F** will open the <u>F</u>ile menu; **ALT, O** will open the F<u>o</u>rmat menu. Although pressing the **ALT** key first to activate a menu bar is the most common convention used to open drop-down menus, you may encounter programs that require you to press **ALT** and the hot key simultaneously to open a drop-down menu.

When the drop-down menu opens, press the hot key to execute the specific command. You do not need to press **ALT** again once the menu is active. If the menu command has a submenu (indicated by a triangle next to the command), press **Right** to open the submenu. Press **Esc** to close the submenu if not needed. Press **Esc** repeatedly to back out of all submenus and menus and return to the working space within the file.

Office 2003 uses Personalized Menus, a feature which displays menus in an abbreviated form. Recently used commands migrate to the top of the menu. The toolbars also adjust to your use by moving recent commands to the left end of the toolbar. I prefer to use static menus and toolbars so that commands are always in the same location. To turn off this feature, right-click in the toolbar area of any Office application and choose *Customize*. Place a check mark at *Always use full menus*. You may also decide to place a check mark at *Show Standard and Formatting toolbars on two rows*. This setting will allow you to see most, if not all, of the commands on both toolbars at all times.

Navigating the Start Menu

The Start menu uses the same keyboarding conventions as other menus. Press the **Logo** key by itself to open the Start menu. In Windows Vista, press **Up** to move out of the Search box and then proceed as below.

- Press the hot key to open an item on the Start menu. If the hot key is used more than once, press again until the item is selected and then press **Enter**. Windows will start selecting items on the left side of the menu first and then move to the right side.

- To go immediately to the right side of the menu, press **Right** and then **Up**.

- Navigate the Program menu by tapping the alpha character or **Up** and **Down**. To open a program group, press **Right**.

- Press **Esc** to close the Program menu and return to the Start menu. Press **Esc** again to close the Start menu.

Navigating Ribbons

Ribbons were introduced with Office 2007, but other software applications have adopted this new approach to accessing commands. It is possible that you will see ribbons used in programs developed by other manufacturers, not just Microsoft. Regardless of the software developer, keyboard access for ribbons has been standardized just like menus and dialog boxes.

Press the **ALT** key to activate the ribbon. KeyTips will display next to each tab, as shown in Figure 3-4. Press the letter or number indicated by the KeyTip to bring the tab to the foreground. KeyTips for each command on the selected tab will be displayed. Continue pressing KeyTips until the command you need is executed. Some KeyTips are actually two letters, so press these sequentially. If the KeyTip is displayed but is dimmed, it will not respond to the keyboard. These commands are not active because the cursor is not in an area of the document where the command can be applied.

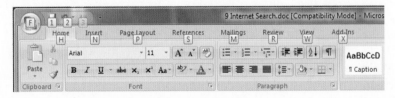

FIGURE 3-4 Press the ALT key to display KeyTips for ribbon Access keys.

Commands with down arrows have drop-down menus associated with them. Press **Down** to select an option from the menu and press **Enter**, or press the underscore character if available. Some drop-down menus have a selection of preset formats (called a gallery). Gallery items have right-click menus associated with them. With the gallery item selected, press **Shift+F10** to display the shortcut menu. Press **Esc** to back out of the current tab. The KeyTips for the tabs will reappear so you can choose a different tab. Press **Esc** again to cancel all KeyTips. You can also press **ALT** at any time to cancel all KeyTips and return to the document workspace.

Word 2007 has retained the majority of Word 2003's key sequences for accessing the drop-down menus on the <u>Menu</u> bar as well as the hot keys on these menus. If you are accustomed to accessing commands in Word 2003 using the keyboard, you can continue to use many of the same key sequences. Press **ALT** followed by the Word 2003 hot key. Word will recognize the key sequence and display a message as shown in Figure 3-5.

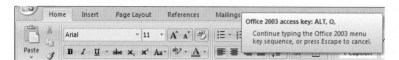

FIGURE 3-5 Word 2007 recognizes Word 2003 key sequences for accessing commands on the Menu bar and drop-down menus.

Managing Individual Windows

Using the keyboard to control windows can significantly increase efficiency. As you learned in Chapter 1, every window has a Control menu with commands corresponding to the control buttons (Minimize , Maximize/Restore , and Close) as shown in Figure 3-6. Press **ALT+Spacebar** to access the Control menu using the keyboard.

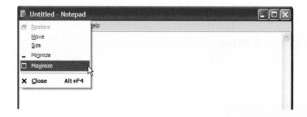

FIGURE 3-6 Press ALT+Spacebar to open the Control menu and then press the underscore character for the command needed.

With the menu open, press **N** to Mi<u>n</u>imize, or press **X** to Ma<u>x</u>imize a window that has been reduced from full screen. This two-stroke key combination (**ALT+Spacebar, N** or **ALT+Spacebar, X**) is the *fastest* way to minimize or maximize a window.

The fastest way to close *any* window, including pop-ups in your web browser, is to press the universal key for Close which is **ALT+F4**.

Switching Between Windows

To switch between open windows using the keyboard, use **ALT+Tab**. Press and *hold* **ALT** while tapping **Tab**. A box will appear with icons for each open window as shown in Figure 3-7. Continue to hold **ALT** and tap **Tab** to move the selection box until the desired window icon is selected. Release both keys to bring the selected window to the foreground, making it the active window. Add **Shift** to the above key combination to move the selection box in the opposite direction. A quick click of **ALT+Tab** will toggle between the current window and the previously viewed window.

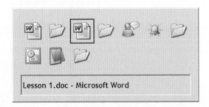

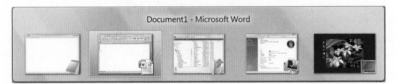

FIGURE 3-7 Use ALT+Tab to switch between windows in Windows XP (top) and Windows Vista (bottom).

Windows Vista has two additional shortcut keys for switching between windows. To flip between windows without holding down **ALT**, press **CTRL+ALT+Tab** to display the list of windows. Press **Tab** until the desired window is selected, then press **Enter**. If you are able to run the slick, new, appearance profile called Aero, press the shortcut key **Logo+Tab** (using the same technique as **ALT+Tab** explained above) to display a live, three-dimensional version of each window. When the desired window is the uppermost window, release the keys.

Working in Windows Explorer

Tab and **F6** are two important keys for navigating within Explorer. **F6** cycles clockwise between distinct panes of a window (toolbar area, left-hand pane, file-list area), and **Tab** will cycle between distinct panes as well as each item within a pane. Press either key repeatedly until the needed area of the window is selected (indicated by the dotted box or shading). Figure 3-8 shows the typical path of the cursor using the **Tab** key in a Windows Vista Explorer window. Within a particular section or pane, use the arrow keys to select items within that area.

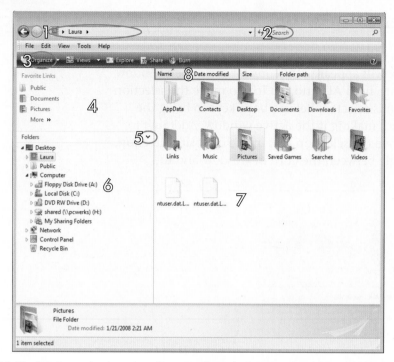

FIGURE 3-8 The Tab key cycles through each pane and its subsections.

Both **Tab** and **F6** are the most common keys for moving between sections within a window, including distinct sections of an application window and of web pages. The cursor typically moves top-to-bottom or clockwise, but the pattern may vary in any given window. For any window divided into panes, try **F6** for navigating *between* panes and **Tab** for navigating *within* panes.

In addition to the navigation commands described above, there are several shortcut keys assigned to specific commands in Explorer. Figure 3-9 shows shortcut keys corresponding to commands on the <u>Toolbar</u> and <u>Address</u> bar.

Navigating the Folder List

Figure 3-10 shows the Folder list in both Windows XP and Windows Vista. Use the following techniques for navigating Folders:

- Press **F6** to move the cursor to the Folder list header then press **Tab** to move into the folder list.
- Press **Down** or tap the **alpha** character to jump to a disk or folder.
- Press **Right** or **Plus** (+ on the number pad) to display subfolders.
- Collapse a folder (hide subfolders) using **Left** or **Negative** (- on the number pad).
- The selected folder's contents will be displayed in the file list area. Press **Tab** to move from Folders to the file list area to select a specific file.

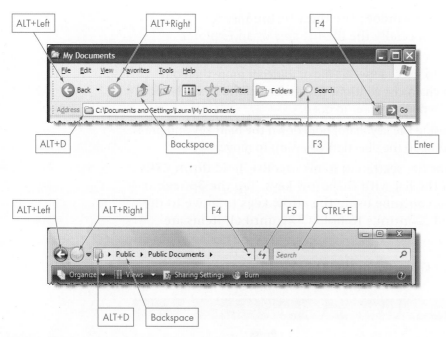

FIGURE 3-9 Shortcut keys used in Windows Explorer.

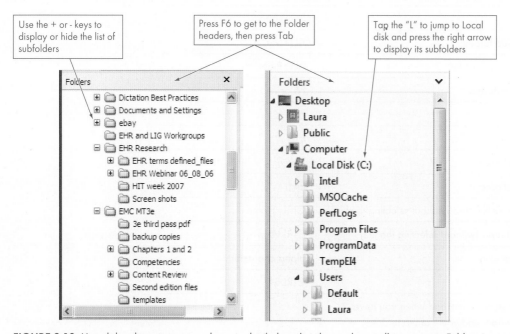

FIGURE 3-10 Use alpha characters, arrow keys, and +/− keys (on the number pad) to navigate Folders in both Windows XP and Windows Vista.

Selecting Files, Folders, and Shortcut icons

Using the keyboard to select items within the file list area of an Explorer window is especially quick and easy because the cursor defaults to the file-list area when you open an Explorer window. Use these techniques for selecting items from any list, especially the file-list area of an Explorer window:

- Press the alpha character to select a specific file or folder. If more than one item has the same alpha character, continue to press the alpha character until the item you need is selected. Press Enter to open.
- To select a range of files using the keyboard, hold down the Shift key and press the arrow key corresponding to the direction you want to move.
- To select noncontiguous (ie, scattered) items in a list, hold down CTRL while moving through the list with the arrow keys. Tap the Spacebar to select a file and then continue using the arrow keys to move to the next item to be selected. Continue to hold CTRL until all items are selected.

Table 3-1 Summarizes shortcut keys used in Windows Explorer.

Table 3-1 Summary of shortcut keys for Windows Explorer.	
To	**Press**
Display the Address bar drop-down list (History)	F4
Select the Address bar	ALT+D
Go up one folder level	Backspace
Go back to a previously viewed folder	ALT+Left
Go forward to a previously viewed folder	ALT+Right
Cycle through distinct areas or panes	F6 or Tab
Search this folder	F3
Open Windows Help	F1
Select the first file in the file-list area	Home
Select the last file in the file-list area	End
Move to the beginning of the file-list area (without selecting the file)	CTRL+Home
Move to the end of the file-list area (without selecting the file)	CTRL+End
Select a file, folder, or shortcut icon	alpha character
Select all items in a folder	CTRL+A
Refresh the current window (use this command when you have made changes to a folder window and you want to update the display or resort the list to include the latest changes).	F5
Rename a file, folder, or shortcut	F2
Open Properties for the selected item	ALT+Enter
Activate the Menu bar (and display when hidden)	ALT or F10
Maximize window and hide toolbars	F11 (toggle to restore)
Delete the selected item(s) and place in the Recycle Bin	Delete

Table 3-1 *(Continued)*	
To	**Press**
Delete the selected item(s) and bypass the Recycle Bin	Shift+Delete
Open shortcut menu for selected item	Application key or Shift+F10
Work within the Folder List	
Expand list of subfolders	+ (Plus) or Right
Collapse folder list	– (Negative) or Left
Expand all subfolders below selected folder	* (Asterisk)
Windows Vista only	
Open the parent window	ALT+Up
Move to Search box	CTRL+E
Search and open the Search pane (while in the Search box)	ALT+Enter
Search in *Internet* Explorer (starting from Search box in *Windows* Explorer)	Shift+Enter
Open another session of the current folder window	CTRL+N

To select most but not all items in a list, press **CTRL+A** to select all and then hold down **CTRL** while clicking items to deselect.

Be careful when using the **CTRL** key to select and deselect items in a list. If you accidentally drag the mouse while clicking, Windows will interpret **CTRL**+drag and *copy* the files that are selected. If this happens, press **CTRL+Z** to delete the copies and begin your selection again.

Navigating Dialog Boxes

Use the **Tab** key to move from one command or option area of a dialog box to the next, or press **ALT+hot key** to move directly to an option. The active spot within a dialog box is indicated by backlighting the text-input box or surrounding the command with a dotted line (see the *All caps* command in Figure 3-11). Since dialog boxes can accept text (ie, they have text input boxes), you must use **ALT+hot key** to indicate a command. (Compare this to a menu, which does not accept text, therefore does not need the **ALT** key to distinguish text from a command.) Study Figure 3-11 for tips on working with dialog boxes. Table 3-2 summarizes shortcut keys used within dialog boxes.

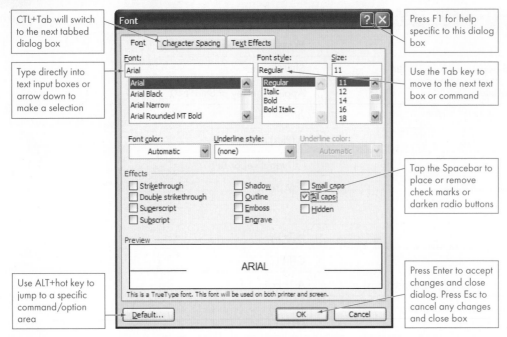

CTL+Tab will switch to the next tabbed dialog box

Type directly into text input boxes or arrow down to make a selection

Press F1 for help specific to this dialog box

Use the Tab key to move to the next text box or command

Tap the Spacebar to place or remove check marks or darken radio buttons

Use ALT+hot key to jump to a specific command/option area

Press Enter to accept changes and close dialog. Press Esc to cancel any changes and close box

FIGURE 3-11 Use Tab to move through dialog boxes or combine ALT with the hot key to select or deselect commands.

Table 3-2	Summary of shortcut keys used in dialog boxes.
To	**Press**
Move left to right and down through a dialog box	Tab
Move up through dialog box	Shift+Tab
Switch to a different tab within the dialog box	CTRL+Tab (add Shift to reverse direction)
Close dialog box without keeping changes	Esc
Accept changes and close dialog box	Enter
Select or deselect a check box or radio button	Spacebar or ALT+hot key
Select from a drop-down list	Type the item name or Down to select, Enter to accept
Open a group of options (eg, the color group in the Font dialog)	F4
Display Help	F1

Navigating Save As and Open Dialog Boxes

Save As and **Open** dialog boxes are actually combinations of dialog boxes and Explorer windows. Many of the techniques used in an Explorer window can be used in these two particular types of dialog boxes. Table 3-3 summarizes the

Table 3-3	Summary of shortcut keys for Save As and Open dialog boxes.
To	**Press**
Move to File Name	ALT+N
Move to Save In or Look in (where available)	ALT+I
Move to Save as type	ALT+T
Open Tools menu (where available)	ALT+L
Open file (Open)	ALT+O or Enter
Save file (Save As)	ALT+S or Enter
Select Places button (where available)	Tab to Places bar, Up or Down to select, Enter
Office 2007 under Windows Vista	
Browse or Hide Folders	ALT+B
Move to Address bar	ALT+D
Display Address bar History	F4
Move to Search text box	CTRL+E

shortcut keys for working with the **Save As** and **Open** dialog boxes. Follow these tips for navigating **Save As** and **Open**:

- Just like Explorer windows, **Tab** and **F6** are used to move through the various areas of the dialog box.
- Like dialog boxes, **ALT+hot key** techniques are used to jump to specific areas marked with an underscore.
- Within any distinct area of a dialog box, such as the Places bar or the toolbar, use the arrow keys to move up, down, left and right, then press **Enter** to select.
- When the dialog box first opens, the cursor location will default to *File name*. Press **Shift+Tab** (once or twice depending on the style of the box) to move to the file-list area, and then use the same techniques as above to select files.

[🔵 start]   When running either version of Office under Windows XP, the **Save As** and **Open** dialog boxes appear as shown in Figure 3-12. You can select the toolbar commands across the top of the dialog box using shortcut keys. Number each command left to right and combine with the **ALT** key. Looking at Figure 3-12, **ALT+1** goes back to the previous folder, **ALT+2** goes up one folder level, **ALT+3** opens your default web browser, etc.

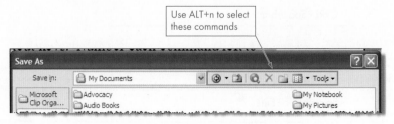

Use ALT+n to select these commands

FIGURE 3-12 Use ALT+n (where n is the number corresponding to the button's position) to access commands across the top of Office 2003 Save As and Open dialog boxes.

Remember, Office 2007 running under Windows Vista uses **Save As** and **Open** dialog boxes that are very much like an Explorer window. Figure 3-13 shows the **Save As** dialog from Word 2007 when running on a Vista computer. The dialog box first opens with the file-list area hidden. To expand the dialog (ie, display Folders and the file list area), press **ALT+B** (Browse Folders).

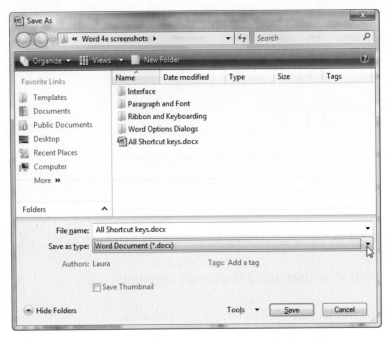

FIGURE 3-13 The Save As dialog box in Office 2007 running under Windows Vista.

Navigating Task Panes

Task panes are used in both Office and Windows itself. Typically they appear along the left or right edge of a window. They function much like dialog boxes, only they remain displayed while working within the main work space. Table 3-4 summarizes shortcut keys for working with task panes. Keys related to specific task panes in MS Word will be mentioned where applicable later in the text.

Table 3-4   Summary of task pane shortcut keys.

To	Press
Open the task pane menu (Office) or a subsection of a task pane (Windows)	CTRL+Spacebar
Cycle cursor between task pane and other panes within the window	F6
Move through commands within a task pane	Tab, Up, Down
Execute the selected command	Spacebar or Enter
Move to the top or bottom of the task pane	Home, End, or CTRL+Home and CTRL+End

Table 3-4	(Continued)
To	**Press**
Additional Task Pane Commands in Word	
Open or close the task pane (Word 2003 only)	CTRL+F1
Move forward or back through previously viewed task panes (Word 2003 only)	ALT+Right and ALT+Left
Close the task pane with task pane selected (Word 2007)	CTRL+Spacebar, C

Universal Shortcut Keys

Many shortcut keys are controlled by Windows and are referred to as **universal keys** because they work in all circumstances. Occasionally, software programmers may (unwisely) overwrite a universal key. Learning these particular shortcut keys proves very helpful since they work in the vast majority of programs and are some of the most common commands used.

Shortcuts Keys Using the Logo Key

Shortcuts using the Logo key are listed in Table 3-5. The Logo key is always active, so you can access items using these shortcut keys at any time. Incorporating these keys into your daily routine will really save you a lot of time and effort.

 You can also select icons from the Desktop using the keyboard. Press Logo+D to display the Desktop then tap the alpha character to select the item you need. Press Enter to open.

 Use the **System Information** dialog (Logo+Pause/Break) to provide information to technical support personnel. This dialog will tell you about your version of Windows, how much RAM is on your PC, the size of your hard drive, and other pertinent information.

Miscellaneous Shortcut Keys

Table 3-6 lists miscellaneous keys that work throughout the Windows environment. Cut, Copy, and Paste are extremely useful for managing text, but are also quite helpful for managing files and folders. Anything that can be selected can be copied to the Windows Clipboard and pasted into another window. Undo (CTRL+Z) is also *very* helpful, especially when you realize you pressed the wrong command. Before you panic, try Undo to see if you can reverse the last command. Some programs will let you press Undo several times to step backward through several commands.

Table 3-5	Shortcut keys using the Logo key.
To	**Press**
Open the Start menu	⊞ (Logo key)
Open Windows Explorer	⊞+E
Display the Desktop (ie, minimize all applications)	⊞+D (Toggle to return to initial program)
Search for files or folders	⊞+F
Open the Run dialog box	⊞+R
Minimize all programs	⊞+M
Restore all minimized programs	⊞+Shift+M
Lock the computer or switch users	⊞+L
Access Windows Help	⊞+F1
Learn about your operating system and your computer	⊞+Pause/Break (located in the upper right-hand corner of your keyboard
Access the Notification Area	⊞+B
Additional Keys for Windows Vista	
Open Ease of Access Center	⊞+U
Open item on Quick Launch bar	⊞+1 (first item), ⊞+2 (second item), etc.
Access the Taskbar	⊞+T
Switch windows using Flip 3-D	⊞+Tab
Bring Windows Sidebar to the front	⊞+Spacebar
Cycle through Sidebar Gadgets	⊞+G
Open Windows Mobility Center (for laptops)	⊞+X

Take special note of the Close command (**ALT+F4**). This command will close any window, including popup windows in a web browser. Using this shortcut key is the safest way to close a popup box so you don't risk activating a hidden download by clicking in the box itself (called a mouse trap). Applications such as Word 2003 use a Multiple Document Interface (MDI), so **ALT+F4** will close the current file unless it is the only file open within that application. If only one file is open within the application, this shortcut will close both the file and the application. This shortcut key will also display the **Shut Down Windows** dialog box if no other window is active.

Shortcut Menus

Shortcut menus, also called right-click menus, are a terrific feature of Windows and all Windows-based programs. Every object displayed in the Windows interface—icons, shortcut icons, files, folders, toolbars, text,

Table 3-6 Miscellaneous shortcut keys used in Windows.

To	Press
Copy	CTRL+C
Cut (Move)	CTRL+X
Paste	CTRL+V
Undo (reverse the last command or the last several commands)	CTRL+Z (repeat to step backwards through several commands)
Delete	Delete
Delete selected item permanently without placing the item in the Recycle Bin	Shift+Delete
Rename files, folders, shortcut icons	F2
Find text (in the current window)	CTRL+F
Select All	CTRL+A
Edit properties for the selected item	ALT+Enter
Copy selected item using the mouse (includes text, graphics, shortcuts, files, and folders)	CTRL while dragging an item to a new location
Create shortcut to selected item using the mouse	CTRL+Shift while dragging an item
Cancel an action, close a menu or a dialog box	Esc
Accept the default (indicated by a dotted box)	Enter Yes
Close any window	ALT+F4
Close the active document but leave the application running	CTRL+F4
Open Task Manager	CTRL+Shift+Esc
Open Security dialog box	CTRL+ALT+Del
Open the Control menu for the active window	ALT+Spacebar
Cycle through Taskbar buttons (in the order they were opened)	ALT+Esc
Toggle Full screen mode (hide toolbars)	F11

graphics, tables, disks, drives, and printers—has a shortcut menu associated with it. Simply right-click any object to display a menu of useful commands. The shortcut menus are specific for each type of object and contain the most common commands needed when working with that particular object. There are too many shortcut menus to describe each one, but some of the most commonly used menus will be described here.

Shortcut menus can also be displayed using the keyboard by pressing the **Application** key.

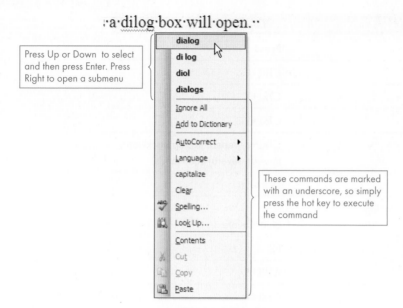

FIGURE 3-14 Use the hot keys or the arrow keys to select commands on a shortcut menu.

Once the shortcut menu is open, you can use the keyboard to navigate the shortcut menu just like any other menu (see Figure 3-14). Press any underscored character to execute that command or press the alpha character. You can also use Up and Down to navigate the menu and press Enter to execute a command. As with other menus, the right arrow next to a menu item indicates a submenu is available and an ellipsis indicates a dialog box will open.

Manage Files and Folders using Shortcut Menus

You can accomplish many file management tasks using shortcut menus. In any folder window, select one or more files and/or folders (see page 43 in XP and page 60 in Vista for instructions on selecting multiple files). Be sure to place the mouse cursor directly over the selection and then click the right mouse button. A shortcut menu will appear that lists the most common commands needed for managing files and folders, including Open, Print, Cut, Copy, Delete, Rename, Send To, and Properties. Figure 3-15 shows the shortcut menu displayed when a file is selected, and Figure 3-16 shows the shortcut menu displayed when a folder is selected. Your shortcut menus may vary somewhat from the examples depending on the type of file(s) selected and software installed on your PC.

The Send To Submenu

The **Send To** submenu, which is available when you right-click a file or folder, has several extremely useful commands. This particular menu can be used to move or copy a file, attach a file to an email message, or to create a shortcut (learn more about creating shortcuts on page 102). Figure 3-17 shows sample Send To menus from two different computers showing different "destinations" (folders and disks) for "sending" the selected files. Removable media, such as a USB thumb drive, will (only) appear on this menu when the media is actually attached to the PC.

Send To either *copies* or *moves* the file or folder depending on the destination selected on the Send To menu. Files are *copied* when the original location and the destination

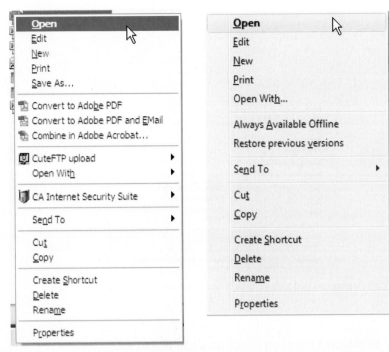

FIGURE 3-15 Examples of the file shortcut menu in Windows XP (left) and Windows Vista (right).

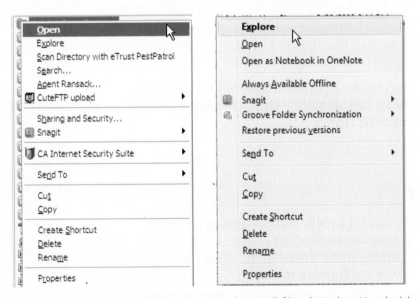

FIGURE 3-16 Examples of the folder shortcut menu in Windows XP (left) and Windows Vista (right).

are on different disks (eg, when sending a file from C:\My Documents to D). Files are *moved* when the original location and the destination are on the *same* disk. To *copy* a file to a different folder *on the same disk* using the Send To menu, hold down the **Shift** key when you click the destination on the Send To menu.

When using the Send To menu to back up or move files, be sure you select actual files and not shortcut icons. Look for the curved arrow to distinguish shortcut icons.

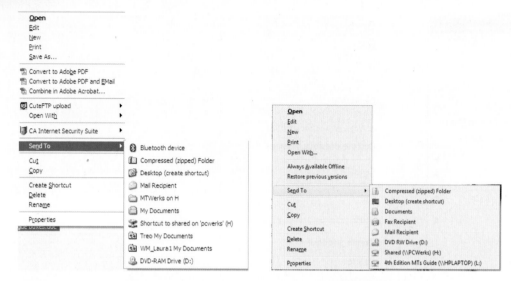

FIGURE 3-17 The Send To menu showing available destinations in Windows XP (left) and Windows Vista (right).

The Send To menu can also be used to attach files to an email message if you are using an email client such as Outlook or Outlook Express (but not web mail like GMail). Follow these steps to email files as an attachment:

1. Select the file(s) you want to attach to an email message.
2. Right-click the selected files to open the shortcut menu.
3. Choose Send To > Mail Recipient.
4. Your default email client (eg, Outlook or Outlook Express) will open a new email message with the selected files already attached. The subject line will contain the name(s) of the attached file(s).
5. Type a recipient's address and click Send.

Common Shortcut Menus

Shortcut menus are ubiquitous, so make it a habit of right-clicking on objects to discover quick, easy ways to accomplish routine tasks. Don't forget you can always use the Application key to open a menu instead of reaching for the mouse. Note the following ideas for using shortcut menus:

- Click within the toolbar area of an Explorer window or an Office application to display a list of available toolbars as well as a command to open a **Customize** dialog box for changing the icons that appear on the toolbars.
- Right-click a blank area on the Taskbar for a menu of commands for managing the Taskbar itself as well as open windows.
- Right-click the Title bar to display the window's Control menu.
- Shortcut menus associated with text (including the text-input boxes of dialog boxes) contain Cut, Copy, Paste, and Delete (or Clear). Occasionally you may encounter a text-input box (in a dialog box) that does not "capture" these keystrokes. In this case, right-click to display these commands on the shortcut menu.

- Properties is one of the most common commands found on shortcut menus. Properties (also called Personalize or Customize on some menus) can be used to change the way an object looks or the way it behaves. Right-click the Desktop, the [Start] button, or the Taskbar and choose Properties/Personalize to reveal dialog boxes for customizing these commonly used Windows elements.

- Right-click a drive name (eg, the C drive in Windows Explorer) and choose Properties to perform maintenance tasks such as Defrag, Disk Cleanup, and Error Checking.

- Right-click an image on a web page for a list of commands including Copy, Save Picture As, Print Picture, Email Picture, etc. Links on web pages also have a shortcut menu with related commands for manipulating the link.

- Right-click in the file-list area of an Explorer Window to display a list of commands for sorting and arranging icons and changing the view (Figure 3-18).

- Right-click in the file-list area of the **Save As** or **Open** dialog box for a list of file-management commands.

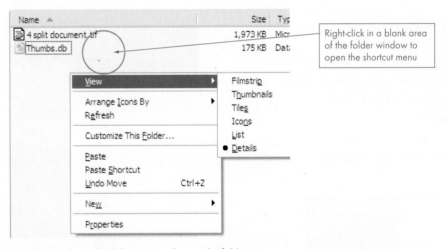

FIGURE 3-18 Use the right-click menu to change the folder view.

 Never hesitate to right-click on an object to discover new ways of performing common, and even not-so-common, tasks. To close the menu without using any commands, simply hit **Esc**.

Shortcut Icons

Shortcut icons are links that take you directly to the item they represent, called the target. Since they are links and not actual files, you can create as many as you like and place them wherever you want. You can even rename them! Using shortcut icons to access the items you use most will increase your productivity and simplify your daily routines.

Shortcut icons can be used to launch a program, open a file or folder, go to a website, start an email message, or access a shared folder or a disk on a network. Shortcut icons can be placed in many different places—on the Desktop, in folders, on toolbars, or on the Start menu—the possibilities are almost endless. You can have unlimited copies of a shortcut icon that points to the same target, and they can each have a different name. For example, you can create a shortcut icon to open Word and place a copy on the Desktop, one on the Start menu, and one on the Quick Launch bar.

It is important to distinguish an object's shortcut icon from the icon that represents the actual object. All shortcut icons have a small curved arrow in the lower left corner. See examples of icons and shortcut icons on page 13.

Creating Shortcuts Icons

As you will see below, there are several ways to create shortcut icons. Begin by learning the different ways to create shortcut icons and then learn how to take advantage of them.

Creating Shortcut Icons for Programs

Follow these steps to create a shortcut to open a program:

1. Open the Program menu (**Start** > Programs or **Start** > All Programs) and locate the program's icon as shown in Figure 3-19.
2. Right-click the program's icon.
3. From the Shortcut menu, choose Send To > Desktop (create shortcut). A shortcut icon for that program will appear on the Desktop.

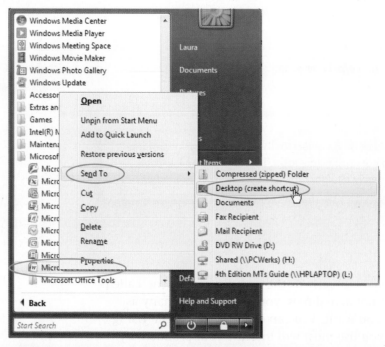

FIGURE 3-19 Right-click the program icon to create a shortcut icon on the Desktop.

Creating Shortcut Icons for Files and Folders

Follow these steps to create a shortcut icon for a file or folder:

1. Press **Logo+E** to open Windows Explorer and locate the file or folder. Do not actually open the file or folder.
2. Right-click the file or folder name and choose Send To > Desktop (create shortcut). A shortcut icon for that program will appear on the Desktop.

Creating Shortcut Icons to Network Drives

If you work with files and folders stored on a network, you can easily access the drive or the files and folders on the drive using a shortcut icon. Follow these steps:

1. Press **Logo+E** to display your computer's folders and drives, including the network drive.
2. Select the drive name and right-click.
3. Choose Create Shortcut.
4. Windows will open a message box confirming that you would like a shortcut placed on the Desktop; answer Yes.

 To quickly create shortcut icons to folders or disks, display the item in Windows Explorer and drag the item's icon from the Address bar onto the Desktop.

Creating Shortcut Icons for Websites

Follow these steps to create a shortcut icon using the drag–and-drop technique.

1. Display the website in Internet Explorer.
2. If the window is maximized (ie, you cannot see any part of your Desktop behind the Internet Explorer window), click Restore (so the window is reduced in size, making part of the Desktop visible behind the Internet Explorer window.
3. Drag the web page's icon (located in the Address bar) as shown in Figure 3-20 and drop it onto the Desktop. You will see a shortcut symbol attached to the mouse pointer while you are dragging.
4. Release the mouse button and a shortcut icon will appear on the Desktop.

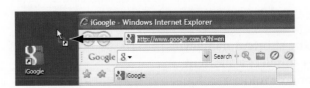

FIGURE 3-20 Drag the website's icon from the Address bar to the Desktop to quickly create a shortcut icon.

Customizing Shortcut Icons

Once you have created a shortcut icon, you may want to customize it by changing its icon or changing its name. Renaming shortcut icons can make the shortcuts more amenable to keyboarding, as will be explained below. The icon associated with the shortcut usually helps to identify the object that it points to, but some icons are rather generic. Changing a generic icon can make the shortcut easier to recognize. Right-click the shortcut icon and choose Properties. In the **Properties** dialog box, click **Change Icon**. Scroll through the available icons as shown in Figure 3-21, select one you like, and click **OK**.

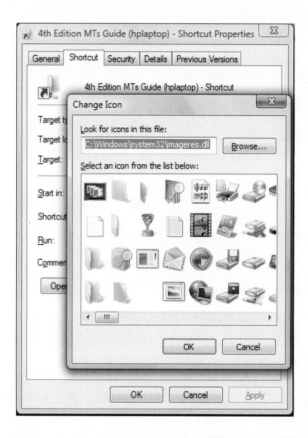

FIGURE 3-21 Change the icon associated with your shortcut icon using the Change Icon dialog.

Naming Your Shortcut Icons

Regardless of how you created your shortcut or where the shortcut is placed, you can rename the shortcut if needed. To change the name of your shortcut, right-click and choose Rename or simply select the icon and press **F2**. Type a new name for your shortcut and press **Enter**. You can name a shortcut anything you like—it will not change the name of the target (ie, the actual object that the shortcut points to).

Hot Keys for Shortcut Icons

Like every other object in Windows, the first character of the shortcut name will be the hot key for selecting that shortcut. To make it easier to select a shortcut using the keyboard, give each shortcut within any one menu or folder a unique first character. You can use numbers and some punctuation marks (comma, semicolon, brackets, hyphen, equal sign, and the single quotation mark) as the first character to control the way the icons sort.

Placing Shortcut Icons

Once you have created a shortcut icon, you will want to place that shortcut icon in strategic places so it is available where you need it. Your options include the Start menu, the Quick Launch bar, commonly used folders, and the Desktop. At first it may be difficult to decide where to place a shortcut icon, but usually ideal places will "reveal" themselves as you are working.

Once a shortcut icon is created, simply drag-and-drop or copy-and-paste the shortcut into folders, onto toolbars, and/or to the Start menu so you have strategic access to that shortcut icon whenever and wherever you need it.

 Since (My) Documents is the default folder for many applications, **Save As** and **Open** always open with this folder listed in the *Save in* or *Look in* box. Place shortcuts in (My) Documents to quickly jump to other commonly used folders when saving or opening files. Name the shortcut so it sorts to the top of the list within the file-list area. Simply click the shortcut within the file-list area to change the *Save in* or *Look in* location.

The Quick Launch bar is located on the Taskbar between the Start button and the program buttons (Figure 1-9). See page 10 for instructions on displaying the Quick Launch bar. Items on the Quick Launch bar are easily accessible with a single mouse click. Simply drag shortcut icons from the Desktop and drop them onto the Quick Launch bar. To remove shortcuts, right-click and choose Delete.

 To quickly open items on the Quick Launch bar using the keyboard, press Logo+n (where n is the number corresponding to the position of the icon on the Quick Launch bar).

 You can expand the height of the Taskbar to accommodate more buttons. With all windows minimized, hover the mouse over the upper edge of the Taskbar until you see a double-headed arrow. Hold down the left mouse button and drag the edge of the Taskbar upward to the desired height.

Deleting Shortcuts

To delete a shortcut icon that you no longer need, simply select the shortcut icon and press Delete. If the shortcut is located on a menu or toolbar, right-click the shortcut icon and choose Delete. Deleting a shortcut will not delete the actual file, folder, or application.

Access Frequently Used Items

A quick way to access applications, files, folders, and websites that you use most often is to place them on the Start menu. This technique works brilliantly for accessing over 30 different items with two quick keystrokes. To minimize keystrokes, this technique requires you to change the Start menu configuration to the Classic single-column style. Although you can still use the double-column Start menu to store shortcuts, it may add one or two more steps to accessing your shortcuts. To convert your Start menu, right-click the Start button and choose Properties > *Classic Start menu*.

The Start menu already includes shortcuts to several items at the bottom of the list (note the underscore letters) but you can add or delete shortcuts above the gray line. Figure 3-22 shows a single-column Start menu with a variety of shortcuts. To add a shortcut, simply drag the shortcut icon from the Desktop and

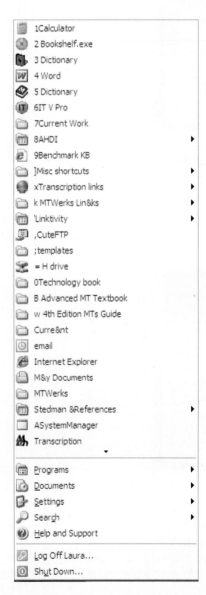

FIGURE 3-22 Add shortcuts to your Start menu and name each with a unique character for two-key access to your most-used programs, files, folders, and websites.

drop it on the Start button. Drag items up and down the menu to arrange in order of preference. Rename your shortcuts (right-click > Rename) so each has a unique first character. To access an item, simply press the **Logo** key followed by the alpha character (sequentially, not at the same time).

You can drag any type of shortcut to the Start menu, including shortcuts to folders, drives or specific folders on networked computers, web pages, applets on the Control Panel (eg, the Sounds applet for adjusting system volume), and accessories such as Windows Calculator. To expand the number of items that are accessible through the Start menu, combine groups of related shortcut icons into a submenu. For example, create a submenu with links to your favorite transcription-related websites so these items can be accessed with three keystrokes (ie, **Logo** key, submenu key, website key). Follow these steps to create a submenu on the Start menu:

1. Right-click the Start button and choose Open. The Start menu will be displayed as an Explorer window.
2. Right-click in an empty area of the Explorer window and choose New > Folder.
3. Name the folder (eg, Transcription links).
4. Open the new folder and drag shortcuts into the new folder.
5. Rename each shortcut so each has a unique alpha character.
6. Close the new folder and the **Start Menu** folder.
7. Press the **Logo** key followed by the folder's hot key to display the folder's contents as a menu. Press the next hot key to open the item listed on the submenu.

Menus and folders are two different methods of displaying the same information. As you can see from above, the Start menu is typically displayed as a menu but can also be displayed as a folder. The Send To menu (described on page 98) can also be displayed as a folder with new shortcuts added. The Desktop is another example of how information can be displayed as a "space" (not a menu or a folder). To display the contents of the Desktop as a folder, right-click the Desktop icon in Windows Explorer and choose Open. Throughout Windows, there are many examples of menus and toolbars that can be displayed as folders, and conversely, folders that can be displayed as toolbars.

Here are a few more tips for managing your Start menu:

- To delete shortcuts from the Start menu, right-click and choose Delete.
- To make the icons smaller so you can fit more shortcuts on the screen, right-click the Start button and choose Properties. On the Start Menu tab, click *Customize* and place a check mark at *Show small icons on Start menu*.

Changing the Start menu to a single column will remove the Search box from the Start menu, but you can still access Search when needed using **Logo+F**. How often you use the Search box may determine how well the single-column menu works for you.

Critical Thinking Questions

1. Explain the difference between a shortcut key written with a plus sign versus a comma.

   _____

   _____

2. Open an Explorer Window. Press F6 to move through each pane of the window. Describe the path of the cursor using the F6 key (write it out or sketch it).

   _____

   _____

3. Repeat the exercise described in #2 using the Tab key.

   _____

   _____

4. Why is learning shortcut keys in Word 2003 a good strategy for a planned migration to Word 2007?

   _____

   _____

5. Think of a particular computer task you do several times a day (eg, opening a document, program, or website). How long (in seconds) does it take? Devise a method for completing this task using the keyboard (create a shortcut icon if necessary). Practice your key sequence and compare the time it takes to complete the task using the mouse.

   _____

   _____

6. Open several windows. Use the different methods described on page 87 for switching between windows. Describe the difference. Now use ALT+Esc to switch between windows. Minimize all the windows (Logo+D) and then press ALT+Esc. How does this method compare to the others? (Hint: watch the Taskbar, note the order that the windows appear and note whether they are minimized or restored/maximized).

   _____

   _____

7. Create a shortcut for accessing Word with the keyboard.

   _____

   _____

8. Press Logo+Pause/Break. Fill in the following information from your own computer:

   Operating system _____

   Version of your operating system _____

   Service pack number _____

   Computer name _____

   Processor speed _____

   RAM _____

9. Use the keyboard to step through the following:

   a. Open Windows Explorer, Word, and one other program of your choice.

   b. Minimize all three windows using Logo+D.

   c. Use ALT+Tab to make Word the active window.

   d. Use the keyboard to minimize Word.

   f. Use ATL+Tab to make the Explorer window active.

   g. Use the keyboard to open the View menu on the Explorer window and change the View to Details.

   h. Use ALT+F4 to close all three windows.

10. Use the keyboard to complete the following tasks:

    a. Open Word.

    b. Open the Font dialog box using the shortcut CTRL+D.

    c. Using the keyboard, change the font settings to Courier New, Italic, 12 pt., all caps.

    d. Type several lines of text using the above font settings.

    e. Select the text you just typed using CTRL+A.

    f. Open the Font dialog box again and change the font back to Times New Roman, Regular, 10 pt., not all caps.

    g. Press CTRL+S to save the document. Name the file Exercise C. Save the document in the folder Word4e Exercises (created in exercise #6 in Chapter 2).

h. Close Word.

i. Open Explorer and use the keyboard to navigate to the folder Word4e Exercises. Locate the file just created. Use the shortcut key to copy the file.

j. Locate (My) Documents and use the shortcut key to paste a copy of Exercise C into that folder.

11. Step through the following:

a. Create a shortcut to your favorite website and place it on the Desktop.

b. Rename the shortcut you just created using the right-click menu.

c. Using Explorer, locate a file or folder that you use frequently. Right-click on the file or folder and create a shortcut on the Desktop.

d. Choose a shortcut on your Desktop and drag it to the Start menu.

f. Rename the shortcut so that the shortcut name starts with a unique character.

g. Open the file or folder using the Logo key and the hot key for that shortcut.

12. Create a shortcut to the Word4e Exercises folder (created in Chapter 2, question #6). Place a shortcut to this folder in at least two different places.

_____

_____

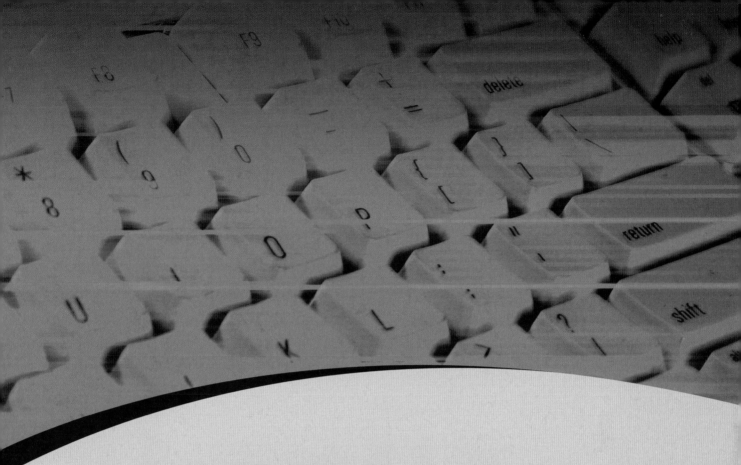

SECTION II

CHAPTER 4

Discovering Word

OBJECTIVES

▸ Identify formatting symbols on the Horizontal Ruler.

▸ Explain the role of the Status Bar in MS Word.

▸ Describe how the commands on Word's menus/ribbons are organized.

▸ Explain how Word's task panes are used and how they compare to dialog boxes.

▸ Describe zoom and view and how Word's various document views affect document appearance.

▸ Describe the role of formatting marks.

▸ Differentiate the various productivity tools available in Word.

The Word 2003 Interface

The Word interface has an incredible amount of detail that can easily be overlooked. Study Figure 4-1 and the images that follow and take note of the many features. Every item on the display has a purpose—either to give information, receive information, or both. Double-click items marked with a mouse icon ⌕ to open a related dialog box and right-click items marked with an ®.

Horizontal Ruler

The **Horizontal Ruler** provides a wealth of formatting information including tab positions, paragraph indents, and page margins. Examine the details of the ruler shown in Figure 4-2.

Status Bar

The **Status Bar**, shown in Figure 4-3, displays information related to the page count, cursor location, and the current "mode." In addition to giving information, all areas of the Status Bar are active and will respond to mouse clicks. Modes change the normal behavior of Word

WORD 2003

Standard and Formatting toolbars ®

Vertical Ruler

Status Bar

Close this document

Horizontal Ruler

Vertical scroll bar

Previous Page/ Object

Browse by Object

Next Page/Object

Horizontal scroll bar

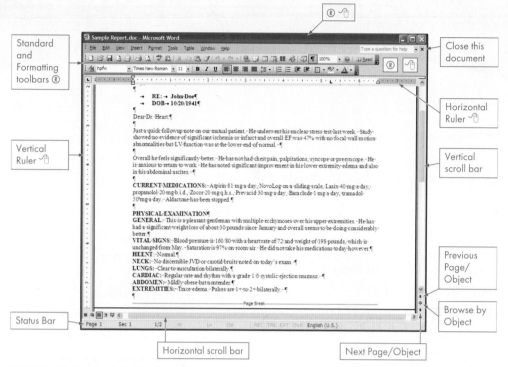

FIGURE 4-1 Details of the Word interface.

Page Margin

Indent marker

Left tab marker

Split document

Tab type indicator

Right indent marker

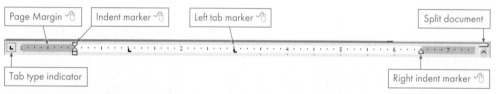

FIGURE 4-2 Details of the Horizontal Ruler.

Page View buttons

Language in use

Current Page & Section

Cursor-location indicators

Mode buttons/indicators
REC macro recorder
TRK Track changes ®
EXT Extend mode
OVR Overtype mode

Spelling and Grammar ®

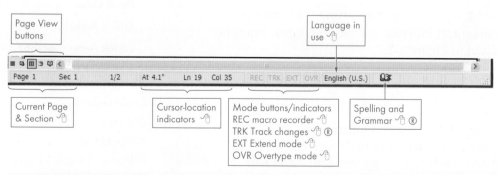

FIGURE 4-3 Details of the Status Bar.

to accomplish a specific task (tracking changes or recording a macro). They also change the way Word responds to the keyboard (eg, Extend and Overtype modes). The label on the mode button becomes black when the mode is active. You can also double-click the cursor-location indicators to open the **Go To** dialog box. Additionally, information related to spelling and grammar is available with a quick glance. A red X (✖) on the Spelling and Grammar icon indicates errors are still present in the document; a red check mark (✓) indicates all errors have been addressed. Double-click the icon to jump to the next spelling or grammar error or right-click the icon to open a shortcut menu.

Toolbars

The two main toolbars in Word are the **Standard toolbar** and the **Formatting toolbar**. By default, these toolbars are displayed on a single row across the top of the document, which makes it difficult to see all the commands available on both toolbars. Since the toolbars not only provide access to commands but also give you instant feedback (at the current position of the cursor), it's a good idea to change the default setting so that both toolbars are displayed in full on two separate rows. To change this setting, follow these steps:

1. Right-click in the toolbar area and choose Customize.
2. Click on **Options**.
3. Place a check mark at *Show Standard and Formatting toolbars on two rows* (see Figure 4-4).

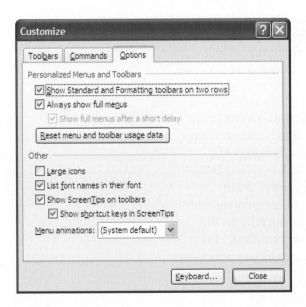

FIGURE 4-4 Change the way menus and toolbars behave using the Options tab on the Customize dialog box.

4. While you have the **Customize** dialog box open, it is a good idea to change the behavior of the menus also. Place a check mark at *Always show full menus*. With this option checked, the menus will drop down from the menu bar with all commands displayed. Otherwise, menus open in an abbreviated form with only your most recent commands displayed.

(Continued)

5. In addition, place a check mark at *Show ScreenTips on toolbars* and *Show shortcut keys in ScreenTips*. With these options checked, you can hover over an icon to display a description of the command and its shortcut key (if available) as in Figure 4-5.

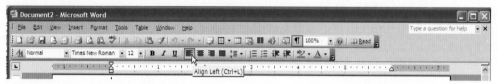

FIGURE 4-5 Hover over an icon to display a description of the command and its shortcut key.

There are many other toolbars available in Word. Some appear automatically when a specific task is being performed (eg, the <u>Header and Footer</u> toolbar appears when editing the header and footer area) and some remain hidden until you display them. Right-click in the toolbar area to see a menu of available toolbars. Place or remove the check mark next to the toolbar to display or hide the toolbar.

Menus

Sometimes the most difficult part of using Word is finding the command you need. The most common commands are typically displayed on the toolbars, but many are found on menus. Spend a few minutes examining the menus that drop down from the <u>Menu</u> bar and noting the patterns and relationships of the commands on each menu. Look at the icons next to the commands, which correlate to the icons on the toolbars. Also note any shortcut keys listed. Review important information about menus on page 17.

Although it may not appear to be so, there really is rhyme and reason to the configuration of the commands on the menus. The drop-down menus found on the <u>Menu</u> bar are very consistent across Office applications and other programs as well (especially Microsoft brand software). File, Edit, View, and Help are used in the vast majority of applications and all have similar if not identical commands. The Insert, Format, and Tools menus are used consistently across the Office applications and contain commands more specific to the application's purpose. The Tools menu in Word is truly your "toolbox" for getting the job done faster and easier. The Tools menu also gives you access to dialog boxes for adjusting your options and customizing Word to work to your best advantage.

Task Panes

Word includes 14 different task panes that can be displayed (one at a time) along the right edge of the document. Task panes allow you to both give and receive information, much like dialog boxes. You can easily move the cursor back and forth between the task pane and the document workspace using **F6**. The **Startup** task pane, shown in Figure 4-6, is automatically displayed when you open Word. Task panes typically contain links (blue, underlined text) that open a related dialog box. For example, the **Reveal Formatting** task pane (shown in Figure 4-6) displays detailed formatting information and provides links to dialog boxes for changing the formatting.

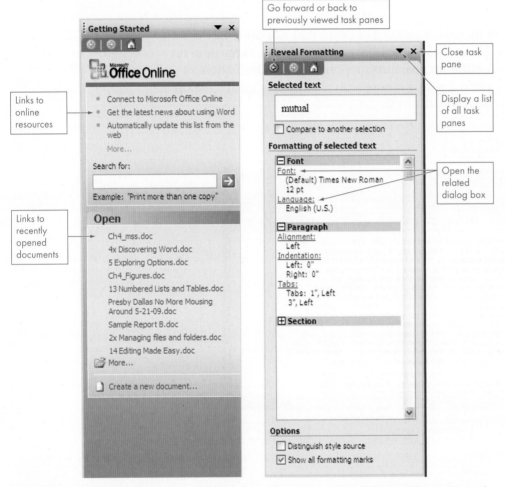

FIGURE 4-6 The Startup task pane (on the left) appears when you open Word. The Reveal Formatting task pane (on the right) provides helpful formatting information and links to dialog boxes to make formatting changes.

Here are a few tips for opening task panes:

- You can open the most recently used task pane at any time using the View menu (View > Task Pane) or the shortcut key **CTRL+F1**.
- Open task panes by selecting one from the drop-down menu (**CTRL+ Spacebar**) at the top of the task pane.
- To open the **Reveal Formatting** task pane, go to Format > Reveal Formatting (**Shift+F1**).
- For the **Format** task pane, choose Format > Styles and Formatting (**ALT, O, S**).

(Continued)

WORD 2007

- To access the **New Document** task pane, go to File > New (**ALT, F, N**).
- Look up a definition or synonym using the **Research** task pane: Tools > Research (**CTRL+Shift+O**).

For more on Word 2003, go to page 122.

The Word 2007 Interface

The Word interface has an incredible amount of detail that can easily be overlooked. Study Figure 4-7 and take note of the many features. Every item on the display has a purpose—either to give information, receive information, or both. Double-click items marked with a mouse icon ⬨ to open a related dialog box and right-click items marked with an ®.

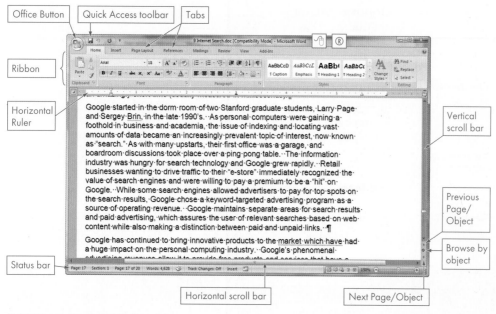

FIGURE 4-7 The Word 2007 interface.

Horizontal Ruler

The **Horizontal Ruler** provides a wealth of formatting information including tab positions, paragraph indents, and page margins. Examine the details of the ruler shown in Figure 4-8. Click the ⎡Show/Hide Ruler⎤ button at the top of the right-hand Vertical Scroll bar to display or hide the ruler.

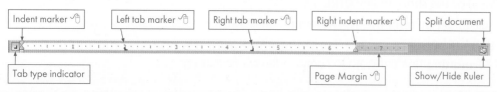

FIGURE 4-8 Details of the Horizontal Ruler.

WORD 2007

Status Bar

The **Status Bar**, as shown in Figure 4-9, displays information related to the page count, cursor location, and the current "mode." In addition to giving information, all areas of the Status Bar are active and will respond to mouse clicks. Modes change the normal behavior of Word to accomplish a specific task (eg, tracking changes or recording a macro). They also change the way Word responds to the keyboard (eg, Extend and Insert/Overtype modes). Double-click the mode buttons to toggle on/off. You can also double-click the cursor-location indicators to open the **Go To** dialog box. Additionally, information related to spelling and grammar is available with a quick glance. A red X (✗) on the Spelling and Grammar icon indicates errors are still present in the document; a blue check mark (✓) indicates all errors have been addressed. Double-click the icon to jump to the next spelling or grammar error or right-click to open a shortcut menu.

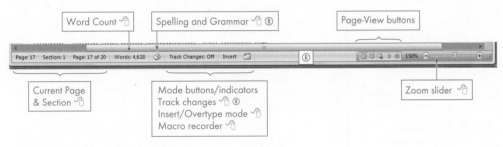

FIGURE 4-9 Details of the Status Bar.

The Status Bar in Word 2007, unlike previous versions, can be customized to show the icons that you are most likely to use. Right-click on the Status Bar to reveal a menu of choices (Figure 4-10). Place a check mark by those items you want displayed on the Status Bar.

Customize Status Bar	
✓ Formatted Page Number	1
✓ Section	1
✓ Page Number	1 of 1
✓ Vertical Page Position	1"
✓ Line Number	1
✓ Column	1
✓ Word Count	0
✓ Spelling and Grammar Check	No Errors
✓ Language	
✓ Signatures	Off
✓ Information Management Policy	Off
✓ Permissions	Off
✓ Track Changes	Off
✓ Caps Lock	Off
✓ Overtype	Insert
✓ Selection Mode	
✓ Macro Recording	Not Recording
✓ View Shortcuts	
✓ Zoom	100%
✓ Zoom Slider	

FIGURE 4-10 Choose options from the Status Bar menu to customize the bar with icons you use often.

WORD 2007

Menus

Word 2007 has one main menu, called the Program menu, which drops down from the **Office Button** in the top left corner. This menu contains many of the same commands as the File menu in previous versions of Word, but it behaves somewhat differently than previous menus. When the menu first opens, the right-hand column of the menu displays a list of recently used documents. This pane is replaced when a submenu is selected. Some commands have two mouse-click areas within the command itself. In Figure 4-11, you can see that the Save As command is divided into two buttons. The left side of the button (pale pink) opens the **Save As** dialog box. Clicking the right-pointing arrow keeps the right-hand submenu open so you can select one of the variations of the main command. Other menus are found throughout the Word 2007 ribbon as drop-down lists and galleries.

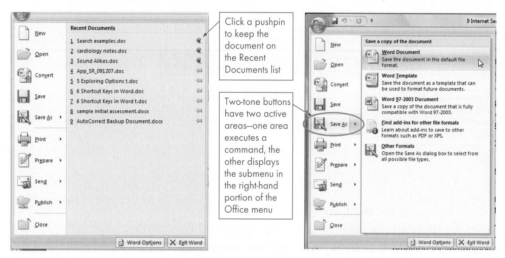

FIGURE 4-11 The Program menu in Word 2007. The image on the left shows the Recent Documents list, and the image on the right shows the Save As submenu.

Ribbon

The ribbon replaces the Menu bar and drop-down menus that have been a staple of Word since the 1990s. The ribbon tabs with buttons and associated drop-down menus contain the majority of commands available in Word. Commands on the ribbon are first divided into tabs and then each tab is further divided into groups. Each group contains a collection of related command buttons. These buttons either execute a specific command or open a drop-down menu of more choices. Hover over a command button to display a ToolTip with an explanation of the command as well as a shortcut key for that command.

Command buttons change size and shape to adjust to the width of the display; they may sit side-by-side or stack on top of each other (as in the Editing group in Figure 4-12) when needed in order to fit within the given width of the window. Command buttons with arrows (▾) next to them will open a drop-down menu of choices related to the command. You can show or hide the ribbon by toggling **CTRL+F1**.

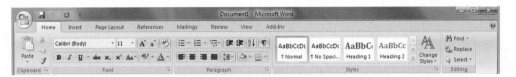

FIGURE 4-12 The ribbon in Word 2007.

Tabs

Sometimes the most difficult part of using Word is finding the command you need. The new ribbon and tab format was designed to make it easier to locate commands by eliminating layers of menus and dialog boxes. But the new interface can be somewhat disconcerting for veteran Word users, since the tabs that are displayed across the top of the ribbon do not exactly correlate to the menu names in Word 2003.

Commands found on the Home tab correspond closely with the commands found on the former Standard and Formatting toolbars. The Insert tab contains commands for inserting blocks of text, tables, graphics, and headers and footers. The Page Layout tab is well-named, as it contains commands for setting up page margins, page size, backgrounds, and watermarks. The Reference tab contains helpful commands for writing (footnotes, citations, tables of contents, and indexes), but not many useful tools for creating medical reports. Mailings includes commands for creating mail merges as well as printing envelopes and labels.

Transcriptionists and editors will find helpful commands on the Review tab, especially tools for spelling and grammar, research, inserting comments, and tracking changes. The View tab closely correlates with the former View menu and provides commands for changing the document view and zoom, displaying formatting marks, and oddly enough, the macro recorder. Word 2007 also uses contextual tabs that are only displayed when needed. For example, the Table tab appears on the ribbon only when the cursor is sitting within a table.

Galleries

A new feature of Word 2007 is the extensive collection of preset formats and styles. Examples include fully formatted header and footer layouts, cover-page layouts complete with graphics and formatted text, font and paragraph styles, and formatted tables. These collections, called galleries, are displayed as drop-down menus with thumbnail images of the preset formats. Gallery options take the guesswork out of creating professional-quality documents, but most of the gallery options are more appropriate for sales and marketing materials and business correspondence as opposed to patient reports. In the context of transcription and editing, you may find limited use for the gallery options.

WORD 2007

Quick Access Toolbar

The only toolbar in Word 2007 is the **Quick Access toolbar** (Figure 4-13). By default, this small toolbar sits just above the ribbon next to the Office Button, but the toolbar can be moved below the ribbon (right-click and choose Show Quick Access Toolbar below the Ribbon). Initially, the toolbar only contains icons for Save, Undo, and Redo, but you can add other commands that you use often. At the right end of the toolbar, click the More icon (down arrow with a line above it) and choose a command from the menu. To add a command found on one of the ribbon tabs, simply right-click the command button and choose Add to Quick Access Toolbar. Learn more about customizing this toolbar on page 400.

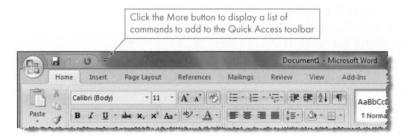

Click the More button to display a list of commands to add to the Quick Access toolbar

FIGURE 4-13 The Quick Access toolbar is positioned next to the Office button and contains icons for Save, Undo, and Redo.

Task Panes

Word includes several task panes that can be displayed along the right or left edge of the document. Task panes allow you to both give and receive information, much like dialog boxes, but unlike dialog boxes, task panes remain open while you work. You can switch back and forth between the task pane and the document workspace (F6). Word 2007 allows you to display more than one task pane at a time. Task panes typically contain links (blue text) that open a related dialog box.

The **Reveal Formatting** task pane, shown in Figure 4-14, displays detailed formatting information and provides links to dialog boxes for changing various aspects of formatting. There is no single way to access the task panes—some open when you click the corresponding dialog box launcher and some open in response to a related command. Two in particular have shortcut keys assigned: **Reveal Formatting** opens with Shift+F1, and **Research** (dictionary and thesaurus) opens with CTRL+Shift+O or Shift+F7.

Viewing Documents

Word offers many ways to display the interface (as described above) as well as various ways of displaying the document itself. Features that change *how* you see a document include document views, white space, and zoom.

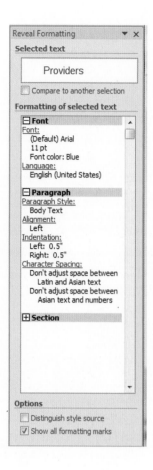

FIGURE 4-14 The Reveal Formatting task pane with (blue) links to dialog boxes for making changes.

Document Views

Document views determine *how the document appears on the display*. Select a view from the View menu (Word 2003)/ View tab (Word 2007) or use the shortcut keys (noted below). You can also click the View buttons located on the Status Bar. Word has several views from which to choose. As always, views allow you to display or hide information to make a particular task easier. The view never affects the way a document will print. Word offers the following views:

Normal view (Word 2003)/ **Draft** view (Word 2007) hides headers, footers, graphics (except those placed in-line with text), and other non-text elements. This view also does not show white space, page margins, or page boundaries. Because the entire document is not displayed, it is very easy to make formatting mistakes or to forget to complete the header and footer area. *Normal view is not recommended for transcribing and editing.* This command is found on the View menu/ View tab, and the shortcut for Normal/Draft view is **CTRL+ALT+N**.

Print Layout view shows text, graphics, headers and footers, and other elements as they will appear on the printed page. Print Layout also displays white space and page boundaries. Print Layout is the *best* view to use while transcribing and editing a document. This command is found on the View menu/ View tab, and the shortcut for Print Layout is **CTRL+ALT+P**.

Print Preview gives the best representation of the document as it will actually print. Use this view as a final check for margins, headers, footers, page breaks, and overall layout. The Print Preview toolbar/tab will automatically appear while in this view. Use **Page Up** and **Page Down** to scroll through the pages. While in Print Preview, the insertion point changes to a magnifying glass that will zoom in and out when clicked over an area of the document. To edit a document while in Print Preview, click the magnifying glass option on the toolbar/tab to toggle the magnifying glass icon to an insertion point. Word 2003 displays an icon for toggling and Word 2007 displays a check box for the Magnifier.

The Print Preview toolbar/tab includes a `Shrink to Fit` button, which will adjust the text size and spacing so that a document with only a few lines of text on the second page will "shrink up" to fit on just one page. You cannot close a document while it is displayed in Print Preview. Click `Close` on the toolbar/tab or change to a different view. Print Preview is found on the File menu in Word 2003. In Word 2007, Print Preview is listed on the Print submenu on the Program menu. In both versions, the shortcut key is **CTRL+F2**.

Reading Layout (Word 2003)/Full Screen Reading (Word 2007) view displays the document as if it were a book with opposing pages. The layout is not true to the actual formatting. This view is meant to facilitate on-screen reading. This is the default view for viewing Word documents received as email attachments. See page 136 (Word 2003) and 160 (Word 2007) for instructions on changing this default setting. This command is found on the View menu/`View` tab.

Outline view displays the document as collapsible headings so you can see the basic structure of the document based on headings. In this context, heading refers to text formatted with Word's built-in heading styles. Learn more about heading styles on page 199. Outline view has limited application in medical documentation, although Outline view can be used to quickly re-order (eg, alphabetize) reports that are transcribed in a single file (see page 463). This view is found on the View menu/`View` tab and the shortcut for Outline view is **CTRL+ALT+O**.

Full Screen view hides all toolbars, menus, ribbons, and other document-interface elements. This view maximizes the space on the screen for displaying the document itself. Press **Esc** to exit Full Screen.

Web Layout is used to display pages formatted in HTML and is not likely to be applicable to transcription.

The document will retain the current view when the document is closed (except for Print Preview and Reading Layout). The next time the document is opened, that same view will be used to display the document. Since some views hide information, you should be aware of the last view used before sending a document to another user, especially if the other user is a novice user—they may presume information is missing or the document is formatted incorrectly. It is best practice to close a document in Print Layout view. To change the view associated with a document, select the view and then make at least one edit to the document before saving and closing. Simply opening a document and changing the view without making any other edits to the document will not permanently change the view. An edit can be as simple as typing a word and then deleting that same word—anything so that Word detects an actual change to the document.

Navigating Documents

There are many ways to move through a document. Short documents can usually be managed easily with the navigation keys (**Up**, **Down**, **Left**, **Right**, **Page Up**, and **Page Down**). Longer documents can be managed using several different tools. The **Go To** dialog box (**CTRL+G**) allows you to jump to a specific page, section, line, or other element. In the **Go To** dialog (Figure 4-15), select the item to "go to" and click Next or Previous. Learn about the **Find** and **Find and Replace** dialog boxes in Chapter 14.

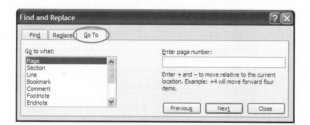

FIGURE 4-15 The Go To tab of the Find and Replace dialog lets you move through a document by jumping to the a particular item in the document.

 Once you have selected a specific go-to item, you can close the dialog box and press **CTRL+Page Down** to "go to" the next occurrence of the selected item. **CTRL+Page Up** goes to the previous item.

Another tool for navigating long documents is the **Browse Object** dialog box (Figure 4-16). Click the dot between the double-arrows at the bottom of the Vertical Scroll bar or click **ALT+CTRL+Home**. Select an object (page, graphic, table, field, list, etc) to jump to the next object of that type. Once you select an object for browsing, the key combinations **CTRL+Page up** and **CTRL+Page Down** change function. These shortcuts will move to the next "browse object" instead of moving to the top of the next or previous page. You can easily tell if the function of the keys has changed by glancing at the **Page Up** and **Page Down** arrows. These double arrows will change from black to blue. To return the function of the keys, open the **Browse** dialog and select the page icon (Browse by Page).

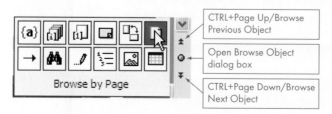

FIGURE 4-16 The Browse Object dialog box lets you jump to the next object using CTRL+Page up and Page down keys. The double arrows at the bottom of the Vertical Scroll bar turn blue when the function of the keys is changed.

Word also allows a document to be split horizontally, allowing you to see two parts of the same document at the same time. This can be helpful if you have a long document with multiple patient reports and a first-page log sheet listing each patient. You can view the list of patients in the upper section of the split and scroll through the reports in the lower section of the split.

Figure 4-17 shows a split document. To split a document, drag the Split Document icon (a small rectangular button located at the top of the Vertical Scroll bar) down until the split screens are the desired size. Drag the line upward to remove the split. You can also press **CTRL+ALT+S** and use the arrow keys to set the position of the split line and then press **Enter**. Press the shortcut again to remove the split.

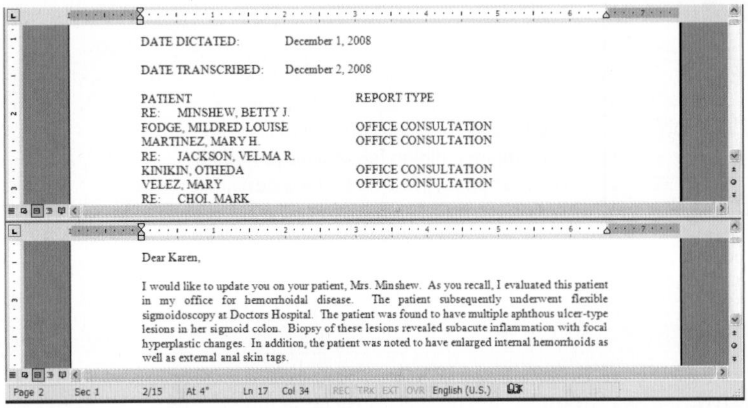

FIGURE 4-17 A split document showing the first page in the upper half of the display and a subsequent page in the lower half.

Zoom

Taking full advantage of the **Zoom** feature in Word will help you transcribe and proof more accurately and with much less eye strain. Zoom makes the document appear larger or smaller on the display but *does not affect the way the document prints*. Enlarge the zoom until a full line of text just fits within the edges of the screen (you don't want to have to scroll left and right to read the text). An easy way to adjust the zoom is to hold down **CTRL** while moving the mouse wheel forward and back.

Be sure to return the zoom setting to 90-100% before closing the document and sending to the client. The zoom setting stays with the document. The next person to open a document with a high zoom setting may misinterpret the zoom as altered formatting (ie, enlarged or bolded font).

If you change the zoom often, record macros and assign shortcut keys to your favorite zoom settings so you can quickly change the zoom with a single keystroke. Learn more about macros in Chapter 12.

White Space

White space refers to the space on the page between the first and last line of text and the top and bottom edge of the page. The white space is always hidden in Normal/Draft view, but is optional in Print Layout view. In Print Layout view, click the gray area displayed between two pages, as shown in Figure 4-18. White space at the bottom and top of pages as well as headers and footers will be hidden from view. Click the black line that separates pages to display the white space. Use a single click in Word 2003 and a double-click in Word 2007. This setting stays with the document, so it is best to display white space before saving and closing a document that will be sent to the client for viewing. Documents displayed at a low zoom (eg, 50-60%) and with white space hidden appear very strange, as if they have irregular paper sizes, since only a part of each page is displayed.

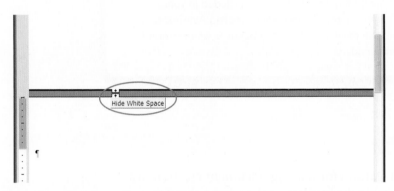

FIGURE 4-18 Click in the imaginary space between two pages to hide white space.

Formatting Marks

Formatting marks are an important part of the Word interface and play a critical role in assuring accurate formatting. Press **CTRL+Shift+8** to reveal formatting marks or click Show/Hide (the paragraph symbol **¶**) on the Standard toolbar/**Home** tab. These marks are displayed on the screen but *do not print*. Word uses the following marks:

- The **paragraph mark** represents the end of a paragraph and is created by pressing **Enter**.
- The right-pointing arrow is inserted when **Tab** is used.
- Dots represent spaces created by pressing the **Spacebar**.
- A curved arrow represents a manual line break (**Shift+Enter**).
- Manual page breaks (**CTRL+Enter**) are noted with a dotted line.

You can decide which formatting marks you would like to use (see page 197). The shortcut key and the Show/Hide icon will toggle between all marks displayed and those specific marks that you choose under **Options** (see page 134 for Word 2003 and page 161 for Word 2007). If you choose to display all marks, Show/Hide will toggle between all marks and no marks displayed. *Displaying all marks at all times is highly recommended.* Remember, these marks will not print and the setting is not saved with the document, so the next person to view the document will not see formatting marks unless they have them displayed on *their* computer. Learn more about formatting marks in Chapter 7.

Transcriptionists and editors should always display formatting marks! It may take time to adjust to the additional markings in and around text, but after working with these marks for a while, you will really come to appreciate them.

Be sure to display formatting marks when creating AutoText and Auto Correct entries. This will help you avoid picking up leading or trailing spaces and paragraph marks that you do not want included in your shortcut. Selecting or avoiding paragraph marks when creating AutoText and AutoCorrect entries will determine how the entry behaves when inserted. Learn more in Chapters 9 and 10.

Productivity Tools

Word comes with many tools and features for making document creation fast, efficient, and consistent. The following list introduces the most helpful features in Word and defines terms that will be used throughout this text. All of these features will be described in greater detail later in this text.

Templates

Many transcriptionists are accustomed to using the term "template" to refer to the basic format of a report (eg, a SOAP note or an H&P template). In Word, a **template** is more than just formatted text; it is an actual file that is used to create a document and to store information about how the document should appear. A template file contains document settings such as font and paragraph styles, page layout, special key assignments, and customized toolbars. Template files also store specific AutoText entries and macros that are only available when that particular template file is being used.

Word uses global templates and document templates. The Normal template (Normal.dot) is the global template and contains settings that are available to *all* documents. The Normal.dot is Word's most important data file and is *always* in use—Word cannot function without it. Document templates are only used when the user specifies. Document templates can contain information unique to that particular type of document. Learn more about template files (dot files) in Chapter 8. Instructions for backing up template files are found on page 71.

Boilerplates

A **boilerplate** contains text that is used repeatedly. A boilerplate refers to the layout of a given report that includes headings and subheadings. Often transcriptionists refer to the standard text layout as a template, but to avoid confusing the term template with Word's use of the term, this text will refer to standard layouts as boilerplates. In this context, a boilerplate refers to just text; templates contain boilerplate text as well as shortcuts, macros, margin settings, AutoText entries, and other settings specific to the type of report.

Macros

Many transcriptionists are accustomed to using the term macro to refer to a method of expanding a few characters (a short form) into words, phrases, or even paragraphs (ie, to expand text). The **Macro** feature in Word, however, is used to record a series of *commands* that can be played back as a single command. For example, a macro can be used to select a disclaimer that is normally part of the standard text and delete that disclaimer—all in a single keystroke. While the macro recorder *can* be used to create shortcuts for inserting text, this is not the best use of the macro feature in Word. AutoText and AutoCorrect are best used for quickly inserting blocks of text.

AutoText

This is a feature built into Word that offers a way to store and quickly insert text, graphics, fields, tables, bookmarks, and other items that you use frequently. AutoText works great for expanding shortcuts into phrases, inserting standard text, normals, and boilerplate text. AutoText is part of the Building Blocks feature in Word 2007. Learn more in Chapter 10.

AutoCorrect

This is a feature of Microsoft Office that is designed to "automatically correct" typos and misspellings. Since AutoCorrect is an Office feature (not just a Word feature), it is also used in Excel and PowerPoint. AutoCorrect entries saved in Word will be available in these other programs as well. Since it was intended to correct typographical errors "automatically" without the user's intervention, it is always active. Many transcriptionists use AutoCorrect as a text expander as well, since it will automatically replace what is typed with the designated replacement text. However, you must use caution when creating shortcuts for expanding text, since the shortcut will expand as soon as you hit the Spacebar or any punctuation key. Learn more in Chapter 9.

Critical Thinking Questions

1. What does the word "browse" mean when referring to the Browse Object dialog?

   _____

   _____

2. Explain how formatting marks and views can help with document layout and formatting.

   _____

   _____

3. List at least six types of information that can be gained from the Horizontal Ruler. List three dialog boxes that can be opened using the Horizontal Ruler.

   _____

   _____

4. (Word 2003 only) Change the behavior of the Standard and Formatting toolbars so they appear on one row and change the behavior of menus and toolbars so they do not change with your ongoing use (Personalized Menu feature). What are the advantages and disadvantages of the Personalized Menus feature in Word? Which method do you prefer?

   _____

   _____

5. (Word 2007 only) Right-click the Quick Access toolbar. Move the toolbar below the ribbon. Hide/display the ribbon using CTRL+F1. What are the advantages and disadvantages to hiding/displaying the ribbon? Which configuration do you prefer?

   _____

   _____

6. (Office 2003 only) Open several applications from the Office suite (eg, Word, Excel, PowerPoint, Publisher). Compare the contents of the File, Edit, and View menus. What commands do they have in common?

   _____

   _____

7. (Office 2007 only) Open several applications from the Office suite (eg, Word, Excel, PowerPoint, Publisher). Compare the contents of the Home, Insert, and View tabs. What commands do they have in common?

   _____

   _____

8. What can you do if a needed command on a menu, toolbar, or ribbon is dimmed?

_____

_____

9. Compare and contrast task panes and dialog boxes. Why do you think these items were named dialog boxes and task panes?

_____

_____

10. Describe each of the four mode buttons available on the Status Bar (Word 2007 users may need to display the mode buttons if they are hidden). How does each change the way Word responds to the keyboard?

_____

_____

11. Describe what happens when you

a. double-click the empty area to the right of the toolbars (Word 2003).

_____

_____

b. right-click in the toolbar area (Word 2003) or the ribbon (Word 2007).

_____

_____

c. double-click the page number of the Status Bar.

_____

_____

d. double-click the spelling and grammar icon on the Status Bar (Word 2003).

_____

_____

e. right-click the spelling and grammar icon on the Status Bar (Word 2003).

_____

_____

f. click the spelling and grammar icon on the Status Bar (Word 2007).

_____

_____

g.   double-click the shaded area of the Horizontal Ruler.

_____

_____

h.   double-click the Title bar.

_____

_____

i.   right-click the Title bar.

_____

_____

12. Open Exercise A (see Critical Thinking see Chapter 2, question #6). Do the following:

a.   Change the view to Normal/Draft and then Print Layout.

b.   Show and hide white space.

c.   Show formatting marks.

d.   Which view do you think is better for transcribing?

_____

_____

e.   Which view do you think is better for proofreading?

_____

_____

f.   How does Print Preview compare to these other views?

_____

_____

13. Give an example of how you might use each of the productivity tools provided in Word.

_____

_____

CHAPTER 5

Exploring Options

OBJECTIVES

▸ Identify and locate key dialog boxes (**Options/Word Options**, **AutoCorrect**, and **Customize**) that determine how Word looks and behaves.

▸ Modify various Word options to suit your style and your work environment to improve your efficiency and reduce your frustration.

▸ Identify options that may impact the quality and accuracy of your documents.

KEYWORDS

Options dialog box (Word 2003)

Word Options dialog box (Word 2007)

AutoCorrect dialog box

You will find that Word is very flexible—maybe even too flexible! It is important to recognize that MS Word is a world-class software application used by hundreds of industries with a wide range of needs. As such, it has tremendous functionality and versatility, necessitating a large number of options and settings. Knowing how to manage your options will help you troubleshoot problems and greatly decrease your frustration, so it is worthwhile to study the dialog boxes described here. This chapter will show you how Word can be adapted to your circumstances to increase your accuracy, efficiency, and satisfaction, and to improve the quality of your documents.

Word 2003 Options

The majority of options in Word 2003 are accessed through the **Options** dialog box (Tools > Options). This particular dialog box brings together 11 different dialog boxes covering a variety of categories. You may encounter some of these individual dialog boxes by clicking icons or related commands throughout the Word interface (eg, the **Spelling and Grammar** dialog can also be accessed using the book icon on the Status Bar). It doesn't matter how you access the dialog—the results will be the same. The **Options** dialog box provides "one-stop shopping" for changing a variety of options. Each individual dialog box will be described below.

WORD 2003

View

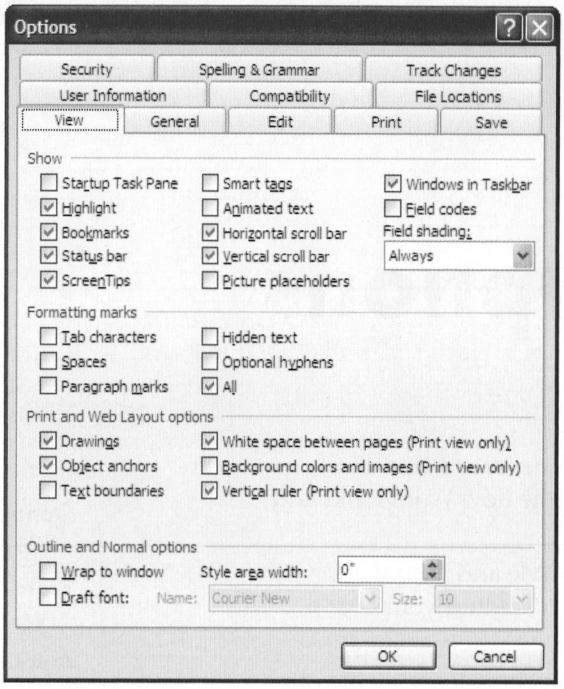

FIGURE 5-1 View Options dialog box determines what is displayed on the screen.

Options on the **View** dialog box control the way documents are *displayed* but do not affect the way your document will *print*.

Startup Task Pane: When selected, the **Startup** task pane automatically appears each time Word is opened (see Figure 4-6).

Highlight: Displays or hides highlighted text (like a Hi-Liter marker) on screen *and* when printed.

Bookmarks: Designates bookmarked text with square brackets.

Status Bar: Displays the <u>Status Bar</u> at the bottom of your workspace (see page 114).

ScreenTips: Displays a popup box when you hover over a Comment, a tracked change, a footnote, or an endnote.

Smart tags: Marks certain types of text (addresses, e-mail addresses, etc) with a purple line to easily identify and add information to other Office programs. Unless you work extensively with Outlook, Excel, or other Office software products, you probably won't use Smart tags.

Horizontal and Vertical scroll bar: Displays scroll bars on the right and across the bottom of the screen. Helpful if you like to use the mouse to navigate documents.

Picture placeholders: Places an empty box within the document in place of graphics. Clear this box if you work with documents containing company logos.

Windows in Taskbar: When selected, each open document will have its own button on the Windows <u>Taskbar</u>. Otherwise, Word will display only one icon on the <u>Taskbar</u> regardless of the number of open documents. In this case, switch between documents using the Window menu on Word's <u>Menu</u> bar.

Vertical ruler: Displays a vertical ruler when the document is displayed in Print view.

Field codes: Displays field codes instead of field results. Toggle this selection using **ALT+F9** (see Chapter 11).

Field shading: Marks fields with shaded gray boxes *Always*, *Never*, or only *When Selected*. Field shading does not print.

Formatting marks: Displays selected formatting marks. Clicking Show/Hide (the paragraph icon) or **CTRL+Shift+8** will toggle between *all* marks and only those selected. If you choose *All*, Show/Hide will toggle between all marks and no marks (learn more in Chapter 7.)

Drawings: When selected, displays graphics while in Print or Web Layout view. Check this box if your documents contain company logos or other images.

Object anchors: Displays an anchor when an object is attached to a paragraph.

Text boundaries: Displays a dotted line showing page margins and columns.

White space between pages (Print view only): Displays the white space between the top of the text and the top of the page. You can also alternate this setting by clicking the narrow gray area between pages (see page 127).

Background colors and images: Displays background images.

Vertical ruler: Displays a ruler down the left side of the page in Print Layout view.

Wrap to window: Allows printed words to fit within the viewable space. Will distort formatting if the window is too narrow.

Style area width: Sets the width of the sidebar in Normal view, which displays the style name for each paragraph.

General

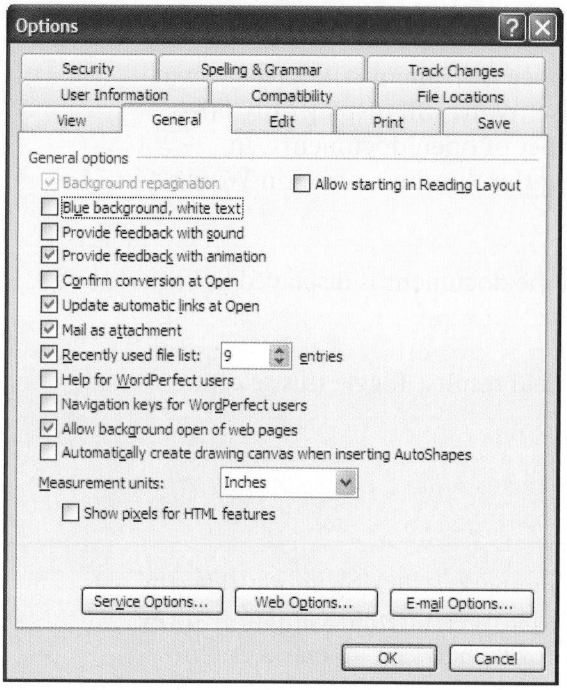

FIGURE 5-2 General Options dialog box contains options that do not fall into any other category.

The **General** dialog box contains options that do not fall under any other category.

Allow starting in Reading Layout: When selected, Word automatically opens documents attached to email in Reading Layout view.

Blue background, white text: Changes screen to appear like Word Perfect 5.1 for DOS.

Provide feedback with sound: Associates sounds with certain events such as error warnings. Sounds may be disturbing or loud when wearing a transcription headset.

Provide feedback with animation: When turned on, Word will use special pointers to indicate certain automated procedures are in progress (eg, background saves).

Confirm conversion at Open: Check if you want to select the converter used to open documents created in other word processing programs.

Update automatic links at Open: Updates information linked to other files when you open a document.

Mail as attachment: Determines whether Word attaches the current file to an e-mail message or inserts text into an e-mail message when you select File > Send to > Mail recipient.

Recently used file list: When checked, Word will keep a list of previously opened documents at the bottom of your File menu. Set the number of entries from 1–9. You can open these documents using **ALT, F, #,** where # corresponds to the file number on the list.

Help for WordPerfect users: When checked, Word displays instructions or demonstrates a Word equivalent when you press a Word Perfect for DOS key combination.

Navigation keys for WordPerfect users: Sets the functions of **Page up**, **Page down**, **Home**, **End** and **Escape** to the WordPerfect equivalent. *This feature is not recommended—it causes more problems than it solves.*

Allow background open of web pages: Allows you to continue using Word while viewing HTML documents on web pages.

Measurement units: Determines which measurement system is displayed on rulers and in some dialog boxes.

The diagrams in this chapter show my suggestions based on my own experience. You may choose to use these suggestions as a starting point for setting your own preferences. These settings are most appropriate for transcriptionists and other healthcare documentation specialists that work with Word as a stand-alone application. Since many transcription companies and hospitals use document management software that incorporates Word, some of the options discussed here may need to be adapted to specific work environments. Follow your employer's specifications where applicable. For simplicity, options that are highly unlikely to be relevant will not be mentioned at all.

• •

Notes

Edit

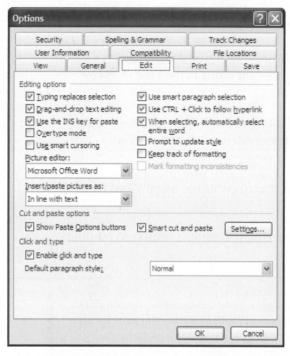

FIGURE 5-3 Edit Options dialog box determines how Word behaves when you are editing including cut and paste routines.

The **Edit** dialog box contains options that control the way Word behaves when you are editing.

Typing replaces selection: Deletes selected text as soon as you begin typing. If you clear this box, Word inserts text in front of selected text but does not delete it.

Drag-and-drop text editing: This allows you to move or copy selected text using the mouse.

Use the INS key for paste: With this box checked, the **Insert** key (next to **Home**) pastes the contents of the Clipboard (Edit > Paste or **CTRL+V**). When not checked, the **Insert** key toggles Overtype mode (see next paragraph).

Overtype mode: This replaces existing text as you type, one character at a time. This may be useful for editing or filling out forms with lines created with underscore characters. You can also toggle on/off by double-clicking OVR on the Status Bar.

Use smart cursoring: With this option checked, your insertion point moves with you as you scroll up or down or when you press an arrow key. The insertion point responds at the page you are currently viewing, not where the insertion point was before you began scrolling.

Use smart paragraph selection: Automatically includes the paragraph mark when you select an entire paragraph.

Use CTRL+Click to follow hyperlink: Allows you to select a hyperlink without actually following the link.

When selecting, automatically select entire word: Allows you to place the cursor at any point in the word to format the entire word. For example, you can italicize a single word without selecting every character in that word.

Prompt to update style: When selected, Word will ask if you want to update a style when manual formatting has been applied.

Keep track of formatting: When selected, Word will track formatting styles as you type.

Mark formatting inconsistencies: When selected, Word will mark formatting inconsistencies (ie, changes in font size in the same paragraph or table) with blue lines. You must also select *Keep track of formatting*.

Show Paste Options buttons: When copying and pasting text, Word will display a button that opens a menu with options for formatting the text that was just pasted.

Smart cut and paste: Automatically adjusts the spacing before and after a sentence to a single space when using cut-and-paste or drag-and-drop editing. *These settings assume that you use one space between sentences.* This setting can also determine font and paragraph style of pasted text.

The cut and paste settings may affect the behavior of third-party text expansion programs, so you may need to tweak these settings if you use other software programs that insert text using text shortcuts (see page 264).

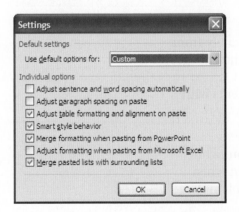

FIGURE 5-4 Additional settings available under Smart cut and paste.

Enable Click and type: Allows you to double-click anywhere in the document and begin typing. The *Default paragraph style* indicates which style to apply to paragraphs inserted using Click and type.

WORD 2003

Save

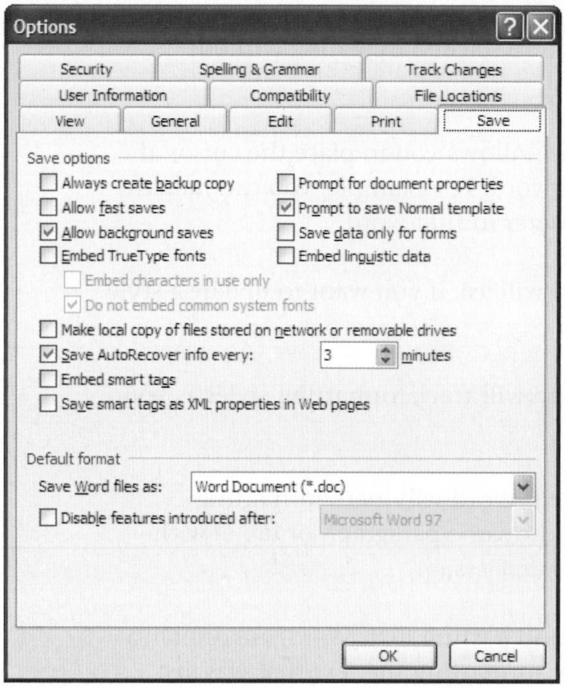

FIGURE 5-5 Save Options dialog box determines how Word saves your documents and what additional information is included in the document file.

These options control the AutoSave feature, backups, and also the standard Save format.

Always create backup copy: When checked, Word creates a backup copy with the extension wbk each time you use the Save command. *Recommended when working on very long or complicated documents that you open and edit many times.* This is not helpful if you create many short documents each day, as most medical transcriptionists do.

Allow fast saves: Select if you want Word to save a list of changes separately from your stored work. You cannot view this list. The idea is to save only the changes and then put all the changes together before closing the document. It is designed to save time when working with long documents or documents with graphics, so this is not likely to be of benefit to transcription. It is also very easy to corrupt the document using this method.

Allow background saves: Select if you want to continue working in Word while saving another document in the background. This would be of benefit when working with documents with graphics or complex tables, but probably not applicable to transcription files.

Prompt for document properties: Opens the **Properties** dialog box the first time you save a file.

Prompt to save Normal template: Prompts you to save changes to the Normal.dot. If you clear this box, changes will automatically be saved (learn more in Chapter 8).

Embed linguistic data: Saves speech and handwriting input data when Word is used to capture voice or handwriting for speech and handwriting recognition. Does not apply to speech recognition files where the audio is captured by dictation equipment and run through a separate speech recognition engine.

Make local copy of files stored on network or removable drives: Temporarily saves a local copy when the original is saved on a network drive or removable media. This option may depend on your transcription platform. If you do not work on a platform, always edit documents on the local drive, not on removable media.

Save AutoRecover info every: Minutes: Enable this option and set the minutes for a short interval such as 1, 2, or 3 minutes. For information about *AutoRecover*, see page 75 "AutoRecover."

Save Word files as: Select the file extension you use most often, most likely *Word 97-2003 Document (*.doc)*. Other document types may be specified by your employer or client.

 It would be very easy to glance at this chapter and become completely overwhelmed with so many details, but memorizing minute details is not the objective. *It is important that you are able to identify and quickly locate key dialog boxes, namely* **Options** (in Word 2003), **Word Options** (in Word 2007), **AutoCorrect,** *and* **Customize**. Read through this chapter to become familiar with the settings and options available so you are familiar with your choices and can easily reference this information when you need to make a specific change. Note how the options within a single dialog box are associated with each other. It's not necessary that you memorize every option; but you will want to pay very close attention to the options that are specifically marked, as these are the options that are most likely to impact your work within healthcare documentation.

Notes

WORD 2003

Spelling and Grammar

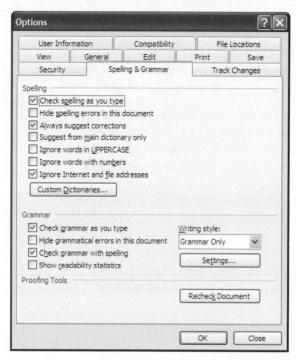

FIGURE 5-6 Spelling and Grammar Options dialog box controls Word's spelling and grammar checking feature.

Options in the **Spelling and Grammar** dialog box determine how Word handles spelling and grammar errors. See Chapter 14 for more detailed information on using the spelling and grammar features.

Check spelling as you type: Marks misspelled or repeated words with a red sawtooth line. Red lines appear as you type.

Hide spelling errors in this document: Misspelled words will not be marked with a red sawtooth line but will still appear in the **Spelling and Grammar** dialog box when you run a spell check.

Always suggest corrections: When checked, Word will offer spelling suggestions in the **Spelling and Grammar** dialog box or the shortcut menu.

Suggest from main dictionary only: If checked, Word will not refer to Custom dictionaries when offering spelling suggestions.

Ignore words in UPPERCASE: Clear this box so headings, drug allergies, and other text typed in all caps will be spell checked. The default setting is to ignore words in uppercase, so it is important to change this setting.

Ignore words with numbers: Clear this box so words with numbers will be spell checked.

Ignore Internet and file addresses: Check to ignore Internet addresses, file paths, or e-mail addresses during a spell check.

Custom Dictionaries: Click this button to select, edit, and create Custom dictionaries. Learn more on page 356.

Check grammar as you type: Check to mark possible grammatical errors with a green sawtooth line. Lines will appear as you type.

Hide grammatical errors in this document: When checked, grammatical errors will not be marked with a green sawtooth line but will appear in the **Spelling and Grammar** dialog box when you perform a spell check.

Check grammar with spelling: With this box checked, grammatical errors will be presented along with spelling errors in the **Spelling and Grammar** dialog box during a spell-check routine.

Show readability statistics: Shows readability statistics after each grammar check. This is not necessary for medical reports.

Settings: Select a writing style or customize the grammar checker to improve grammar checking. The option to check *Grammar only* (as opposed to grammar and style) is more useful in the context of medical documentation. Adjusting settings in the **Grammar** settings dialog is more helpful than disabling grammar checking altogether. Learn more on page 358.

Check/Recheck Document: Click to begin a spell check or to repeat a spell check after changing spell-check options or if spell checking a document that was previously checked on another PC. Quality Assurance editors can use this command to repeat the spell-check routine on documents previously checked by the MT. Learn more on page 361.

You will want to keep track of your changes so you can evaluate the consequences of your selections and decide whether to keep the change or go back to a previous setting. The best way to document your settings before making changes is to use the Print Screen feature in Windows. Display the dialog box to be changed and click **Print Screen** (to capture the entire display) or **ALT+Print Screen** (to capture the active window). This will take a "snapshot" of your display and place that image on the Windows Clipboard. Paste the image (**CTRL+V**) into a Word document and print. Jot down the date along with any notes about the changes you made and place your notes in a binder.

WORD 2003

Print

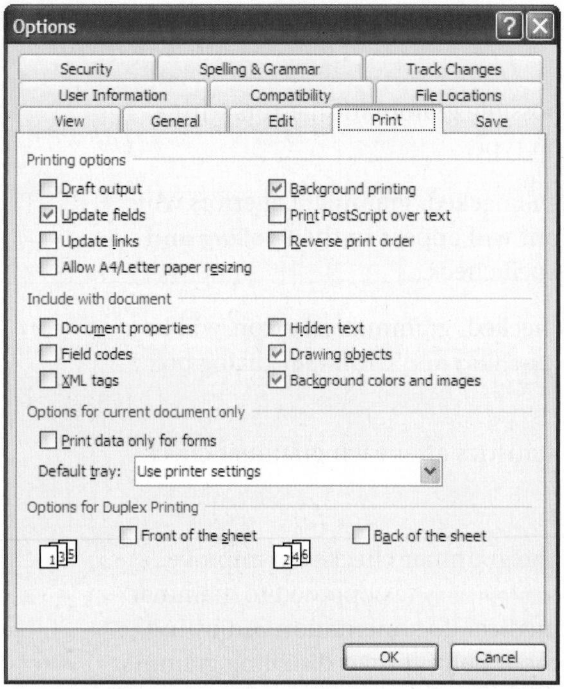

FIGURE 5-7 Print Options dialog box determines what and how a document prints.

Options found on the **Print** dialog box control how and what will print.

Draft output: Prints faster by omitting graphics (drawing objects and pictures).

Update fields: Updates fields before printing.

Background printing: Allows you to work while printing.

Reverse print order: Outputs document starting with the last page.

Hidden text: Prints hidden text with a dotted underline.

Background colors and images: Prints backgrounds and images when applicable.

Default tray: Selects paper tray for current document only. Will override Windows' setting in the printer's **Properties** dialog box on the Control Panel.

• •

Notes

Track Changes

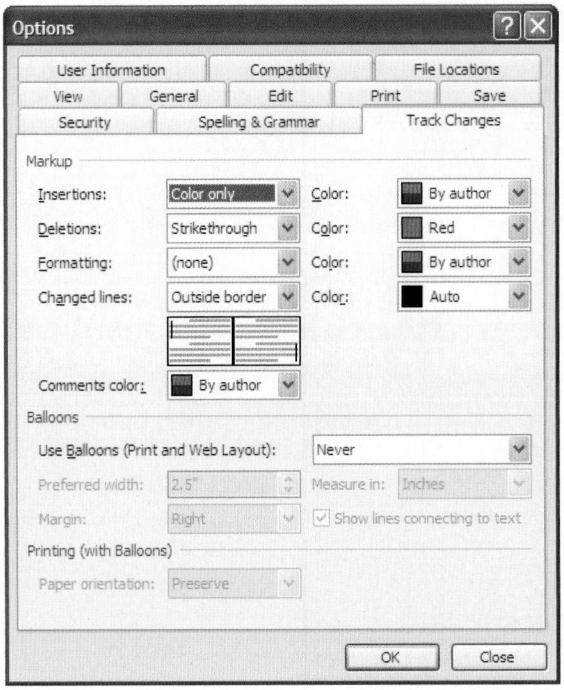

FIGURE 5-8 The Track Changes Options dialog box allows you to determine how edits are marked for tracking purposes.

These options control Track Changes and Comments, also referred to as Reviewing.

Use this dialog box to set preferences for the Track Changes feature (also called Revisions). You might use this feature for feedback during training or quality assurance review, but it is not applicable to routine transcription. Each type of edit can be color coded to indicate the type of change and the person who made the change.

Changed lines: Places a vertical line in the margin to mark a paragraph that contains changes. This helps call attention to paragraphs that have very small changes that might otherwise go unnoticed.

Use Balloons (Print and Web Layout): Select *Never*, *Always*, or *Only for comments/formatting* to determine if and when balloons are displayed. This setting affects both tracked changes and comments (learn more about comments on page 375 and on the accompanying CD).

If balloons are enabled, set the size and position (right or left margin) of the balloons.

It's surprisingly easy to accidentally invoke Track Changes (the shortcut key is **CTRL+Shift+E**). If text is suddenly marked with red and/or blue underlines or strikeouts, you have inadvertently turned on revision marks. Press **CTRL+Shift+E** to toggle off or click TRK on the Status Bar. Use **CTRL+Z** to reverse the changes made while track changes was enabled or click Accept Changes (blue check mark) on the Reviewing toolbar that appears when Track Changes is enabled. Learn more about Track Changes on the accompanying CD.

WORD 2003

User Information

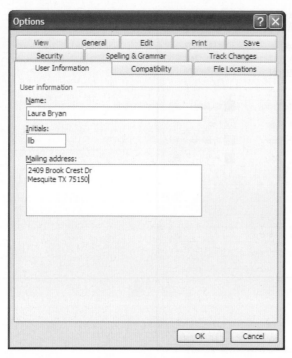

FIGURE 5-9 The User Information dialog box stores information that is used by other features in Word.

The **User Information** dialog box sets the username, return address information, and user initials. Be sure to fill in this information on your copy of Word.

Name: Type your name. This information is referenced when completing Document Properties and in letters and envelopes. Learn more about Document Properties in Chapter 11.

Initials: Word uses these initials to identify the user who inserted comments, endnotes, foot notes, and tracked changes.

Mailing address: Sets the default return address for envelopes.

Notes

Compatibility

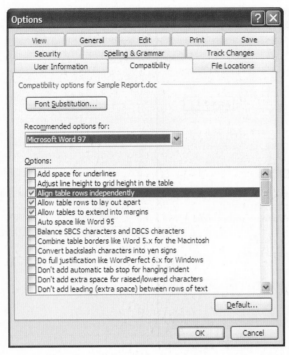

FIGURE 5-10 The Compatibility Options dialog box determines how documents created in other word processing programs are displayed in Word.

The **Compatibility** dialog box allows you to change the way Word interprets documents that have been created in other word processing programs. These settings do not actually change formatting codes (so the document will still appear correctly if opened in the other word processing program), but will allow the document to more closely resemble the appearance of the original document *when displayed in Word.*

Click on *Recommended options for* and select the appropriate program.

Notes

Security

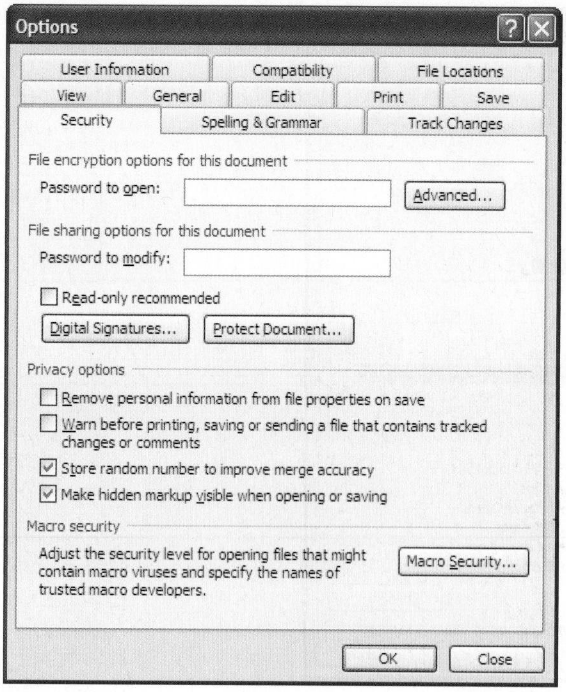

FIGURE 5-11 The Security Options dialog box allows you to set security and privacy options for a document as well as control macro security options.

The **Security** dialog box sets passwords, privacy features, and macro handling procedures.

Password to Open: Assign a password that will be required to open this document. Passwords are case sensitive.

Advanced: Allows you to select a level of encryption. This must be done for each document when the document is saved by choosing Tools > Security Options from the **Save As** dialog box.

Password to Modify: When a password is assigned, another user cannot save changes to the document unless they supply the correct password. To work around this, they can save the file using a different name and then make changes.

Read-only recommended: Suggests that the user review the document without making changes, although they do actually have the ability to save changes.

Digital Signatures: To verify the authenticity of the author of the document, a digital signature can be added. Digital signatures can be purchased from third-party companies such as VeriSign.

Protect Document: Allows the author to limit the types of changes that can be made to the document by subsequent users.

Remove personal information from this document on save: When selected, all personal information, including the user's name, initials, address, company name, and other information stored in Properties is removed.

Warn before printing, saving, or sending a file that contains tracked changes or comments: Word warns the user before closing or printing any document that still contains tracked changes or comments.

Store random number to improve merge accuracy: Word uses a numbering system to help improve the accuracy of comparing documents. Clearing this box decreases the accuracy of document comparison, but this is probably not an issue for transcriptionists.

Make hidden markup visible when opening or saving: If the previous user tracked changes and then hid markup (revision marks such as strikethrough), this setting assures that markup is displayed when opened on this computer.

Macro Security: This does not detect viruses and does not replace virus-checking software; rather, this option determines whether macros are enabled. Options include *Low*, *Medium*, *High*, and *Very High*. *Very High* only enables macros that are contained in documents or templates stored in your trusted locations. *High* disables macros contained in documents and templates if the macros are not signed with a digital certificate or if the certificate is not on your list of trusted sources. If you choose the *Low* setting, all documents or templates from other users will open with macros enabled. *Medium* is probably the most reasonable setting. This option may never be of concern to you as a transcriptionist, especially if you place all templates in the **Templates** folder (see page 236 for an explanation of the Templates folder).

• •

Notes

WORD 2003

File Locations

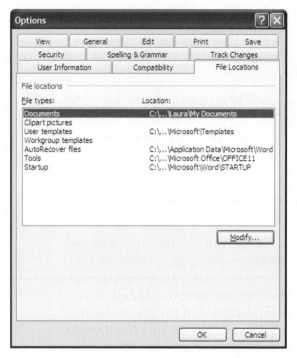

FIGURE 5-12 The File Locations dialog box determines where important program files are stored.

The **File Locations** dialog box specifies folder locations for specific types of files used by Word. Use this dialog box to change the default working folder (see page 33 for XP and 29 for Vista). Office 2003 installs with **(My) Documents** as the default working folder. Other than changing the *Documents* setting, no other changes in this dialog box are recommended (unless your employer specifies).

Follow these steps to change the default working folder (this change will affect all Office applications):

1. Open the **File Locations** dialog box.
2. Select *Documents*.
3. Click **Modify**.
4. Browse your computer and select a different folder.
5. Click **OK**.
6. Close the **File Locations** dialog box.

Now, each time you use the Office **Save As** or **Open** dialog box, your selected folder will automatically appear (instead of **My Documents**).

Refer to this dialog box to identify file paths for important Word program files. To see the complete path name, select a *File Type* from the list and click **Modify**. The path name will appear in the *Folder name* box. Use **Esc** to back out without saving changes.

Office Assistant

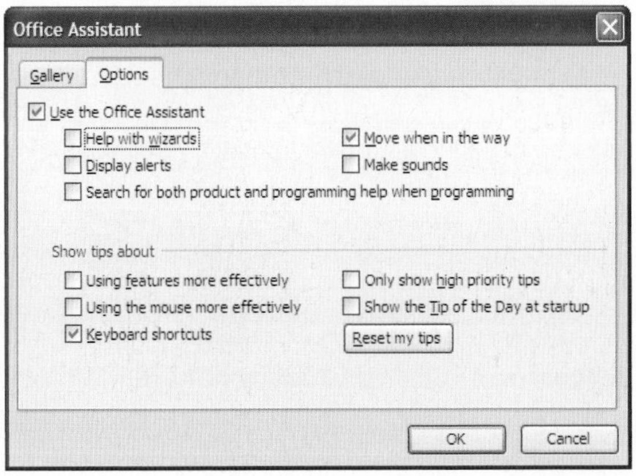

FIGURE 5-13 Change the way the Office Assistant provides help in the Office Assistant dialog box.

The Office Assistant is part of the Microsoft Office help system. The Office Assistant (a paperclip called Clippit) will show up to help you at certain cues. You can change *when* and *if* the character appears to help you.

Choose Show Office Assistant from the Help menu on the main Menu bar. Right-click on the character and choose Options. This opens the **Office Assistant** dialog box as shown in Figure 5-13. If you do not want the character to appear under any circumstances, clear the check box at *Use the Office Assistant*. Otherwise, choose when you would like the assistant to provide help or feedback.

To choose a different assistant, click on the Gallery tab. Your choices include a cat, dog, professor, robot, and a few others. You may need the Office install disc to use characters other than Clippit.

One other option is to set the Office Assistant to "animate." In this mode, the character will stay on the screen and perform silly maneuvers or play charades while you work. To animate a character, place the check mark at *Use the Office Assistant* (you can disable all the individual help features if you only want the character to entertain you). Click OK to close the dialog. Right-click on the character and choose Animate on the shortcut menu.

Notes

Customize

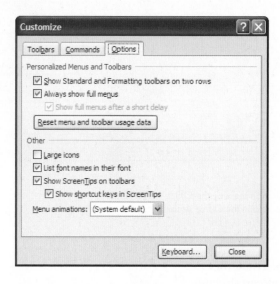

FIGURE 5-14 The Customize dialog box.

The **Customize** dialog box as a whole manages all customizations, including the appearance and behavior of menus and toolbars, custom key assignments, custom toolbars, and menu modifications. The **Options** dialog will be described here. **Toolbars** and **Commands** within the **Customize** dialog box will be described in Chapter 15. The **Customize** dialog box can be found on the Tools menu (Tools > Customize).

The **Options** dialog box is used to control menus and toolbars. *Personalized Menus and Toolbars* is a feature in Microsoft Office that changes the location of commands on menus and toolbars based on your actual use. When the feature is enabled, recently used menu items migrate to the top of each drop-down menu found on the main <u>Menu</u> bar. The menus initially open in an abbreviated form and after a few seconds open to display all available commands. Toolbar icons migrate to the left as you use them, while infrequently used icons drift to the right (out of sight). While the idea is to make common commands more easily accessible, it often creates confusion and makes infrequently used commands difficult to find.

To change this behavior, place a check mark at *Always show full menus*. With this option checked, the menus will drop-down from the <u>Menu</u> bar with all commands displayed. Place a check mark at *Show Standard and Formatting toolbars on two rows* so you can see all icons on both toolbars. Otherwise, these two toolbars share a single row, which abbreviates both toolbars and hides many of the icons. To return the menus and toolbars to their native configuration, click <u>Reset menu and toolbar usage data</u>.

Large icons will display larger buttons on the <u>Standard</u> and <u>Formatting</u> toolbar. The option to *List font names in their font* will display the fonts in their actual style in the Font drop-down box on the <u>Formatting</u> toolbar. This will make it easy to quickly identify the font you need.

Place a check mark at *Show ScreenTips on toolbars* and *Show shortcut keys in ScreenTips*. With these options checked, you can hover over an icon to display a description of the command and its shortcut key (if available).

AutoCorrect Options

The AutoCorrect dialog box (Tools > AutoCorrect) consists of several tabbed dialog boxes that control the productivity-enhancing features available in Word, including AutoText, AutoCorrect, and Word's automatic formatting features. More detailed information is given for AutoCorrect and AutoText in Chapters 9 and 10. AutoFormat and Smart Tags are not covered in this text.

AutoText

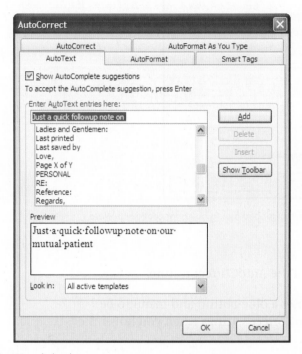

FIGURE 5-15 The AutoText dialog box.

See Chapter 10 for a complete description of this feature. To enable ToolTips for this feature, place a check mark at *Show AutoComplete suggestions*. This will allow you to insert AutoText entries using the **Enter** key.

(Continued)

Notes

AutoCorrect

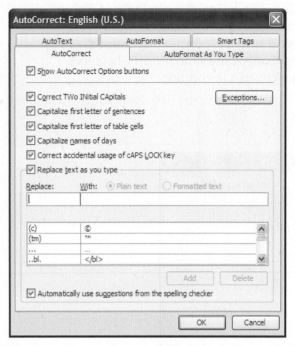

FIGURE 5-16 The AutoCorrect dialog box contains several tabbed dialog boxes for controlling Word's productivity features.

Use the **AutoCorrect** dialog box to control the AutoCorrect feature.

Show AutoCorrect Options buttons: This causes a blue button and menu to be displayed with options for changing AutoCorrect settings when you hover the mouse over text affected by AutoCorrect.

Correct TWo INitial CApitals: Automatically changes text to title case when capitalization errors are created by holding down the **Shift** key too long.

Capitalize first letter of sentences: Capitalizes the first character after a period. If the sentence ends in a digit, Word will not capitalize the next word.

Capitalize first letter of table cells: Automatically capitalizes the first word in a table cell.

Capitalize names of days: Automatically capitalizes names of the days of the week.

Correct accidental usage of the cAPS LOCK key: Turns the CAPS LOCK key off and corrects the word to title case if you press the **Shift** key while CAPS LOCK is on.

Replace text as you type: Automatically replaces text listed in the *Replace* column with text in the *With* column. AutoCorrect is invoked with the **Spacebar** or any punctuation key, so the replacement will always occur. Learn more in Chapter 9.

Automatically use suggestions from the spelling checker: Word will automatically replace a misspelled word with a word from the dictionary. Learn more about this feature on page 269.

Exceptions > *Automatically add words to list (all three tabs)*: Automatically adds words to the exception list if you use the **Backspace** key to immediately correct a word that was changed by the AutoCorrect feature. I recommend turning this off on all three **Exceptions** tabs. Learn more on page 272.

AutoFormat As You Type

This dialog controls features that change your formatting as you are typing based on specific cues. The settings under **AutoFormat As You Type** can create a few "sticky" spots for MTs. AutoFormat As You Type does just that—automatically makes formatting changes while you are typing. AutoFormat As You Type can be useful if you know how to manage the changes. A similar feature, called AutoFormat, makes formatting changes in one pass (after the document is typed) and must be invoked using Format > AutoFormat. AutoFormat is not particularly useful for transcription.

Until you become familiar with managing *Automatic numbered lists*, you may want to disable this option. Automatically numbered lists tend to create as many problems as they solve. A full explanation of this feature is given in Chapter 13.

Be sure you are familiar with all the options in the AutoFormat As You Type dialog box.

Any of these automatic formatting changes can be reversed right away using Undo (**CTRL+Z**).

Notes

WORD 2003

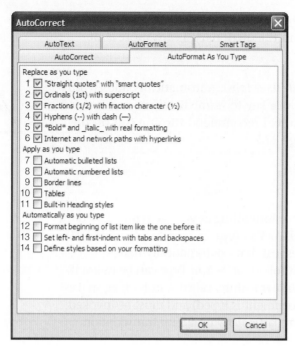

FIGURE 5-17 The AutoFormat As You Type dialog box controls automatic formatting features in Word.

The following table describes what happens when you use the AutoFormat As You Type feature. The numbers in Figure 5-15 refer to the option numbers in Table 5-1.

Table 5-1	Explanation of AutoFormat As You Type features	
Option	**When you type:**	**Word does this:**
1 Straight quotes with smart quotes	straight quotation marks (' and ")	changes the quotation marks to smart (curly) quotes (' and ").
2 Ordinals (1st) with superscript (1st)	an ordinal number, such as 1st, 2nd, 3rd, and 4th	changes the entry to 1st, 2nd, 3rd, and 4th.
3 Fractions 1/2 with fraction character ½	fractions 1/4, 1/2, or 3/4	changes the entry to ¼, ½, or ¾. Use superscript and subscript to create other fractions.
4 Hyphens (--) with dash (–)	text, a space, one hyphen (-), one or zero spaces, and more text, eg, 3-10	changes the spaces and hyphen to an en dash (–), eg, 3–10.
4 Hyphens (--) with dash (—)	two words separated by two hyphens (no spaces)	changes the hyphens to an em dash (—).
5 *Bold* and _italic_ with real formatting	text with an asterisk at the beginning and end such as *HISTORY*	formats text as bold.

Table 5-1   Explanation of AutoFormat As You Type features (*Continued*)

Option	When you type:	Word does this:
5 *Bold* and _italic_ with real formatting	text with underscore at the beginning and end such as _in situ_	formats the text with italic formatting
6 Internet and network paths with hyperlinks	an Internet, network, or e-mail address, such as http://www.MTWerks.com	formats the address as a hyperlink.
7 Automatic bulleted lists	an asterisk, one or two hyphens, a greater-than sign (>), or an arrow created by a greater-than sign preceded by a hyphen or equal sign (-> or =>)	formats a bulleted list.
7 Automatic bulleted lists	a symbol inserted with the Symbol command, followed by two or more spaces or an inline picture (must be within 1.5 times the height of the line), then text	formats a bulleted list where the symbol or picture is the bullet.
8 Automatic numbered lists	a number followed by a period, hyphen, closing parenthesis, or greater than sign (>), followed by a space or tab and then text	formats a numbered list.
9 Border lines	three or more hyphens, underscores, equal signs, asterisks, tildes (~), or number signs (#) above a paragraph	places a border above the paragraph: a thin line for hyphens, a single, thick line for underscores, a double line for equal signs, a dotted line for asterisks, a single wavy line for tildes, or a decorative line for number signs.
10 Tables	a plus sign, a series of hyphens, another plus sign, and so on, and then press ENTER, such as +—+———+————+	inserts a table, where the plus signs become the column borders, and the number of hyphens determines the column width.
11 Built-in Heading styles	text on a single line	applies one of Word's built-in heading styles
12 Format beginning of list item like the one before it	a list item that starts with a bullet, asterisk, or similar character, followed by bold, italic, or underlined text, followed by a delimiter (period, colon, hyphen, em dash, question mark, exclamation point, or similar character), then a space or tab, and then plain text. For example: • **LESI**: L4-L5, L5-S1 • **CESI**: C4-C5, C5-C6	repeats the same formatting to the lead-in text of the next list item. Word does not format the delimiter.
13 Set left- and first-indent with tabs and backspaces	the tab at the beginning of a paragraph, or press backspace at the beginning of a paragraph that is indented.	converts a tab to an indent command when the Tab is typed at the beginning of a paragraph and at the beginning of the second line of the paragraph. Removes the indent command from a paragraph when Backspace is pressed at the beginning of the paragraph.
14 Define styles based on your formatting	a document and apply custom formatting to paragraphs.	creates new style definitions automatically based on manual formatting applied to paragraphs.

WORD 2003

Automatic numbering and bulleting do not always convert well when the document is opened in other text applications. Also, if your documents will be imported into an electronic record system that uses plain text (`txt` files) or rich text format (`rtf` files), you should disable most of the features in the **Auto-Format As You Type** dialog box. The characters produced by the auto-formatting features (eg, superscripts, subscripts, single-space fractions) are not compatible with all applications and the final report may display boxes or nonsense characters in place of "smart quotes," ordinals, and single-space fractions. Check with your client or employer about compatibility issues.

If you have tried to draw a line for the doctor's signature using the **Underscore** key, you may have discovered the line continues across the entire page! This is because Word is automatically formatting a border. You can immediately reverse the action by pressing **CTRL+Z**, or you can turn this feature off by removing the check mark at *Borders*.

• •

Notes

Word 2007 Options

The vast majority of options in Word 2007 are accessed through the **Word Options** dialog box. To access this dialog box, click the `Office` button and choose `Word Options`. This dialog box brings together nine different dialog boxes covering a variety of categories. To access a dialog box, click the name listed in the left-hand column of the **Word Options** dialog. The **Advanced** dialog box is further divided into ten sections or categories of options. Each individual dialog box will be described below.

The diagrams in this chapter show my suggestions based on my own experience. You may choose to use these suggestions as a starting point for setting your own preferences. These settings are most appropriate for transcriptionists and other healthcare documentation specialists that work with Word as a stand-alone application. Since many transcription companies and hospitals use document management software that incorporates Word, some of the options discussed here may need to be adapted to specific work environments. *Follow your employer's specifications where applicable.* For simplicity, options that are highly unlikely to be relevant will not be mentioned at all.

It would be very easy to glance at this chapter and become completely overwhelmed with so many details, but memorizing minute details is not the objective. *It is important that you are able to identify and quickly locate key dialog boxes, namely* **Options** (in Word 2003), **Word Options** (in Word 2007), **AutoCorrect,** *and* **Customize.** Read through this chapter to become familiar with the settings and options available so you are familiar with your choices and can easily reference this information when you need to make a specific change. Note how the options within a single dialog box are associated with each other. It's not necessary that you memorize every option; but you will want to pay very close attention to the options that are specifically marked, as these are the options that are most likely to impact your work within healthcare documentation.

• •

Notes

Popular

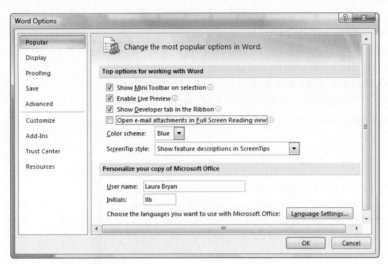

FIGURE 5-18 Popular Options dialog box.

Show Mini Toolbar on selection: The Mini Toolbar floats in the middle of the document just above the selected text. Place a check mark here if you would like to use the toolbar. It's mostly useful but may at times get in the way.

Enable Live Preview: Shows potential changes to the document as you move the mouse over gallery items. The changes are not permanent until you actually click the option.

Show Developer tab in the Ribbon: Places the **Developer** tab on the ribbon with commands for recording macros and working with XML and forms.

Open e-mail attachments in Full Screen Reading view: Documents received as email attachments (in Outlook or Windows Mail) are automatically displayed in Full Screen Reading view. Remove the check mark to display these documents in Print Layout. Full Screen view is easy to read, but the formatting and page breaks do not display correctly.

Color scheme: Choose a color scheme to apply to Word (blue, silver, or black).

ScreenTip style: This option allows you to choose whether Word displays helpful information when you hover the mouse pointer over a command. *Don't show ScreenTips* disables all screen tips. *Don't show feature descriptions* displays a simple screen tip with only the command name. *Show feature descriptions in ScreenTips* gives the command name as well as an enhanced description of the command.

User name: Type your name as you want it to appear in Document Properties (learn more about document properties in Chapter 11). Be sure to complete this information.

Initials: These initials identify you as the author of comments, footnotes, and tracked changes. Be sure to complete this information.

Choose the languages you want to use with Microsoft Office: Select the primary language to be used. Word uses this information for spell checking, grammar checking, and some AutoCorrect features.

Display

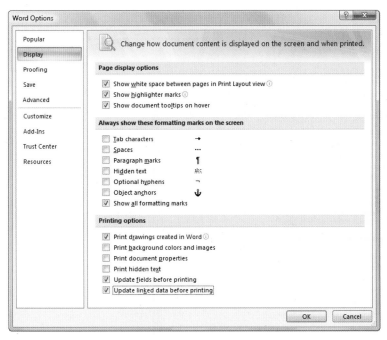

FIGURE 5-19 Display Options dialog box.

This dialog determines how your document is displayed and which elements are included in the document's view. It also lists several printing options.

Show white space between pages in Print Layout view: Displays the white space between the top of the text and the top of the page. You can also alternate this setting by double-clicking the narrow gray area between pages (see page 127).

Show highlighter marks: Displays or hides highlighted text (like a Hi-Liter marker) on the screen *and* when printed.

Show document ToolTips on hover: Displays a popup box when you hover over a comment, a tracked change, a footnote, or an endnote.

Always show these formatting marks on the screen: Displays selected formatting marks. The Show/Hide ¶ button on the ribbon and/or the shortcut key **CTRL+Shift+8** will toggle between *all* marks and only those selected here in this dialog box. If you choose *All*, Show/Hide will toggle between *all marks* and *no marks* (see also page 197.)

Print drawings created in Word: Check if your documents include graphics (eg, a logo in the letterhead).

Print background colors and images: Displays background images.

Print document properties: Prints document properties at the end of document printing.

Print hidden text: Prints text formatted as hidden with a dotted underline.

Update fields before printing: Updates fields before printing. Learn more about fields in Chapter 11.

Update linked data before printing: Updates links in other documents before printing.

Proofing

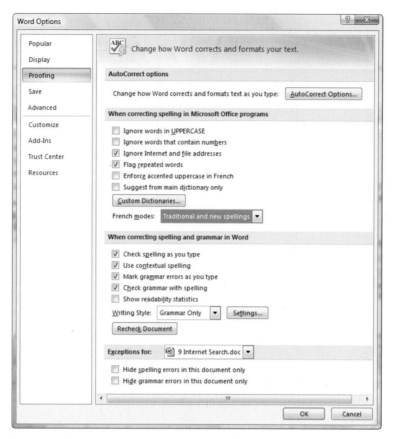

FIGURE 5-20 Proofing Options dialog box for controlling spelling and grammar.

See AutoCorrect Options on page 178.

The **Proofing** dialog controls how Word performs a spelling and grammar check.

Ignore words in UPPERCASE: Clear this box so headings, drug allergies, and other text typed in all caps will be spell checked. The default setting is to ignore words in uppercase, so it is important to change this setting.

Ignore words that contain numbers: Clear this box so words with numbers will be spell checked.

Ignore Internet and file addresses: Check to ignore Internet addresses, file paths, or e-mail addresses during a spell check.

Flag repeated words: Check to flag words that are typed twice in a row.

Suggest from main dictionary only: If checked, Word will not refer to Custom dictionaries when offering spelling suggestions.

Custom Dictionaries: Click this button to select, edit, and create Custom dictionaries. Learn more in Chapter 14.

Check spelling as you type: Marks misspelled or repeated words with a red sawtooth line. Removing this check mark does not disable spell check; words will be identified as misspelled in the **Spelling and Grammar** dialog box during a spell-check routine.

Use contextual spelling: Check to have Word mark homonyms that are potentially spelled wrong based on context (eg, their, there, and they're). These words are marked with a blue dotted line.

Mark grammar errors as you type: Check to mark possible grammatical errors with a green sawtooth line (see also *Check spelling as you type* above).

Check grammar with spelling: With this box checked, grammatical errors will be presented along with spelling errors in the **Spelling and Grammar** dialog box during a spell-check routine.

Show readability statistics: Shows readability statistics after each grammar check.

Writing Style: Click **Settings** to select a writing style or customize the grammar checker. The option to check *Grammar only* (as opposed to grammar and style) is more useful in the context of medical documentation. Adjusting settings in the **Grammar settings** dialog is more helpful than disabling grammar checking altogether. Learn more on page 358.

Check/Recheck Document: Click to begin a spell check or to repeat a spell check after changing spell-check options or if spell checking a document that was previously checked on another PC. Quality Assurance editors should use this command routinely to repeat the spell check routine on documents previously checked by the MT. Learn more on page 361.

Hide spelling errors in this document only: Misspelled words will not be marked with a red sawtooth line but will still appear in the **Spelling and Grammar** dialog box when you run a spell check.

Hide grammar errors in this document only: When marked, grammatical errors will not be marked with a green sawtooth line but will appear in the **Spelling and Grammar** dialog box when you perform a spell check.

You will want to keep track of your changes so you can evaluate the consequences of your selections and decide whether to keep the change or go back to a previous setting. The best way to document your settings before making changes is to use the Print Screen feature in Windows. Display the dialog box to be changed and click **Print Screen** (to capture the entire display) or **ALT+Print Screen** (to capture the active window). This will take a "snapshot" of your display and place that image on the Windows Clipboard. Paste the image (**CTRL+V**) into a Word document and print. Jot down the date along with any notes about the changes you made and place your notes in a binder.

WORD 2007

Save

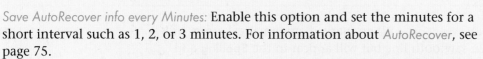

FIGURE 5-21 Save Options dialog box allows you to choose how documents are saved.

This **Save** dialog determines the default format for documents when they are saved as well as locations for saving files and recovered files.

Save files in this format: Select the file extension you use most often. Unless instructed otherwise by your employer, use Word Document (*.docx). If you routinely send documents to others who use previous versions of Word, you may prefer to save all your documents in the previous document format that is compatible with all versions of Word. In this case, choose *Word 97-2003 Document (*.doc)*. Learn more about document formats on page 70.

Save AutoRecover info every Minutes: Enable this option and set the minutes for a short interval such as 1, 2, or 3 minutes. For information about *AutoRecover*, see page 75.

AutoRecover file location: Specifies where Word stores recovered files until the user decides to use or discard them. Most likely, there is no need to change this file location.

Default file location: The default file location specifies the default working folder. Office installs with **(My) Documents** as the default working folder (see page 33 for XP and page 49 for Vista). Follow these steps to change the default working folder for all Office applications:

1. Next to *Default file locations*, click **Browse**.
2. Browse your computer and select a different folder.
3. Click **OK**.

Now, each time you open the Office **Save As** or **Open** dialog box, your selected folder will automatically appear (instead of **Documents**).

Customize

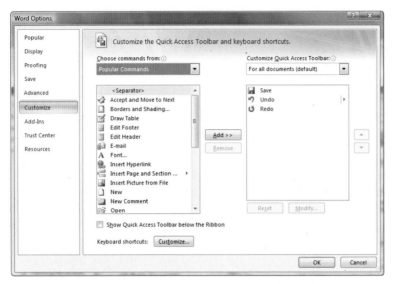

FIGURE 5-22 The Customize dialog box allows you to customize the Quick Access toolbar.

Use the **Customize** dialog box to tweak the <u>Quick Access</u> toolbar and to access the **Customize Keyboard** dialog box.

A full explanation of the **Customize** dialog box can be found in Chapter 15. If you prefer to display the <u>Quick Access</u> toolbar below the ribbon, place a check mark at *Show Quick Access Toolbar below the Ribbon*.

Add-Ins

Add-ins are programs that may be installed on your computer that run in tandem with Word. Add-ins are not covered in this text.

• •

Notes

Trust Center

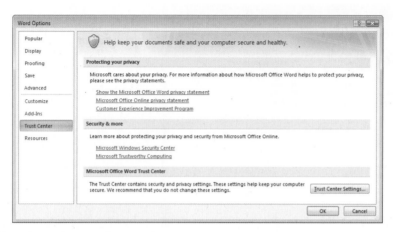

FIGURE 5-23 The Trust Center information box.

The **Trust Center** provides information about Windows security and Word's macro security features.

This dialog provides information about Microsoft's security policies as well as links to Windows' security settings. To increase or decrease security related to macros, click `Trust Center Settings`. Increasing your macro security settings is probably not necessary in the context of medical documentation. It would be important if you routinely receive documents that contain macros from unknown users. By default, documents and templates with the extension .dotx will have macros disabled. Files with the extension docm and dotm will have macros enabled automatically if they are stored in the **Templates** folder (learn more about the **Templates** folder on page 236). Other documents and templates with the docm and dotm extension that are stored outside the **Templates** folder will prompt the user to enable or disable macros. Learn more in Chapters 8 and 12.

● ●

Notes

Resources

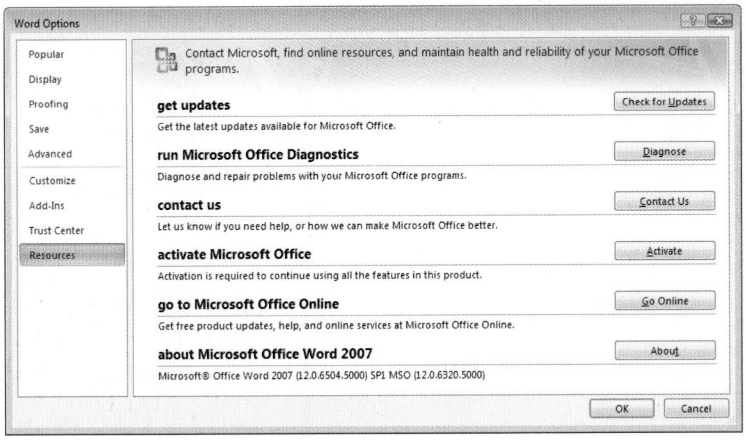

FIGURE 5-24 Resources area for accessing help and information.

Resources provides information for getting help and learning about your copy of Word/Office.

This dialog provides access to software updates and diagnostic tools. This dialog generally replaces the Help menu in previous versions. Click About to learn about your copy of Word (version number, build, and service packs installed) as well as which Office suite is installed on your PC.

Notes

Advanced Options

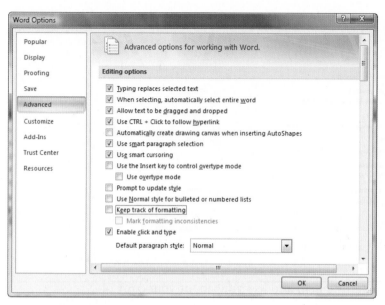

FIGURE 5-25 Advanced Editing Options dialog box.

The **Advanced Options** dialog box has many smaller sections with a mind-boggling selection of options. The most relevant options for medical documentation will be mentioned here.

Editing Options

Editing Options determines how Word behaves when editing and copy/pasting text.

Typing replaces selected text: Deletes selected text as soon as you begin typing. If you clear this box, Word inserts text in front of selected text but does not delete it.

When selecting, automatically select entire word: Allows you to place the cursor at any point in the word to format the entire word. For example, you can italicize a single word without selecting every character in that word.

Allow text to be dragged and dropped: This allows you to move or copy selected text using the mouse.

Use CTRL+Click to follow hyperlink: Allows you to select a hyperlink without actually following the link.

Use smart paragraph selection: Automatically includes the paragraph mark when you select an entire paragraph.

Use smart cursoring: With this option checked, your insertion point moves with you as you scroll up or down or when you press an arrow key. The insertion point responds at the page you are currently viewing, not where the insertion point was before you began scrolling.

Use the Insert key to control overtype mode: Check this box to be able to toggle Overtype mode on and off using the **Insert** key.

Use overtype mode: Overtype mode replaces existing text as you type, one character at a time. This may be useful for editing or filling out forms with lines created with underscore characters. You can also toggle on/off by double-clicking Insert on the Status Bar (to display the Insert icon, right-click the Status Bar and choose Overtype).

Prompt to update style: When selected, Word will ask if you want to update a style when manual formatting has been applied and then the style re-applied.

Use Normal style for bulleted or numbered lists: Applies the Normal style to lists instead of the Paragraph list style.

Keep track of formatting: When selected, Word will track formatting styles as you type.

Enable click and type: Allows you to double-click anywhere in the document and begin typing. The *Default paragraph style* indicates which style to apply to paragraphs inserted using Click and type.

• •

Notes

WORD 2007

Cut, Copy, Paste

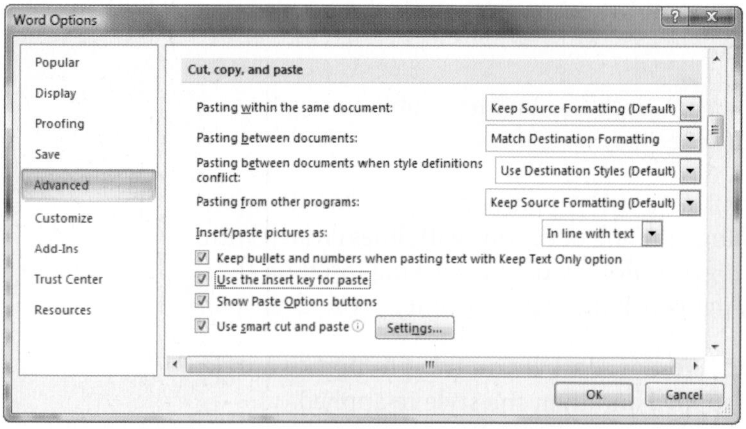

FIGURE 5-26 Cut, Copy, and Paste options found on the Advanced dialog box.

This dialog determines how Word inserts text when using cut and paste.

Paste options behavior: Set each of the options that you want to automatically apply to cut and paste routines. To use a different option when you actually paste an item, click the Paste Options button (that appears in the document at the time you paste an object) to modify the paste behavior for that instance only.

Insert/paste pictures as: Determines the default text wrapping (*inline with text, square, behind, in front,* etc) when a picture is inserted. This is probably not applicable to medical transcription.

Keep bullets and numbers when pasting text with Keep Text Only option: When you paste a collection of text and images, you can choose to paste the text only (eg, when pasting from a web page). This option retains bullet points when pasting text only.

Use the Insert key for paste: With this box checked, the **Insert** key (next to the **Home** key) carries the Paste command (**CTRL+V**).

Show Paste Options buttons: When copying and pasting text, Word will display a button that opens a menu with options for formatting the text that was just pasted.

Use smart cut and paste: Determines exactly how text is inserted when cut and pasted is used. Click **Settings** to adjust.

Settings: If you choose *Adjust sentence and word spacing automatically and Adjust paragraph spacing on paste*, Word will eliminate extra spaces between sentences and extra paragraph marks between paragraphs when you use cut and paste or drag-and-drop editing. *These settings assume that you use one space between sentences.* These settings may affect the behavior of text expansion programs, so you may need to tweak these settings if you use other software programs that insert text as you transcribe.

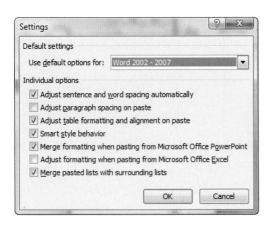

FIGURE 5-27 Use the Settings dialog box to determine how Word adjusts text when using copy and paste.

• •

Notes

WORD 2007

Show Document Content

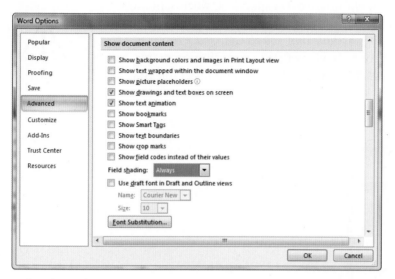

FIGURE 5-28 The Advanced Document Content area determines what you see displayed on the screen.

Document Content determines what elements of your document are displayed on the screen.

Most of these options are not applicable to medical documents. Pertinent options are listed here. All options determine what is *displayed*; none of these affect the way the document prints.

Show bookmarks: Designates bookmarked text with square brackets.

Show Smart Tags: Marks certain types of text (addresses, e-mail addresses, etc) with a purple line to easily identify and add information to other Office programs. Unless you work extensively with Outlook, Excel, or other Office software products, you probably won't use Smart tags.

Show field codes instead of their values: Displays field codes instead of field results. Toggle this selection using **ALT+F9** (see Chapter 11).

Field shading: Marks fields with shaded gray boxes *Always*, *Never* or only *When Selected*. Field shading does not print. Learn more about fields in Chapter 11.

Notes

Display

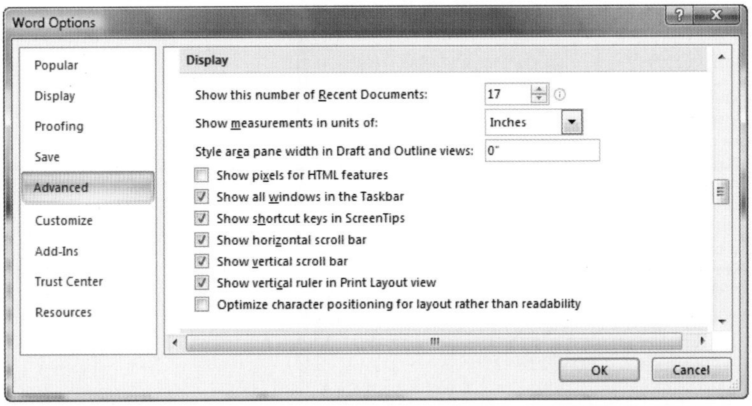

FIGURE 5-29 The Advanced Display options determine which elements of the Word interface are displayed.

The **Display** dialog box determines which Word elements are displayed.

Show this number of Recent Documents: Determines the number of documents displayed on the right side of the Program menu. Click the pushpin next to a document to keep that document on the Recent Documents list.

Show measurements in units of: Determines which measurement system is displayed on rulers and in some dialog boxes.

Style area pane width in Draft and Outline views: Sets the width of the sidebar in Draft or Outline view, which displays the style name for each paragraph.

Show all windows in the Taskbar: When selected, each open document will have its own button on the Windows Taskbar. Otherwise, Word will display only one icon on the Taskbar regardless of the number of open documents; to switch between documents, go to **View** > Window > **Switch Windows**.

Show shortcut keys in ScreenTips: With this option checked, you can hover over an icon to display a description of the command and its shortcut key (if available). This can be very helpful when learning shortcut keys.

Show horizontal scroll bar: Displays a scroll bar across the bottom of the screen. This is helpful if you like to use the mouse to navigate documents.

Show vertical scroll bar: Displays a scroll bar on the right side of the screen. This is helpful if you like to use the mouse to navigate documents.

Show vertical ruler in Print Layout view: Displays a ruler down the left side of the page in Print Layout view.

Optimize character positioning for layout rather than readability: Select this option to display character positioning accurately, as it will appear in the printed document with respect to blocks of text. Spacing between characters may be distorted when this option is turned on. For best readability on the screen, turn this option off.

General

FIGURE 5-30 General Options under the Advanced dialog box.

Options that do not fit any other category fall under **General**.

Provide feedback with sound: Associates sounds with certain events such as errors. Sounds may be disturbing or loud when wearing a transcription headset.

Provide feedback with animation: When turned on, Word will use special pointers to indicate certain automated procedures are in progress (eg, background saves).

Mailing address: Complete this box with your mailing address (or that of your client's) if you print envelopes using Word's envelope feature.

File Locations

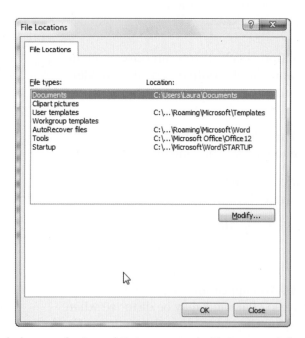

FIGURE 5-31 Click the button under General Options to open the File Locations dialog box.

Click **File Locations** to open the **File Locations** dialog. **File Locations** sets the default file locations for documents, templates, recovered files, etc. These defaults tell Word where to look for the specified information. Other than changing the *Documents* setting, no other changes are recommended (unless your employer specifies). To change *Documents* (the default working folder), see page 164 (**Save** dialog box, *Default file location*).

Refer to this dialog box to identify file paths for important Word program files. To see the complete path name, select a *File Type* from the list and click **Modify**. The path name will appear in the *Folder name* box. Use **Esc** to back out without making changes.

Compatibility

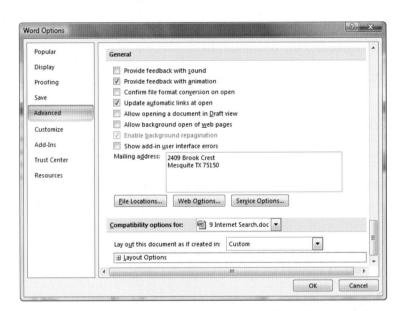

FIGURE 5-32 Compatibility options are found at the bottom of the Advanced Options dialog.

These options determine how documents created in other brands of word processing software are handled by Word 2007.

When working with documents created in other word processors or other versions of Word, you can make adjustments to control the way the documents appear. This dialog allows you to change the way Word interprets documents that have been created in other word processing programs. These settings do not actually change formatting codes (so the document will still appear correctly if opened in the other word processing program), but will allow Word to display the document in a way that more closely resembles the appearance of the original document.

Print

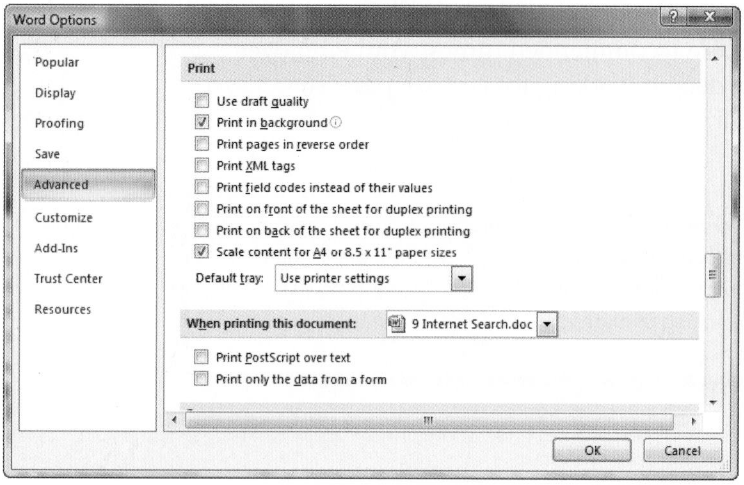

FIGURE 5-33 Print Options dialog box.

Print options determine how the printer handles the document to be printed.

Use draft quality: Prints faster by omitting graphics (drawing objects and pictures).

Print in background: Allows you to work while printing.

Print pages in reverse order: Outputs document starting with the last page.

Print on front of sheet for duplex printing/back of sheet: Determines how pages print when printing on both sides of the page when the printer does not have duplex capability.

Default tray: Selects paper tray for current document only. It will override Windows' settings in the printer's **Properties** dialog box on the Control Panel.

Print only the data from a form: Prints only the data entered in form fields. Allows you to print on preprinted forms.

• •

Notes

Save

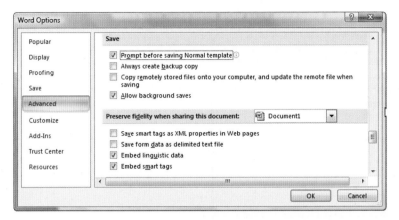

FIGURE 5-34 Additional Save options are found under the Advanced dialog box.

This dialog determines how Word saves elements within the document as well as backup copies and the Normal template.

Prompt before saving Normal template: Prompts you to save changes to the Normal.dotm. If you clear this box, changes will automatically be saved (learn more in Chapter 8).

Always create backup copy: When checked, Word creates a backup copy with the extension `wbk` each time you use the Save command. This setting is *recommended only when working on very long or complicated documents that you open and edit many times*. This is not helpful if you create many short documents each day, as most medical transcriptionists do.

Copy remotely stored files onto your computer and update the remote file when saving: Moves a temporary copy to the local hard drive when working on files stored on a remote computer. This is helpful if you lose a connection while working on a document. *Check with your employer before checking this option if you work on documents stored on a server.*

Allow background saves: Select if you want to continue working in Word while saving another document in the background. Again, this would be of benefit for documents with graphics or complex tables, but probably not applicable to transcription files.

Notes

AutoCorrect Options

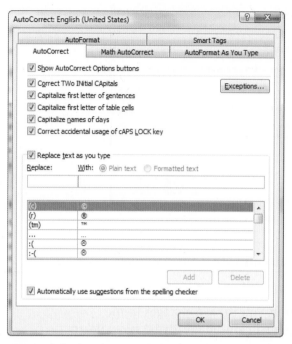

FIGURE 5-35 The AutoCorrect dialog box contains tabs for controlling the productivity features in Word.

The **AutoCorrect** `Office` `Word Options` `Proofing` `AutoCorrect Options` dialog consists of several tabbed dialog boxes that control the productivity features available in Word. Options for AutoCorrect will be covered here, and more detailed information is given on how to use AutoCorrect in Chapter 9. The AutoFormat As You Type feature is described below, but Math AutoCorrect, AutoFormat, and Smart Tags are not covered in this text.

The following options are available on the **AutoCorrect** dialog box under the `AutoCorrect` tab. You will find most of these features to be very helpful.

Show AutoCorrect Options buttons: When you hover the mouse over text affected by AutoCorrect, this setting displays a blue button and menu with options for changing AutoCorrect settings.

Correct TWo INitial CApitals: Automatically changes text to title case when capitalization errors are created by holding down the **Shift** key too long.

Capitalize first letter of sentences: Capitalizes the first character after a period. If the sentence ends in a digit, Word will not capitalize the next word.

Capitalize first letter of table cells: Automatically capitalizes the first word in a table cell.

Capitalize names of days: Automatically capitalizes names of the days of the week.

Correct accidental usage of the cAPS LOCK key: Turns the CAPS LOCK key off and corrects the word to title case if you press the **Shift** key while CAPS LOCK is on.

Replace text as you type: Automatically replaces text listed in the *Replace* column with text in the *With* column. AutoCorrect is invoked with the **Spacebar** or any punctuation key, so the replacement will always occur. Learn more in Chapter 9.

Automatically use suggestions from the spelling checker: Word will automatically replace a misspelled word with a word from the dictionary. Learn more about this feature on page 269.

Exceptions: *Automatically add words to list* (*all three tabs*): Automatically adds words to the exception list if you use the **Backspace** key to immediately correct a word that was changed by the AutoCorrect feature. I recommend turning this off on all three **Exceptions** tabs. Learn more on page 272.

AutoFormat As You Type

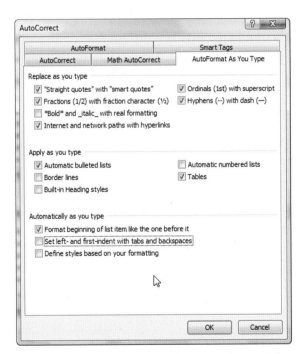

FIGURE 5-36 AutoFormat As You Type dialog box controls automatic formatting features in Word.

Refer to pages 155-158 under Word 2003 for details of the AutoFormat As You Type feature.

Critical Thinking Questions

1. Describe the recently-used file list. How can you change the number of documents displayed on this list?

_____

_____

2. Name two possible functions of the Insert key.

_____

_____

3. If your reports require words or phrases to be typed in uppercase, how can you make sure Word spell checks these words?

_____

_____

4. Explain how you can turn off Automatic numbered lists.

_____

_____

5. Which three fractions will automatically be formatted as single-space fractions?

_____

_____

6. Explain how each of the following automatic features will affect your document if you have checked the boxes in the AutoFormat As You Type dialog box.

Built-in Heading styles

_____

_____

Border lines

_____

_____

Automatic numbered lists

_____

_____

7. List the dialog box related to the following options:

Display field codes and shading

_____

_____

Select which formatting marks are to be displayed

_____

_____

Set user initials and return address for envelopes

_____

_____

Set left- and first-indent with tabs and backspaces

_____

_____

AutoRecover settings

_____

_____

Prompt to save normal template

_____

_____

Change grammar settings

_____

_____

Check and recheck spelling

_____

_____

8. Where would you go to:

Disable the Startup Task Pane (in Word 2003)

_____

_____

Disable Smart Tags

_____

_____

Settings for Automatic Capitalization and TWo INitial CAps

_____

_____

Turn off the AutoCorrect feature that automatically adds exceptions to the
AutoCorrect list

_____

_____

9. Step through the following:

   a.   Set the Recently used file list to 9.

   b.   Close the dialog box.

   c.   Open 3 different Word documents. Use the File menu and the Recently used file list to switch between these three files.

   d.   Close the files and use the keyboard and the Recently used file list to open one of the files.

10. Make sure AutoRecover is enabled and change the interval to every 3 minutes.

11. Remove the check mark at Ignore words in UPPERCASE.

12. Which option would be helpful for learning shortcut keys?

   _____

   _____

13 (Office 2007 only) Explain how and why you would change the default file format used to save new documents created in Word 2007.

   _____

   _____

14. (Word 2003 only) Describe Personalized Menus. Explain which option you prefer and why.

   _____

   _____

15. Describe the AutoFormat As You Type feature. Explain why you may be required to disable many of the autoformat features.

   _____

   _____

CHAPTER 6

Shortcut Keys in Word

OBJECTIVES

▸ Use shortcut keys to move throughout a document, select text, apply formatting, and edit text.

▸ Use shortcut keys to save, print, open, close, and start new documents.

▸ Use resources for referencing and printing shortcut keys.

This chapter includes a reference list of the most useful shortcut keys in MS Word, categorized several different ways. This list includes the shortcut keys that are assigned when Word is first installed. You can always reassign shortcut keys if you do not like the native assignments. See page 394 (Word 2003) or page 403 (Word 2007) for instructions on assigning and reassigning shortcut keys in Word. Review keyboarding concepts in Chapter 3.

Print a List of Shortcut Keys

You may find it very helpful to keep a list of shortcut keys. You can create a document that lists all of Word's built-in shortcuts and then print a hard copy for reference. Follow these steps:

1. Press **ALT+F8**.
2. In the *Macros in* box, select *Word commands*.
3. In the *Macro name* box, select *ListCommands*.
4. Click Run.
5. In the **List Commands** dialog box, click *Current menu and keyboard settings*, or choose *All Commands* for a list of all possible Word commands.

This procedure creates a document with *all of Word's commands* listed in a table, along with any assigned shortcut keys. You can save this document as you would any other document and then print a copy. This list is helpful for identifying the hundreds of commands available in Word.

It is possible that you may work with Word combined with other transcription or document management software. In some cases, shortcut keys may be overwritten or altered. Many of the most common commands in Word have multiple shortcut key assignments, so it is possible that if the primary or most popular key assignment has been changed, there will be an alternate key. Use the list described above to reference alternate keys when necessary.

Print a List of Custom Macro Keys

If you have made changes to shortcut key assignments, the changes will be included in the above list of shortcut keys, but shortcut keys that you have assigned to macros will not (learn more about macros in Chapter 12). To print a list of key assignments for macros, use the **Print** dialog box. Open a document (using the desired template if applicable) and press **CTRL+P**. In the bottom left corner, open the *Print what* box and select *Key assignments*.

Here is a tip for memorizing the shortcut keys: Choose three or four shortcuts that you would like to memorize. Write them on a sticky note and place it on your computer monitor. Every few days, as you memorize these keystrokes, replace your sticky note with another list of three or four keystrokes. Soon you will have memorized enough keys to nearly banish the mouse!

Helpful Shortcut Keys

Remember, the "key" to using shortcuts is to have your cursor in the right place when you give the command. To format a single word, simply place the insertion point anywhere within the word; it is not necessary to select the entire word. (Be sure to choose *Automatically select entire word* as described on page 139 for Word 2003 and 168 for Word 2007.) You can format paragraphs by simply placing the cursor anywhere in the paragraph. For other commands, select the text that you want to affect before pressing the shortcut keys. (The list on the following pages is not the same list that will print with either of the above instructions.) Those marked with a ✓ may be especially useful to a transcriptionist.

Function Keys

	F1	Get online Help or the Office Assistant
	F2	Move text or graphics
✓	F3	Insert an AutoText entry
✓	F4	Repeat the last action

	F5	Choose the Go To command
	F6	Go to next pane or frame
	F7	Start Spelling and Grammar check
✓	F8	Extend a selection
	F9	Update selected fields
	F10	Activate the Menu bar or the ribbon
✓	F11	Go to the next field
✓	F12	Choose the Save As command

Shift+Function Key

✓	Shift+F1	Start context-sensitive Help or reveal formatting
✓	Shift+F2	Copy text
✓	Shift+F3	Change the case of letters
	Shift+F4	Repeat a Find or Go To action
✓	Shift+F5	Move to a previous revision (cycles through the last three locations)
✓	Shift+F6	Go to the previous pane or frame
	Shift+F7	Look up the current word in the Thesaurus
	Shift+F8	Shrink a selection
	Shift+F9	Switch between a field code and its result
	Shift+F10	Display a shortcut menu
	Shift+F11	Go to the previous field
	Shift+F12	Save command

CTRL+Function Key

✓	CTRL+F2	Print Preview
	CTRL+F3	Cut to the Spike
✓	CTRL+F4	Close the window
	CTRL+F5	Restore the document window size
	CTRL+F6	Go to the next window
	CTRL+F7	Move the current window (Control menu, Word 2003 only)
	CTRL+F8	Size the current window (Control menu, Word 2003 only)
✓	CTRL+F9	Insert an empty field
	CTRL+F10	Maximize or Restore the document window
	CTRL+F11	Lock a field
	CTRL+F12	Open a document (Open dialog box)

CTRL+Shift+Function Key

CTRL+Shift+F3	Insert the contents of the Spike
CTRL+Shift+F5	Edit a bookmark
CTRL+Shift+F6	Go to the previous window
CTRL+Shift+F7	Update linked information in a Word source document
CTRL+Shift+F8	Extend a selection or block (then press an arrow key)
CTRL+Shift+F9	Unlink a field
CTRL+Shift+F11	Unlock a field
CTRL+Shift+F12	Print the current document

ALT+Function Key

	ALT+F1	Go to the next field
✓	ALT+F3	Create an AutoText entry
✓	ALT+F4	Close the current document or close Word if only one document is open
	ALT+F5	Restore the program window size
	ALT+F6	Move between document and an open dialog box (eg, Find)
✓	ALT+F7	Find the next misspelling or grammatical error
✓	ALT+F8	Run a macro
✓	ALT+F9	Switch between all field codes and their results
	ALT+F10	Maximize the program window
	ALT+F11	Display Microsoft Visual Basic code

ALT+Shift+Function Key

	ALT+Shift+F1	Go to the previous field
	ALT+Shift+F2	Save document
	ALT+Shift+F9	Run GoToButton or MacroButton from the field that displays the field results
✓	ALT+Shift+F10	Display a menu or message for a smart tag or Paste Options button

Change or Resize the Font

CTRL+Shift+F	Change the font
CTRL+Shift+P	Change the font size
CTRL+Shift+>	Increase the font size

	CTRL+Shift+<	Decrease the font size
	CTRL+]	Increase the font size by 1 point
	CTRL+[	Decrease the font size by 1 point

Apply Character Formats

✓	CTRL+D	Open Font dialog box
✓	Shift+F3	Change the case of letters (toggle key)
✓	CTRL+Shift+A	Format letters as all capitals
✓	CTRL+B	Apply bold formatting
✓	CTRL+U	Apply an underline
	CTRL+Shift+W	Underline words but not spaces
	CTRL+Shift+D	Double-underline text
	CTRL+Shift+H	Apply hidden text formatting
✓	CTRL+I	Apply italic formatting
	CTRL+Shift+K	Format letters as small capitals
✓	CTRL+Equal Sign	Apply subscript formatting
✓	CTRL+Shift+Plus Sign	Apply superscript formatting
✓	CTRL+Spacebar	Remove manual character formatting
	CTRL+Shift+Q	Change the selection to the Symbol font

View and Copy Text Formats

✓	CTRL+Shift+8	Display Formatting characters
✓	Shift+F1	Reveal formatting or get context-sensitive help
✓	CTRL+Shift+C	Copy formats
✓	CTRL+Shift+V	Paste formats

Set Line Spacing

	CTRL+1*	Single-space lines
	CTRL+2*	Double-space lines
	CTRL+5*	Set 1.5-line spacing
	CTRL+0 (zero)*	Add or remove one line space preceding a paragraph

*Use the number keys across the top of the keyboard, not the number pad.

Align Paragraphs

✓	CTRL+E	Center a paragraph
✓	CTRL+J	Justify a paragraph

✓	CTRL+L	Left-align a paragraph
✓	CTRL+R	Right-align a paragraph
✓	CTRL+M	Indent a paragraph from the left
✓	CTRL+Shift+M	Remove a paragraph indent from the left
✓	CTRL+T	Create a hanging indent
✓	CTRL+Shift+T	Reduce a hanging indent
✓	CTRL+Q	Remove manual paragraph formatting

Apply Paragraph Styles

CTRL+Shift+S	Apply a style
ALT+CTRL+K	Start AutoFormat
CTRL+Shift+N	Apply the Normal style
ALT+CTRL+1	Apply the Heading 1 style
ALT+CTRL+2	Apply the Heading 2 style
ALT+CTRL+3	Apply the Heading 3 style
CTRL+Shift+L	Apply the List style (bullets)

Delete Text

✓	Backspace	Delete one character to the left
✓	CTRL+Backspace	Delete one word to the left
✓	Delete	Delete one character to the right
✓	CTRL+Delete	Delete one word to the right
✓	CTRL+X	Cut selected text to the Clipboard
✓	CTRL+Z	Undo the last action
	CTRL+F3	Cut to the Spike

Copy and Move Text and Graphics

✓	CTRL+C	Copy text or graphics
✓	CTRL+C, CTRL+C	Display the Clipboard
✓	CTRL+V	Paste the Clipboard contents
	CTRL+Shift+F3	Paste the Spike contents
	ALT+Shift+R	Copy the header or footer used in the previous section of the document

Insert Special Characters

✓	CTRL+F9	A field
✓	Shift+Enter	A line break

✓	**CTRL+Enter**	A page break
	CTRL+Shift+Enter	A column break
	CTRL+Hyphen	An optional hyphen
✓	**CTRL+Shift+Hyphen**	A nonbreaking hyphen
✓	**CTRL+Shift+Spacebar**	A nonbreaking space
	ALT+CTRL+C	The copyright symbol
	ALT+CTRL+R	The registered trademark symbol
	ALT+CTRL+T	The trademark symbol
	ALT+CTRL+period	An ellipsis
	ALT+CTRL+negative	Em dash
	CTRL+negative	En dash

✓ ## Move the Insertion Point

Left	One character to the left
Right	One character to the right
CTRL+Left	One word to the left
CTRL+Right	One word to the right
CTRL+Up	One paragraph up
CTRL+Down	One paragraph down
Shift+Tab	One cell to the left (in a table)
Tab	One cell to the right (in a table)
Up	Up one line
Down	Down one line
End	To the end of a line
Home	To the beginning of a line
ALT+CTRL+Page Up	To the top of the window
ALT+CTRL+Page Down	To the end of the window
Page Up	Up one screen (scrolling)
Page Down	Down one screen (scrolling)
CTRL+Page Down	To the top of the next page (or to the previous browse object)
CTRL+Page Up	To the top of the previous page (or to the next browse object)
CTRL+End	To the end of a document
CTRL+Home	To the beginning of a document
Shift+F5	To a previous revision or to the location of the insertion point when the document was last closed

✓   **Select Text (Extend selection)**

Shift+Right	One character to the right
Shift+Left	One character to the left
CTRL+Shift+Right	To the end of a word
CTRL+Shift+Left	To the beginning of a word
Shift+End	To the end of a line
Shift+Home	To the beginning of a line
Shift+Down	One line down
Shift+Up	One line up
CTRL+Shift+Down	To the end of a paragraph
CTRL+Shift+Up	To the beginning of a paragraph
Shift+Page Down	One screen down
Shift+Page Up	One screen up
CTRL+Shift+Home	To the beginning of a document
CTRL+Shift+End	To the end of a document
ALT+CTRL+Shift+Page Down	To the end of a window
CTRL+A	To include the entire document
ALT+drag	Select a column of text (not in a table)

Tip: If you know the key combination to move the insertion point, you can select the text by using the same key combination while holding down **Shift**. For example, **CTRL+Right** moves the insertion point to the next word, and **CTRL+Shift+Right** selects the text from the insertion point to the beginning of the next word.

Extend a Selection

✓	**F8**	Turn extend mode on
✓	**F8 x2**	Selects the word
✓	**F8 x3**	Selects the sentence
✓	**F8 x4**	Selects the paragraph
	Shift+F8	Reduce the size of a selection
	Esc	Turn extend mode off

Pressing **F8** followed by any letter or navigation key will extend the selection to the next occurrence of that letter in the document. See page 365 for a more detailed explanation.

Move Around in a Table

Tab	Next cell in a row
Shift+Tab	Previous cell in a row
ALT+Home	First cell in a row

ALT+End	Last cell in a row
ALT+Page Up	First cell in a column
ALT+Page Down	Last cell in a column
Up	Previous row
Down	Next row
CTRL+Shift+Enter	Split a table above the insertion point

Insert Paragraphs and Tab Characters in a Table

Enter	New paragraphs in a cell
CTRL+Tab	Tab characters in a cell

Create, View, and Save Documents

✓	CTRL+N	Create a new document
✓	CTRL+O	Open a document
✓	CTRL+W	Close a document
	ALT+CTRL+S	Split the document window
	ALT+Shift+C	Remove the document window split
✓	CTRL+S	Save a document

Find, Replace, and Browse Through Text

✓	CTRL+F	Find text, formatting, and special items
	Shift+F4	Repeat find (after closing Find and Replace dialog)
	CTRL+H	Replace text, specific formatting, and special items
	CTRL+G	Go to a page, bookmark, footnote, table, comment, graphic, or other location
	ALT+CTRL+Z	Go back to a page, bookmark, footnote, table, comment, graphic, or other location
	ALT+CTRL+Home	Browse through a document (opens the Browse Object dialog box in lower right corner)

Undo and Redo Actions

✓	Esc	Cancel an action
✓	CTRL+Z	Undo an action
✓	CTRL+Y	Redo or repeat an action
✓	Any Arrow Key	Deselect text without deleting or replacing text

Switch to Another View

✓	ALT+CTRL+P	Switch to Print layout view
	ALT+CTRL+O	Switch to Outline view
	ALT+CTRL+N	Switch to Normal view in Word 2003 or Draft view in Word 2007
✓	CTRL+F2	Switch to Print Preview

Keys for Working with Fields

	ALT+Shift+D	A Date field (see caution on page 307).
	ALT+CTRL+L	A ListNum field
	ALT+Shift+P	A page field
	ALT+Shift+T	A time field
✓	CTRL+F9	An empty field
	CTRL+Shift+F7	Update linked information in a Word source document
	F9	Update selected fields
	CTRL+Shift+F9	Unlink a field
	Shift+F9	Switch between a field code and its result
✓	ALT+F9	Switch between all field codes and their results
	ALT+Shift+F9	Run GoToButton or MacroButton from the field that displays the field results
✓	F11	Go to the next field
✓	Shift+F11	Go to the previous field
	CTRL+F11	Lock a field
	CTRL+Shift+F11	Unlock a field

Keys for Working in Task Panes

	F6	Move to the Task Pane
	CTRL+Tab	When a menu or toolbar is active, move to the Task Pane. Press **ALT** first to activate the Menu bar.
	Tab	Moves down through a task pane when active
	CTRL+Down	Display all the commands on the task pane
	CTRL+Home or CTRL+End	Move to the top or bottom of the task panes
	CTRL+Spacebar, C	Close the task pane in Word 2007

Critical Thinking Questions

1. How can you print a list of shortcut keys assigned to macros?

   _____

   _____

2. What happens when you press the Shift key along with any navigation key?

   _____

   _____

3. Explain how the CTRL key affects the navigation keys.

   _____

   _____

4. Open a document with several paragraphs of text. Set the insertion point anywhere in the middle of the document. Give the position of the insertion point after pressing the following keys:

   a. Home

   _____

   b. End

   _____

   c. CTRL+Home

   _____

   d. CTRL+End

   _____

   e. CTRL+Up

   _____

   f. CTRL+Del

   _____

   g. CTRL+Backspace

   _____

   h. Page Up

   _____

   i. Page Down

   _____

5. List three ways to close a document using the keyboard.

_____

_____

6. Give the shortcut keys for:

a. Save As

_____

b. Increase font size by 1 point

_____

c. Run Spelling and Grammar check

_____

d. Copy formatting

_____

e. Print Preview

_____

f. Format letters as all capitals

_____

g. Insert a page break

_____

h. Open a shortcut menu (two possible keys)

_____

7. Describe what happens when you press the F8 key twice, three times, and then four times.

_____

_____

8. Make a list of CTRL keys assigned to the 26 letters of the alphabet along with their command.

_____

_____

9. What happens when any arrow key is pressed when text is selected?

_____

_____

CHAPTER 7

Formatting

OBJECTIVES

▸ Identify and use formatting marks.

▸ Recognize the role of styles in MS Word and manage the Normal style.

▸ Apply character formatting using the Font dialog box and shortcut keys.

▸ Use the Paragraph dialog box, Horizontal Ruler, and shortcut keys to format paragraphs.

▸ Format a typical SOAP note.

▸ Use headers and footers for letterhead and patient demographic information.

▸ Use section breaks to manage headers and footers and page margins.

KEYWORDS

default font
default tab stop
direct formatting
Font dialog box
formatting marks
hanging indent
header and footer
horizontal alignment
indent
line spacing
Normal style
Paragraph dialog box
paragraph mark
Reveal Formatting task pane
section break
set tab
style

Shortcut keys
Shift+F1
CTRL+L
CTRL+R
CTRL+E
CTRL+J
CTRL+M
CTRL+Shift+M
CTRL+T
CTRL+Shift+T
CTRL+D

Formatting Basics

Understanding fundamental concepts and techniques related to formatting will increase your productivity and accuracy and create professional looking documents that are easy to edit. Word processors are designed to lay out text consistently and efficiently using standard paragraph formats and formatting commands. One of the most common mistakes a user can make is to treat their document-creation software like an old manual typewriter! Software is *so much smarter* than typewriters. MS Word is a high-powered, world-class application with a tremendous set of features and functionality for efficiency, accuracy, and productivity. Using actual formatting commands (instead of repeatedly pressing Tab or Spacebar) can save hundreds of keystrokes over the course of a day of transcribing and make editing infinitely easier. Table 7-1 defines important formatting terms used in word processing.

The Insertion Point

The mouse pointer appears as an I-beam whenever it overlies an area that accepts text input. Clicking the I-beam in a given position sets the

Table 7-1	**Formatting Terms Used in Document Creation Software.**
Indent	(noun) The space between the left and right margin and the edge of the text. (verb) To move text away from the right or left margin.
Hanging indent	A format in which the first line of a paragraph is closer to the left margin compared to the second and subsequent lines of the paragraph. This format is typically used in a numbered list where the number is at the left margin and the text is lined up ¼ to ½ inch from the number.
Center	A command that aligns text in the center of the margins.
Header and Footer	The space at the upper and lower edge of a document that typically contains the letterhead, page number, and patient demographic information. The header and footer space is separated from the body of the document so the text within the body of the report can be edited without affecting the placement of the text contained within the header and footer.
Hard page break	A forced page break inserted by the user (*cf* soft page break).
Soft page break	A page break which occurs automatically when the text reaches the lower margin of the page.
Justify	A command that aligns text even with both the right and left margins.
Template	A file that is used as the basis of a new document for a given document type or report type. A template contains formatted headings and other text that appears on all documents of that type.
Set Tab	A defined position on a line that determines where the insertion point will stop when the Tab key is pressed. Pressing Tab typically moves the cursor ½ inch, but a set tab stop will move the cursor to the exact position on the line defined by the tab stop.
Right-aligned	Text which is formatted even with the right margin (instead of the left margin).

cursor. The cursor (also called the insertion point) *blinks* to help locate its position. In MS Word, the cursor "rules." In other words, the cursor determines what information is displayed on toolbars, menus, and ribbons and also determines where formatting commands will be applied.

Formatting information is "given back" to the user by the toolbars, ribbons, rulers, and the Status Bar based on the location of the cursor. For example, buttons (icons) become clear or change color when the cursor rests at a location where the corresponding command has been applied. The Horizontal Ruler also displays information based on the location of the cursor. A lot of information can be gleaned from a quick glance at the toolbar/ribbon area. The toolbars and ruler displayed in Figure 7-1 indicate that (at the location of the cursor) the text is formatted in the Normal style, Times New Roman 12 pt, with bold and automatic numbering. The paragraph is left-aligned with an indent set at ¼ inch, a left-aligned tab stop at ½ inch, and a hanging indent applied. The left and right page margins are 1¼ inches. Formatting marks are displayed and the Zoom is set at 100% (not displayed in Word 2007's ribbon).

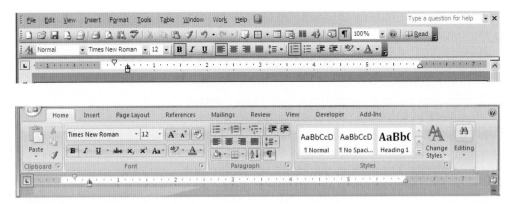

FIGURE 7-1 The Formatting toolbar and the Home ribbon with formatting commands.

Formatting Marks

Formatting marks are an important feature of MS Word to aid in formatting, editing, and troubleshooting formatting problems. These marks, as shown in 7-2, are displayed on the screen but *do not print*. The **paragraph mark** represents the end of a paragraph and is created by pressing **Enter**. The right-pointing arrow is inserted when **Tab** is pressed. The dots represent spaces created by pressing the **Spacebar**. A curved arrow represents a manual line break (**Shift+Enter**). Manual page breaks (**CTRL+Enter**) are noted with a dotted line. Press **CTRL+Shift+8** to reveal formatting marks (or click the paragraph symbol ¶ on the <u>Standard</u> toolbar/<u>Home</u> tab).

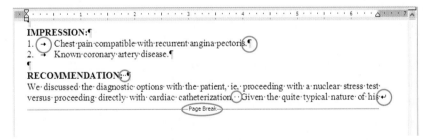

FIGURE 7-2 Formatting marks display on the screen to indicate spaces, tabs, line and page breaks, and paragraphs.

A new, blank document will contain a single paragraph mark. *The paragraph mark contains all the formatting information for the text immediately preceding the mark.* Pressing **Enter** inserts a new paragraph and therefore a new paragraph mark. The paragraph mark will also change in appearance to indicate character formatting such as font size and type, bold, italic, or colored.

When a paragraph mark is deleted, the formatting information is transferred to the next available paragraph mark and the remaining text will take on the formatting of the *deleted* paragraph mark. In other words, when you merge several paragraphs by deleting the paragraph marks that separate them, the text will retain the formatting of the first paragraph. If you include a paragraph mark in a copy-paste routine, you will bring formatting information along with the selected text and insert a hard return at the point where the text is pasted.

Commands associated with paragraph formatting (and therefore stored in the paragraph mark) can be found in the **Paragraph dialog box** as shown in Figure 7-13. Displaying paragraph marks, especially while editing, helps you manage formatting by giving you visual clues as to where your paragraphs begin and end as well as the type of formatting applied to the paragraph mark. You may find the formatting marks distracting when you first begin to use them, but after a while you will come to depend on them. Formatting marks are *very* important and it is worthwhile to become accustomed to working with them displayed.

Blank pages at the end of a document are usually the result of "leftover" paragraph marks. These paragraph marks are inadvertently created while typing and editing a file. Displaying formatting marks will reveal the trailing paragraph marks so they can easily be deleted, thereby getting rid of the blank page.

It's easy to demonstrate how a paragraph mark actually "carries" formatting information. Selecting and copying a paragraph mark (without any text) and pasting it in a new location will apply the formatting information stored in that mark to the text immediately preceding the paragraph mark.

In addition to the formatting marks that are displayed within the document space, the rulers and toolbars also convey helpful information to aid in formatting and editing:

- The shaded areas at each end of the ruler indicate the page margins.
- The "stacked" pointers on the ruler indicate the formatting applied to the *selected* paragraph (ie, the paragraph containing the cursor).
- The top, downward pointer indicates the position of the first line of a paragraph and the lower, upward pointer indicates the position of subsequent lines of the paragraph.
- The square at the base of the pointers indicates the paragraph's indention.

You can easily determine the formatting of a paragraph by examining the position of the indicators on the ruler—even if there is no text associated with the paragraph mark.

Word has a reputation for making "mysterious" formatting changes, but these changes are not as inexplicable as they may first appear. The key to successfully formatting and editing is an understanding of how paragraph marks are handled and the consequences of retaining or deleting these marks. You will experience far less frustration with Word if you develop a habit of displaying formatting marks, especially when editing and troubleshooting formatting.

Applying Formatting Commands

Whereas paragraph formatting is stored in the paragraph mark, font formatting is applied directly to the character (*including spaces created by the Spacebar*). The formatting remains with the character no matter where the character is moved within the document.

Formatting can be applied in two different ways. When typing new text, font formatting can be "turned on" just before typing the text and then "turned off" when no longer needed. For example, to type a bold heading such as **HISTORY**, press **CTRL+B** H I S T O R Y **CTRL+B**. On the other hand, if the text is already typed (ie, you are editing), first select the text and then press the formatting command. The formatting will only be applied to the selected text. To make editing easier, a single word can be formatted by simply placing the insertion point *anywhere within the word*.

Likewise, paragraphs can be formatted before or after typing the text, and the insertion point can be *anywhere in the paragraph* when the command is applied. To apply formatting to more than one paragraph at a time, a portion of text (or the paragraph mark) from each paragraph must be selected before the command is applied. In Figure 7-3, any paragraph formatting command given would apply to all three paragraphs even though only a few words from the first and third paragraph are selected. Note that this figure displays *three* paragraphs, because even a paragraph mark with no associated text constitutes a paragraph.

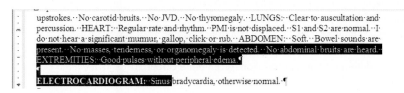

FIGURE 7-3 A portion of the text from each paragraph must be selected to apply format commands to more than one paragraph.

When you press **Enter** to end one paragraph and begin another, the resulting paragraph will have the same characteristics as the previous one. For example, to make all paragraphs in a report left-aligned and single-spaced, you only have to set those attributes for the first paragraph and continue pressing **Enter** to create each new paragraph. The exception to this rule is if Word has applied a specific style that includes a command to change the formatting of the following paragraph (see below under Introduction to Styles).

Introduction to Styles

A **style** is a defined set of formatting commands. Styles simplify formatting tasks by bundling formatting commands into a single definition, allowing you to apply several commands to a paragraph or a word in one step. For example, instead of taking four separate steps to apply justified alignment, hanging indent, tab stops at 1 inch and 2 inches, you could apply a single paragraph style predefined with those attributes. In addition to formatting commands, styles may include commands that specify the formatting of the paragraph that immediately follows it (eg, if you apply Heading 1 style to a line of text and press **Enter**, the new paragraph will be formatted in the Body Text style).

Styles are also the basis of many of Word's features such as Document Map and automated tables of contents. Styles can be used to designate text within a document for searching, replacing, reformatting, indexing, updating, organizing, and reorganizing text with a few quick keystrokes. See the special project on page 465 to learn how to use styles to create an automated log sheet.

A complete understanding of styles is not absolutely necessary in the context of transcription because transcriptionists typically work with documents containing consistent and repetitive formatting. Rarely does a single medical report require a variety of fonts, font sizes, headings of various sizes, or a variety of paragraph formats. Transcription also does not typically require the creation of reference tables (such as a table of contents) or outlines. As far as transcription is concerned, it is important to understand the basics of styles and how to troubleshoot formatting problems when styles are involved.

Personally, I do not make extensive use of styles while transcribing (although they are indispensable when writing an article, a report, or a book). Instead, when starting a new account, I set up template files and apply as much formatting as possible to the template so there are very few formatting changes to make during routine transcription. Learn more about templates in Chapter 8.

There are two types of styles: paragraph styles and character styles. A paragraph style controls all aspects of a paragraph's appearance, such as font, alignment, indention, tab stops, line spacing, and borders. See a complete list of paragraph attributes on page 208. A character style contains only character-level attributes (ie, any of the attributes in the **Font** dialog box). Character styles can be applied to selected text within a paragraph if that particular text needs to be formatted differently than the rest of the paragraph. Word installs with an extensive list of styles. The most important paragraph styles are Normal, Heading 1, Heading 2, and Heading 3. Every paragraph in Word has a style assigned to it—either by default or by the user.

The **Normal style** is the default style used by Word. All new documents open with a single paragraph mark with the Normal style applied. The Normal style in Word 2003 is defined as Times New Roman, 12 point, single-spaced and left-aligned. Word 2007 installs with the Normal style defined as

Calibri, 11 point, left-aligned with line spacing at 1.15, and the space after paragraphs equal to 10 points. Learn how to change the definition of the Normal style below.

Styles themselves typically do not cause formatting problems, but Word's automated features related to styles may create unexpected formatting changes. For example, if the *Built-in Headings Style* option (**AutoFormat As You Type**) is active, Word will automatically apply a Heading style when you type bold, centered text without a period at the end. In addition, Word's built-in heading styles are set to automatically format the paragraph immediately following the heading with the Body Text style (instead of carrying the same style forward as normally occurs when you hit **Enter**). To prevent styles from making unwanted changes, disable the two options related to styles in the **AutoFormat As You Type** dialog box (page 157).

Styles work the same way in both Word 2003 and Word 2007. Word 2003 has a style drop-down list on the <u>Formatting</u> toolbar, and Word 2007 has an extensive selection of style buttons in the <u>Style</u> group on the **Home** tab. Both versions use the **Styles** task pane (Figure 7-4) to manage styles. To apply a style, set the cursor in the paragraph to be formatted and click the style name.

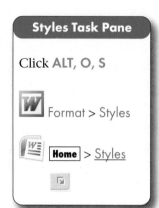

Styles Task Pane

Click **ALT, O, S**

Format > Styles

Home > Styles

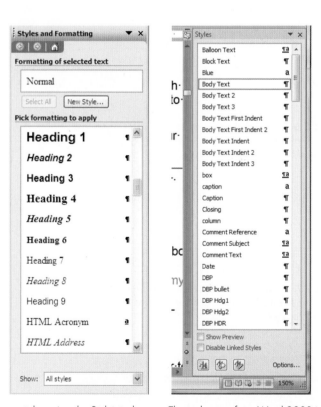

FIGURE 7-4 Manage styles using the Styles task pane. The task pane from Word 2003 is shown on the left and Word 2007's is shown on the right.

Hover the mouse pointer over a style name in the **Styles** task pane to see a ToolTip describing the style (see Figure 7-5).

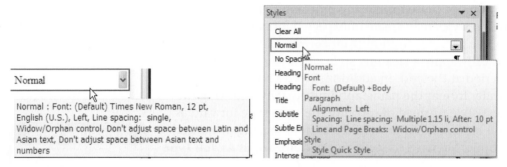

FIGURE 7-5 Hover the mouse pointer over the style name to see a ToolTip describing the attributes of the style.

Right-click the style name in the **Styles** task pane to reveal a menu of commands for managing styles (Figure 7-6). In Word 2007, you can also right-click the style's button in the Style group to reveal a menu (Figure 7-7).

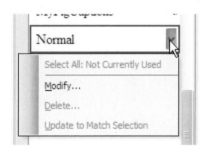

FIGURE 7-6 Right-click the style name listed in the Styles task pane to display a menu of commands for managing that particular style.

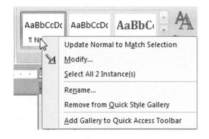

FIGURE 7-7 In Word 2007, right-click the style button in the Styles group to display a menu of commands for managing that particular style.

The definition of the Normal style in Word 2007 has proven to be problematic for many. The Normal style in Word 2007 is set to create "space after" each paragraph (ie, the style includes the command to automatically place space after a paragraph). You can easily revert to Word 2003's set of styles. As shown in Figure 7-8, click **Change Styles** > Style Set > Word 2003. Open the menu again and click Set as Default. To change the font associated with the Normal style, see directions under Font Formatting below.

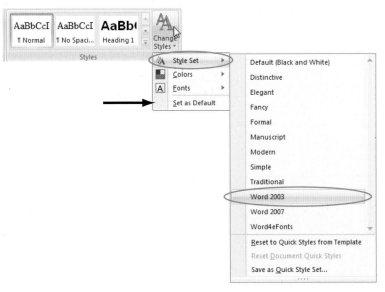

FIGURE 7-8 Use the Change Styles button to change the Style set in Word 2007 to Word 2003's style set.

Font Formatting

Applying format changes to fonts is quite easy. Click the command before you start typing and repeat the command to stop applying the format. To edit, select the text and click the command to be applied. If applying font changes to a single word, simply place the cursor within the word; you don't have to select the entire word to apply a font change. The most commonly used font commands are found on the Formatting toolbar/**Home** tab. The **Font dialog box** (**CTRL+D**), shown in Figure 7-9, is also very useful for making font changes, but nothing beats shortcut keys for utmost efficiency. The most commonly used character commands, Bold, Italic, and Underline, have easy-to-use shortcut keys already assigned (**CTRL+B**, **CTRL+I**, and **CTRL+U** respectively). See a list of other shortcut keys that correspond to options in the **Font** dialog box on page 187.

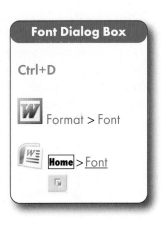

Font Dialog Box

Ctrl+D

Format > Font

Home > Font

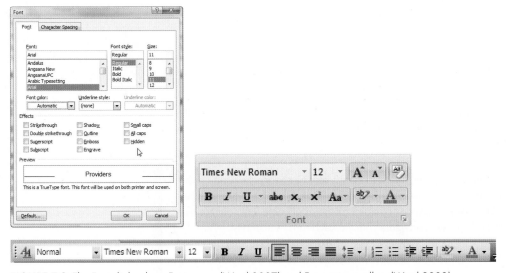

FIGURE 7-9 The Font dialog box, Font group (Word 2007) and Formatting toolbar (Word 2003).

You can also access the **Font** and the **Paragraph** dialog boxes using the shortcut menu. Right-click text to display the shortcut menu, as shown in Figure 7-10.

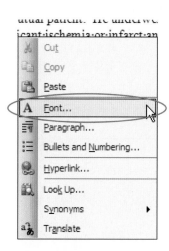

FIGURE 7-10 Right-click text to reveal a shortcut menu.

Word 2007 offers a mini formatting toolbar that floats within the document space. To reveal this toolbar, select some text and move the mouse pointer over the "ghost" image of the toolbar. You can also right-click on a word (without selecting the word) and the toolbar as well as a shortcut menu will appear, as shown in Figure 7-11.

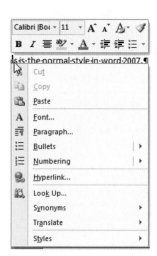

FIGURE 7-11 In Word 2007, right-click on text to reveal a mini toolbar and a shortcut menu for editing and formatting text and paragraphs.

To make a single font change, I almost always use the shortcut key, but I prefer to use the **Font** dialog box when making several character-level changes at one time. The **Font** dialog box contains all the applicable font commands in one place and is easy to navigate with the keyboard. You can type directly into the *Font, Font Style,* and *Size* boxes, using **Tab** to jump between them. Press **Enter** to accept the change and close the dialog box.

Note the *All Caps* command listed on the right in the middle of the **Font** dialog box. This is the perfect command to use in areas of a document that use all caps (such as the allergy section or the pre- and postdiagnosis sections of a surgical report). Apply this command to the specific area of your template. Text typed in this space will always insert in caps without having to press **Caps Lock**. Remember, if you continue typing from this point (and press the **Enter** key), you will continue to insert text in all caps.

Default Font

When you open a new, blank document in Word, the text always starts out in the Normal style, and the Normal style, by definition, uses the **default font**. This means the font face, font style, and font size will be determined by the current definition of the Normal paragraph style. If you have worked in Word for a while, you have probably noticed that even though you change the font when you create a document, the font sometimes reverts back to the original font within the same document, and it always reverts to the same font when starting a new document. Simply changing the font or font size on the toolbar or the **Font** dialog box *does not* change the default font settings—it only changes the font at that point in the document and continues as long as you type in that same text string. Any spaces within your document that were *not selected* when you changed the font setting will still carry the default font settings. If you begin typing in one of these "spots," the font will appear in the default format. Displaying formatting marks will make this problem easier to diagnose.

If your particular work does not use the same font as the (default) Normal style, you will find yourself changing the font with each new document (a frustrating task to repeat over and over). You can change the default font associated with the Normal style so that you do not have to constantly change your formatting as you work. There are several ways to change the default font, but the method that is consistent among all versions of Word uses the **Font** dialog box. Follow these steps:

1. Open the **Font** dialog box (CTRL+D).

2. Select the font attributes that you would like to use as the primary font in the majority of your documents. Click Default in the left lower corner of the **Font** dialog box (Figure 7-9).

3. You will be asked to change the font for all *new* documents based on the Normal template. Click Yes. (Note: the Normal template is the default template and the one used unless otherwise specified. Learn more in Chapter 8.)

Now, all *new* documents based on the Normal template will start with this font. This change will *not* reformat any documents that have already been typed, and it will not change (update) any text that is already in the document (unless the text was selected when you made the font change). When closing Word, you may be asked if you want to save changes to the Normal.dot; answer Yes.

Superscript and Subscript

Superscript and subscript characters can be formatted using shortcut keys or the **Font** dialog box. To format subscript text, as in H_2O, use the shortcut **CTRL+=** (equal sign). The shortcut for superscript formatting, as in cm^2, is **CTRL+Shift+=** (equal sign). Just before typing the character, press the command, then type the character. Return to normal text by pressing the command again (ie, these are toggle commands). You may also type and select the character first then apply the command using the shortcut key or by opening the **Font** dialog box (**CTRL+D**) and choosing *Subscript* (**ALT+B**) or *Superscript* (**ALT+P**).

Since superscripts and subscripts are cumbersome to format, create Auto-Correct entries for items you use often (see Chapter 9).

Superscript and subscript characters are not compatible with all medical record systems, especially those that import text in plain-text format. Check with the provider or facility to determine which formatting characters are compatible with their document management system.

Fractions

The fractions ¼, ½ and ¾ will automatically format as single-space fractions if you have selected this option in the **AutoFormat As You Type** dialog box (see page 156). Simply type 1/4, 1/2 or 3/4 and the fraction will reformat to a single-space fraction when you hit the **Spacebar**. Additional fractions can be found on the **Symbols** dialog box in the *Subset: Currency* (see below).

To create other fractions, use subscript and superscript numbers (as described above). Change the upper number to superscript and the lower number to subscript. Create AutoCorrect entries for uncommon single-space fractions that you happen to use on a routine basis (learn more about AutoCorrect in Chapter 9).

Creating compound fractions such as 1½ can be cumbersome because you have to type a space after the whole number in order for AutoFormat As You Type to recognize 1/2 as the trigger for ½. This requires you to backspace to close up the space between the whole number and the fraction (ie, change 1 ½ to 1½). To quickly create compound fractions such as 1½, use AutoCorrect to create a shortcut for inserting the single-space fraction following the whole number. The trick is to create an Auto-Correct entry that closes the space between the whole number and the single-space fraction. See page 266 for an explanation.

Single-space fractions are not compatible with all medical record systems, especially those that import text in plain text format. Check with the provider or facility to determine which formatting characters are compatible with their document management system.

Symbols

Word includes an extensive collection of symbols. Set the cursor where you want to insert a symbol and follow these steps:

1. Open the **Symbol** dialog box.
2. Locate the symbol on the grid (Figure 7-12) and click to select. You may need to change the *Font* or the *Subset* to find the exact symbol you need.

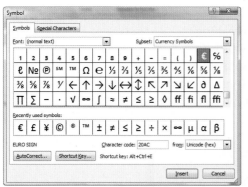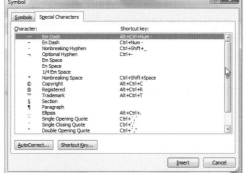

FIGURE 7-12 The Symbol dialog box has an extensive list of symbols available in all the font sets.

3. The shortcut key (if any) will appear below the grid when the symbol is selected. Note the shortcut key for future use. Click **Insert** to place the symbol in your document.
4. If you use the symbol routinely, click **AutoCorrect**, which will open the **AutoCorrect** dialog box so you can save the symbol as an AutoCorrect entry (see page 268), or click **Shortcut Key** to assign a shortcut key to the symbol (see page 394 in Word 2003 and page 403 in Word 2007). More characters are listed on the **Special Characters** tab. Some potentially useful characters include an em dash, en dash, optional hyphen, and ellipsis.

Use AutoCorrect to effortlessly insert the degree symbol. See page 269 for an explanation.

> **Symbol Dialog Box**
>
> ALT, I, S
>
> Insert > Symbol
>
> **Insert** > Symbols
>
> > **Symbol** > More
>
> Symbols

Symbols may not be compatible with all medical record systems, especially those that import text in plain text format. Check with the provider or facility to determine which formatting characters are compatible with their document management system.

Nonbreaking Spaces and Nonbreaking Hyphens

Nonbreaking characters prevent adjacent words from separating across a line break. For example, a title and surname should remain together on the same line (ie, `Mr.` should not end one line and `Smith` start the next). Use a nonbreaking space between words that should not separate. Word will treat the two words as if they were a single word, but a space will be displayed for readability. The trick is to use the nonbreaking space command *instead* of the **Spacebar**. With formatting characters displayed, a nonbreaking space will appear as a degree symbol, so `Mr.°Smith` will appear as `Mr. Smith`. The shortcut key for a nonbreaking space is **CTRL+Shift+Spacebar**.

Nonbreaking hyphens are applied the same way. Substitute a nonbreaking hyphen for a regular hyphen when you do not want hyphenated words to separate, as in `Mrs.°Smith-Jones`. With formatting characters displayed, a nonbreaking hyphen will appear as an em dash (ie, longer than a hyphen), but the hyphen will print normally. The shortcut key for a nonbreaking hyphen is **CTRL+Shift+Hyphen**.

Create a shortcut using AutoText to automatically insert a nonbreaking space after the title `Dr.` See page 281 for Word 2003 and page 291 for Word 2007 for an explanation.

Paragraph Formatting

MS Word does not define a paragraph in the same way as your 8th grade English teacher. As far as Word is concerned, a paragraph is anything (or nothing) that immediately precedes a paragraph mark (¶). Every time you strike the **Enter** key, you create a paragraph mark. This means a blank line containing a paragraph mark is technically a paragraph, as well as a single word, a three-word heading, or a group of sentences. Displaying paragraph marks gives you a visual demarcation of each paragraph and makes formatting and editing much easier. Review formatting marks on page 197.

Commands that are associated with the paragraph mark are found in the **Paragraph** dialog box (Figure 7-13).

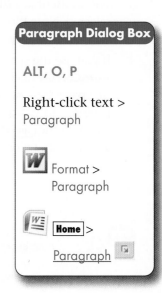

Paragraph Dialog Box

ALT, O, P

Right-click text >
Paragraph

Format >
Paragraph

Home >
Paragraph

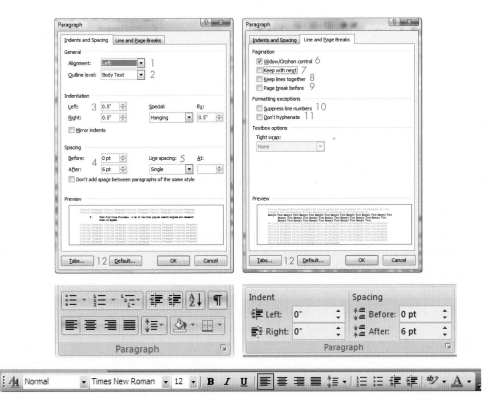

FIGURE 7-13 The Paragraph dialog box, the Paragraph groups (Word 2007) and the Formatting toolbar (Word 2003).

The following list describes the commands found in the **Paragraph** dialog box and therefore associated with the paragraph mark:

Alignment refers to the horizontal placement of text. Paragraphs can be aligned even with the left side of the page, the right side of the page, both sides (justified), or centered between the margins. *Note*: Except within the cell of a table, vertical alignment is not part of the paragraph formatting but is considered part of the page setup.

Outline level relates to the built-in Heading styles (numbered 1-9). This attribute is important when working in Outline view, but is generally not relevant to transcription.

Indention refers to the distance of the text from the left and/or right *margins*. There are five types of indention: Left, right, negative left, and special (including first line and hanging indent).

Spacing Before and *After* refers to the amount of space automatically inserted between paragraphs, either before or after the paragraph. Using before and after spacing, you can change the space between paragraphs without inserting blank lines (ie, paragraph marks).

Line spacing, such as single or double spacing, refers to the amount of space between lines within a paragraph.

Widow and orphan control prevents a single line of a paragraph from separating from the remainder of the paragraph across a page break.

Keep with next ensures that the first line of the next paragraph will remain on the same page as the preceding paragraph to which this formatting is applied, as in the case of a heading, which should always remain on the same page as the text it introduces.

Keep lines together prevents the lines within a paragraph from separating across a page break. If necessary, Word will force all lines to the next page, potentially leaving a large white space at the bottom of a page.

Page break before ensures that the text will always start a new page, as in a major heading or a new chapter heading.

Suppress line numbers prevents line numbering of the selected paragraph if line numbering has been turned on. Line numbering is set in the **Page Setup** dialog box and is predominantly used by the legal community. These line numbers *do* appear in the printed document.

Don't hyphenate prevents text in the applicable paragraph from using automatic hyphenation. Normally, automatic hyphenation is set for the entire document as part of the Language settings, but this setting overrides the document setting for the given paragraph.

Tabs opens the **Tabs** dialog box. Set tabs are used to define specific points for aligning text horizontally across a page. They are also used to control the indent commands. Learn more about tabs on page 213.

> Using actual formatting commands and paragraph-control commands (instead of forcing line and page breaks with manual breaks and other workarounds) is far more efficient and creates a more professional document. You never have to worry about orphans, widows, and stranded headings and signature lines when documents are formatted with paragraph-control commands. Plus, editing is much simpler and much faster when the document layout does not have to be reviewed and corrected each time an edit is made.

Alignment

Horizontal alignment determines the orientation and appearance of the left and right edges of a paragraph. Alignment commands include Left-aligned (**CTRL+L**), Right-aligned (**CTRL+R**) Centered (**CTRL+E**) and Justified (**CTRL+J**). To change the alignment, place the cursor anywhere in the paragraph and press the corresponding shortcut key or click the icon on the formatting toolbar/ribbon. A left aligned paragraph (Figure 7-14), the most common alignment, aligns the left edge of the paragraph with the left margin and leaves the right edge "ragged."

¶
REVIEW OF SYSTEMS: No significant change of weight, fever or chills, easy fatigability, blurred vision, chronic headaches, history of glaucoma or cataracts, orthopnea, or paroxysmal nocturnal dyspnea. No peripheral edema. No palpitations. No history of asthma, chronic cough, hemoptysis, hematemesis, melena, or hematochezia. Gastroesophageal reflux is well controlled on Prevacid. Stable nocturia one time per night. No urgency or frequency. She has arthritis principally in her hands. No myalgias. No history of diabetes or thyroid disorder. No history of seizure or stroke. No easy bruising or bleeding diathesis.¶
¶

FIGURE 7-14 A left-aligned paragraph with a "ragged" right edge and the corresponding icon on the toolbar/ribbon.

A justified paragraph (Figure 7-15) is aligned even with both the left and right margins. It is essentially a left-aligned paragraph with a flush-right edge.

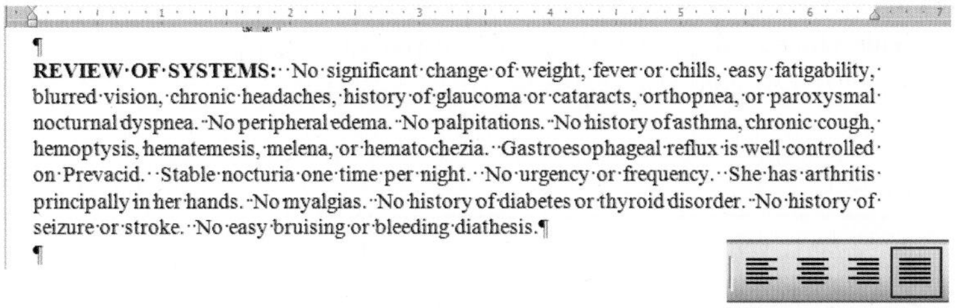

FIGURE 7-15 A justified paragraph and the corresponding icon on the toolbar/ribbon.

Centered paragraphs are used mostly for titles, especially at the top of a page. Right-aligned paragraphs are rarely used for actual paragraphs, but are typically used to align the date or some other single line of information flush with the right margin. A right-aligned paragraph does not work well if you also have text that needs to align with the left margin and/or the center of the same line. Learn how to format a line containing left-, center- and right-aligned text on page 215.

Line Spacing

Line spacing determines the amount of vertical space between lines of text *within* a paragraph. By default, lines are single spaced in Word 2003 (ie, the default setting in the Normal style is single spacing). The default spacing in Word 2007 is 1.15. You can use the Indents and Spacing tab (**Paragraph** dialog box), the icons on the toolbar/ribbon (Figure 7-16), or shortcut keys to set your line spacing. Line spacing commands use the CTRL key and the number keys across the top of the keyboard (not the number pad). For single-line spacing, press CTRL+1, for double spacing press CTRL+2, and for 1.5 line spacing press CTRL+5.

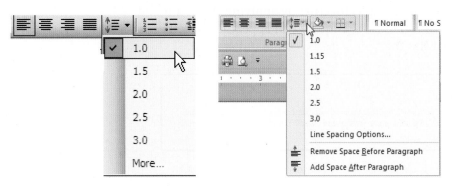

FIGURE 7-16 Click the down arrow next to the Line spacing icon to display spacing options. The menu for Word 2003 is shown on the left and Word 2007 on the right.

Paragraph Spacing

Word also includes the paragraph commands *Space Before* and *Space After*. These commands add space before and after paragraphs without using the **Enter** key to insert blank lines (Figure 7-17). You can specify the amount of space to add before or after a paragraph using the **Indents and Spacing** tab of the **Paragraph** dialog box. Also, the shortcut key **CTRL+0** will add/remove the equivalent of a blank line above a paragraph.

This·paragraph·is·formatted·with·Space·after·set·at·12·points.¶

Notice·there·is·space·between·the·lines·of·text·and·the·space·was·not·created·using·the·Enter·key·(ie,·there·are·no·paragraph·marks·between·the·paragraphs).¶

FIGURE 7-17 Space before and Space after commands create space between paragraphs without using the Enter key.

The default paragraph style in Word 2007 is set to automatically insert 10 points of space after the paragraph. See page 202 for instructions on resetting the default paragraph style in Word 2007.

Paragraph Breaks

When text reaches the end of the page, Word automatically continues it on the next page (a soft page break). To keep lines together on a page or to prevent widows and orphans, use the **Line and Page breaks** tab in the **Paragraph** dialog box. A widow is the last line of a paragraph that appears by itself at the top of a page. An orphan is the first line of a paragraph that appears by itself at the bottom of a page.

To break a paragraph at a given point without creating a new paragraph (ie, break the line without pressing the **Enter** key), press **Shift+Enter**. This can be helpful when you want to control the paragraphing at the bottom of the page or for controlling automatic numbered lists (see page 331).

Use the *Keep with next* command to keep headings with the text that it introduces. You can keep several paragraphs together by applying the command to each paragraph. As shown in Figure 7-18, a square will appear in the left margin of each paragraph that has the *Keep with next* command applied.

PHYSICAL·EXAMINATION¶
GENERAL:··This·is·a·pleasant·gentleman·with·multiple·ecchymoses·over·his·upper·extremities.··He·has·had·a·significant·weight·loss·of·about·30·pounds·since·January·and·overall·seems·to·be·doing·considerably·better.¶

FIGURE 7-18 A small square appears in the left margin when Keep with next has been applied to the paragraph.

Apply *Keep with next* to headings such as REVIEW OF SYSTEMS or PHYSICAL EXAMINATION so that headings will not end up at the bottom of one page and the corresponding text start at the top of another page. Add this same command to the last paragraph and each line of the signature to prevent the signature line from being stranded on the last page of a report.

Vertical Alignment

Vertical alignment determines the paragraph's position relative to the top and bottom margins. This is useful, for example, when you are creating a title page, because you can position text precisely at the top or center of the page. Setting vertical alignment makes it very easy to center several lines of text in the middle of a page or to justify the paragraphs so they are spaced evenly down the page. Double-click in the margin area of the <u>Ruler</u> to open the **Page Setup** dialog box (see page 224 for more information on the **Page Setup** dialog box). On the ⬛**Layout**⬛ tab, select the appropriate option under *Vertical Alignment*.

If your document contains a cover page with the vertical alignment centered but additional pages with the vertical alignment set to *Top* (the usual setting), you will need to insert a section break to be able to use more than one vertical alignment setting in the same document. Learn more about section breaks on page 229.

Setting Tab Stops

Word has a **default tab stop** at ½-inch intervals. This is the distance the cursor travels each time the **Tab** key is pressed. Simply pressing the **Tab** key has the same result as pressing the **Spacebar** about five times. These are not actual tab "stops" since these tabs will move as you insert text to the left of them. To create a *set tab stop*, you must specify the exact location of the tab stop using the <u>Horizontal Ruler</u> or the **Tab** dialog box. A **set tab** stabilizes column formatting and also guides the indent commands (see below). Paragraphs with set tabs will have tab indicators displayed on the <u>Horizontal Ruler</u>. Default tabs do not appear on the <u>Horizontal Ruler</u>.

Tab stops are part of paragraph formatting and do not apply to the entire document. Each paragraph can have a unique set of tab stops.

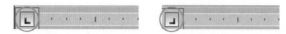

FIGURE 7-19 Click the Tab Type indicator at the far left of the Horizontal Ruler to select the type of tab. Left and right tab indicators are shown here.

The `Tab type indicator` button at the far left of the <u>Horizontal Ruler</u> (Figure 7-19) cycles through five types of tabs (left, right, center, decimal, or bar) plus the first-line indent marker and the hanging-indent marker. To set a tab stop, follow these steps:

1. Place the insertion point in the paragraph in which you want to set a tab.
2. Click the indicator button until it changes to the type of tab needed.
3. Left-click on the lower margin of the <u>Horizontal Ruler</u> where you want to set a tab stop. A tab marker will appear on the ruler corresponding to the type and location of the tab. Drag tab markers left and right on the <u>Horizontal Ruler</u> to adjust tabs as needed.
4. Hold down the **ALT** key while dragging a tab indicator left and right on the ruler. This will display additional markings on the ruler for more precise placement of the tabs.

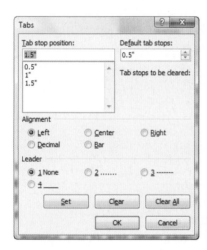

FIGURE 7-20 Tabs dialog box

> **Tabs Dialog Box**
>
> **ALT, O, T**
>
> **W** Format > Tabs
>
> **W** `Home` > <u>Paragraph</u> ⌐ > `Tabs`

You can also set tab stops using the **Tab** dialog box (Figure 7-20). Follow these steps:

1. Set the insertion point in the paragraph to contain the tabs.
2. Open the **Tabs** dialog box.
3. In the *Tab stop position* box, type the position (in inches) where you want to set a tab.
4. Select the *Alignment* (*Left*, *Center*, *Right*, *Decimal*, or *Bar*).
5. Select a *Leader* if you need to insert lines or dots to span the distance of the tab (as in a table of contents).
6. Click `Set` (**ALT+S**).
7. If needed, type another tab position and click `Set`. Each tab stop will appear in the larger box below the *Tab stop position* box.

8. If you need to clear one or all of the tabs, select the tab(s) from the list in the larger box and click **Clear** or **Clear All**.

9. When you are finished adding or clearing tabs, click **OK** or press **Enter**.

When tabs are set, the cursor will jump to the exact position of the tab when the **Tab** key is pressed. Tabs work well for aligning text in the center of a line (center tab) or at the right margin (right tab), especially when there is other text on the same line that requires a different alignment.

To set text at the left, center, and right margins (eg, the patient name at the left, chart number centered, and the date at the right margin), format a left-aligned paragraph with a center tab in the middle and a right-aligned tab at or near the right margin. As you can see from Figure 7-21, using default tabs and the **Spacebar** requires more keystrokes than using set tab stops.

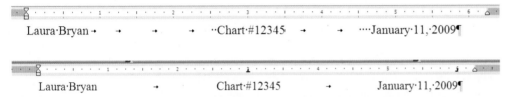

Laura·Bryan →   →   →   →   ··Chart·#12345⟩   →   →   ····January·11,·2009¶

Laura·Bryan   →   Chart·#12345   →   January·11,·2009¶

FIGURE 7-21 Use set tabs to align text at the left, center, and right on the same line. Compare formatting marks, including tab markers on the ruler, in the top diagram to the formatting marks in the bottom diagram.

To remove a set tab, simply drag the tab marker off the ruler using the mouse.

If you have to press the **Tab** key more than once to accomplish the desired formatting, either set the tabs or use a table—avoid pressing the **Tab** key several times in a row. A line that uses multiple tabs across the page is more difficult to control than placing the text within a table. Learn more about tables in Chapter 13.

Applying Indents

Indents can be the most frustrating aspect of paragraph formatting. Many users mistakenly use the **Tab** key to move text off the left margin to give the appearance of an indent, but this method can be fraught with problems. When formatting complex paragraphs (as in the SOAP note), using the **Tab** key to move text in from the left margin can be time-consuming and tedious and can create formatting problems, especially if the paragraph is subsequently edited.

Compare the paragraphs in Figure 7-22 and note the arrows (formatting marks) indicating use of the **Tab** key. Paragraph #3 shows the results of editing paragraph #2. After editing, the tab characters become scattered throughout the paragraph and the indent is lost.

---

1. → This·paragraph·has·a·hanging·indent·applied·and·does·not·require·the·use·of·the·Tab· key.··As·the·text·wraps·to·the·next·line,·it·automatically·indents.¶

2. → This·paragraph·does·not·have·a·hanging·indent·applied.··The·Tab·key·is·used·to·insert·
   → the·indent.··Each·time·the·text·approaches·the·end·of·the·line,·I·must·carefully·watch·
   → to·know·when·to·insert·the·tab·character.··This·slows·down·my·typing·and·requires·
   → more·keystrokes.¶

3. → This·is·the·same·paragraph·with·text·inserted·at·the·beginning.··This·paragraph·does· not·have·a·hanging·indent·applied.··The·Tab·key·is·used·to·insert· → the·indent.··Each·time·the· text·approaches·the·end·of·the·line,·I·must·carefully·watch·→·to·know·when·to·insert·the·tab· character.··This·slows·down·my·typing·and·requires·more·keystrokes.¶

FIGURE 7-22 Formatting a paragraph indent using the Tab key (paragraph #2) can create formatting problems if the paragraph is edited (paragraph #3).

The value of using shortcut keys and formatting commands simply cannot be overstated. Remember, computers are not typewriters with mechanical parts to move about the page, so do not treat your computer like a typewriter! Software is so much smarter than typewriters. Using actual commands instead of repeated use of the **Tab** key and the **Spacebar** can save hundreds of keystrokes over the course of a day of transcribing. Equally as important is the ease of editing—any changes required to the text will not require an overhaul of the paragraph formatting.

See page 372 for instructions on quickly cleaning up a paragraph with scattered tab characters (as shown in Figure 7-22).

Left Indent

An **indent** moves text away from the page margin. To format a paragraph with a left indent, as shown in Figure 7-23, choose one of these methods:

- Click the [**Increase Indent**] icon ⊞ on the Formatting toolbar/Paragraph group. Click again to increase the indent.
- Press **CTRL+M**. Repeat the command to increase the indent. If there is no tab set, the indent command will move the paragraph in by ½ inch (the distance of the default tab) each time the command is applied.
- Drag the [**Left Indent**] marker on the Horizontal Ruler to the desired position.
- To decrease/remove the indent, press **CTRL+Shift+M** or click the [**Decrease Indent**] icon ⊞.

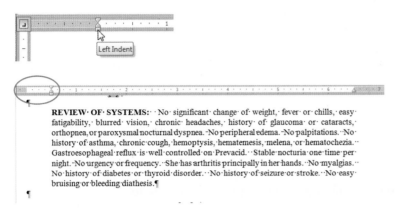

REVIEW· OF· SYSTEMS:· ·No· significant· change· of· weight,· fever· or· chills,· easy· fatigability,· blurred· vision,· chronic· headaches,· history· of· glaucoma· or· cataracts,· orthopnea,· or paroxysmal nocturnal dyspnea.· ·No peripheral edema.· ·No palpitations.· ·No· history· of· asthma,· chronic· cough,· hemoptysis,· hematemesis,· melena,· or· hematochezia.· · Gastroesophageal· reflux· is· well· controlled· on· Prevacid.· ·Stable· nocturia· one· time· per· night.· ·No· urgency· or frequency.· ·She· has arthritis principally in her hands.· ·No· myalgias.· · No· history· of· diabetes· or· thyroid· disorder.· ·No· history· of· seizure· or· stroke.· ·No· easy· bruising· or· bleeding· diathesis.¶

FIGURE 7-23 The left indent marker indicates the paragraph has been indented and shows the depth of the indent relative to the left page margin (indicated by the blue shaded area on the ruler).

A negative left indent is not typically used in healthcare documentation. This format allows a paragraph to start to the *left* of the page margin. It may be useful for making a title or a specific paragraph stand out since it will extend to the left of any other paragraphs.

The AutoFormat As You Type feature includes the option to *Set left and first-indent with tabs and backspaces.* When this feature is enabled, you simply press **Tab** at the beginning of the first and second line of a paragraph to apply an indent. The tabs are converted to an actual indent command. This feature works well for simple first-line indents and indented paragraphs, but neither of these styles is common in medical transcription. I find the feature to cause more problems than it solves, especially when working with hanging indents (which *are* common in transcription). I prefer to clear the check box in **AutoFormat As You Type.**

Right Indent

A right indent prevents text from going all the way to the right margin. Use the Horizontal Ruler to slide the `Right Indent` marker to the desired position, or type in a value in the **Paragraph** dialog box (Figure 7-24). The indent icons on the toolbar/ribbon are only applicable to a left indent, and there is no preset shortcut key for a right indent.

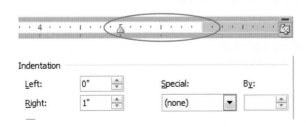

FIGURE 7-24 Slide the right indent marker away from the right margin to set a right indent or open the Paragraph dialog box and type a number into the Right indent box.

First-Line Indent

A first-line indent marks a new paragraph by indenting the first line only. This style is not commonly used in medical documentation. This particular indent is most easily accomplished by simply pressing **Tab** at the beginning of the first line of each new paragraph.

Hanging Indent

The **hanging indent** is one of the most common formats used in transcription. In this format, the first line of a paragraph is closer to the left margin than subsequent lines (Figure 7-25).

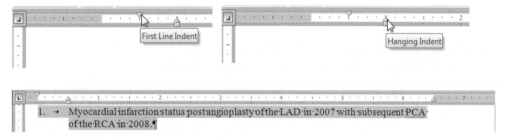

FIGURE 7-25 The Indent markers on the ruler will indicate the location of the first and subsequent lines of the paragraph when a hanging indent is applied.

Use any of these methods to create this format:

- Press **CTRL+T**. Press again to increase the depth of the hang. Setting tab stops will tell Word exactly how deep to hang the indent; otherwise, the "hang" will increase by ½ inch (the distance of the default tab) each time the command is applied.
- Open the **Paragraph** dialog box and choose *Hanging* in the *Special* drop-down box. Type the depth of the hang in the *By* box.
- Slide the [**Indent markers**] on the <u>Horizontal Ruler</u>.
- Press **CTRL+Shift+T** to decrease/remove the hanging indent.

Adjusting the hanging indent using the <u>Horizontal Ruler</u> can be frustrating at times. If you slide the hanging indent marker, the first-line indent marker moves with it. First drag the hanging-indent marker then readjust the first-line indent marker as needed. It's usually easier to increase or decrease the hang using the shortcut key **CTRL+T** and **CTRL+Shift+T**.

Word's built-in numbered list styles often conflict with established numbered list styles used in transcription, so you may prefer to turn off numbered lists and simply format lists "manually." Learn more about managing numbered lists in Chapter 13.

Formatting a SOAP Note

The SOAP note is deceptively difficult to format correctly. Using the **Tab** key to indent paragraphs is probably the most common method, but this approach requires the most work and creates problems if the paragraphs need to be edited. These notes are often short and dictated in high volume, so any time spent streamlining this process will be returned many times over.

Below is a method for formatting the SOAP note using indent and hanging indent commands. Chapter 13 offers an alternative method using tables. Using the correct formatting commands, you can type each paragraph within the SOAP note without hitting **Tab** at the beginning of each line or forcing line breaks using the **Enter** key. Simply type within each paragraph space and the text will flow to the next line and indent appropriately.

This SOAP note format (Figure 7-26) uses both indents and hanging indents in the same paragraph, making it essential to set tab stops. You will have better success with this format if you remove the check mark at *Automatic numbered lists* and *Set left- and first-indent with tabs and backspaces* as described on page 157.

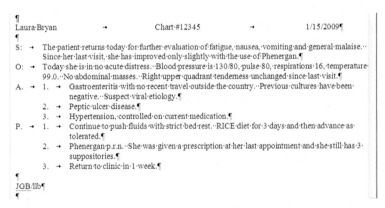

FIGURE 7-26 A sample SOAP note formatted with indents and hanging indents. Notice that the Tab key was never used to move text off the left margin.

The Subjective (S) and Objective (O) sections are simple hanging-indent paragraphs and do not typically present problems. Simply set a tab stop at ½ inch (or the depth of the hang) and press **CTRL+T** to apply a hanging indent to the Subjective paragraph. Press **Enter** to carry the formatting forward and type the Objective section.

The Assessment and Plan sections, on the other hand, do present problems if there is an indented numbered list as in Figure 7-26. Items 1 and 2 under Assessment represent two different types of paragraphs, so we will format each one separately.

Number 1 under Assessment is a left-aligned paragraph with two set tabs and a hanging indent. To format this paragraph, follow these steps:

1. Set a second tab stop at 1 inch. Since the Objective paragraph already has a tab set at ½ inch with a hanging indent, these paragraph settings will carry forward to the Assessment when you press the **Enter** key.

2. Press **CTRL+T** to increase the hanging indent to the 1-inch tab stop.

3. Type your text and press **Enter** to proceed to Assessment #2.

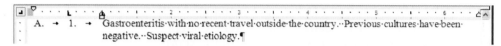

> A. → 1. → Gastroenteritis·with·no·recent·travel·outside·the·country.··Previous·cultures·have·been· negative.··Suspect·viral·etiology.¶

Assessment #2 is an *indented* paragraph with a hanging indent.

1. Tab stops are already set, as they carried forward from previous paragraphs.

2. Press **CTRL+M** to indent to the first tab stop at ½ inch.

3. Press **CTRL+Shift+T** to reduce the hanging indent by one tab stop.

4. Assessment #3 is formatted the same as #2, so simply press **Enter** to continue until you get to the Plan.

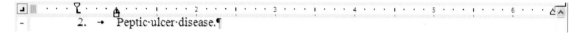

> 2. → Peptic·ulcer·disease.¶

Next, format the Plan:

1. The first line of the Plan is not indented, so press **CTRL+Shift+M** to remove the indent (ie, move the paragraph back to the left margin).

2. Press **CTRL+T** to adjust the hanging indent.

3. Repeat steps under Assessment #2 for Plan #2.

4. When finished with the Plan, press **Enter** for a new paragraph and then press **CTRL+Q** to remove all formatting (tabs, indents, and hanging indents) and return to a left-aligned paragraph.

Once you have successfully formatted the Assessment, use the Format Painter to copy the formatting from the Assessment section to the Plan section. To do this, place the insertion point within Assessment #1 and press **CTRL+Shift+C** (copy format). Move the insertion point to the first item in the Plan and press **CTRL+Shift+V** (paste format). These shortcut keys copy only the formatting, not the actual text. Repeat for Assessment #2 and Plan #2.

Once you have successfully formatted a SOAP note, save the format as a boilerplate to use repeatedly without having to apply formatting. To do this, display paragraph marks. Carefully delete *only the text*, preserving the numbers and the paragraph marks, including the very last paragraph mark. As long as the paragraph marks remain, the formatting will "stick." Insert "jump points" using empty fields (see Chapter 11). An example is shown in Figure 7-27. Select the entire format and save as either a template (see Chapter 8) or a boilerplate using AutoText (Chapter 10). If you typically transcribe multiple reports in a single Word file, copy/paste the boilerplate, one right after the other, until you have enough copies of the boilerplate to transcribe a typical day's work. Save the collection of boilerplates as a template.

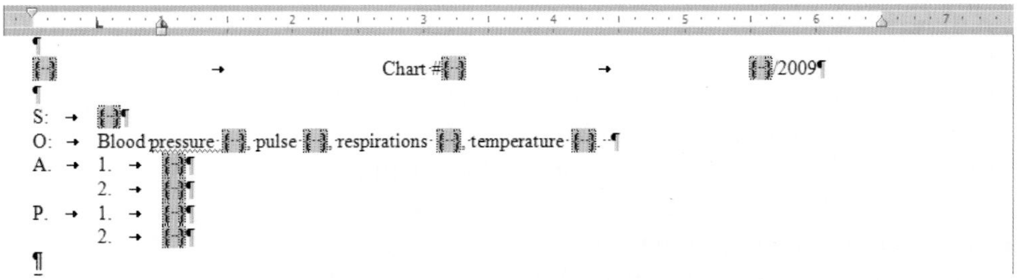
[ ] Chart #[ ] [ ]/2009

S: [ ]
O: Blood pressure [ ], pulse [ ], respirations [ ], temperature [ ].
A. 1. [ ]
2. [ ]
P. 1. [ ]
2. [ ]

FIGURE 7-27 A sample SOAP note boilerplate with formatting and jumps. Each shaded bracket represents a jump point for quickly placing the insertion point.

This same SOAP note formatting is commonly used for operative notes, only the indents and hanging indents are deeper. Figure 7-28 shows a sample operative note using indents and hanging indents. Formatting is applied in the same way as the SOAP note, only the tabs are set at different depths. See more sample formats in Chapter 16.

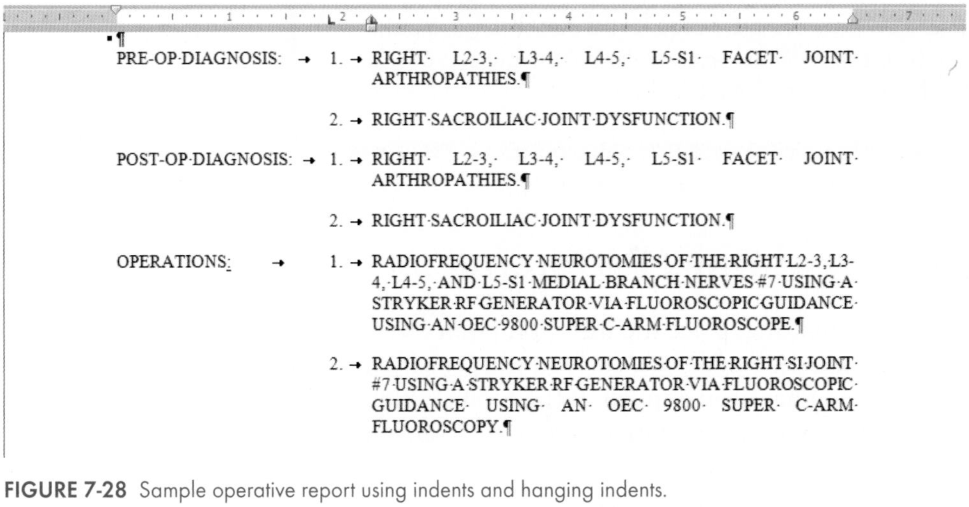
PRE-OP DIAGNOSIS: 1. RIGHT L2-3, L3-4, L4-5, L5-S1 FACET JOINT ARTHROPATHIES.
2. RIGHT SACROILIAC JOINT DYSFUNCTION.
POST-OP DIAGNOSIS: 1. RIGHT L2-3, L3-4, L4-5, L5-S1 FACET JOINT ARTHROPATHIES.
2. RIGHT SACROILIAC JOINT DYSFUNCTION.
OPERATIONS: 1. RADIOFREQUENCY NEUROTOMIES OF THE RIGHT L2-3, L3-4, L4-5, AND L5-S1 MEDIAL BRANCH NERVES #7 USING A STRYKER RF GENERATOR VIA FLUOROSCOPIC GUIDANCE USING AN OEC 9800 SUPER C-ARM FLUOROSCOPE.
2. RADIOFREQUENCY NEUROTOMIES OF THE RIGHT SI JOINT #7 USING A STRYKER RF GENERATOR VIA FLUOROSCOPIC GUIDANCE USING AN OEC 9800 SUPER C-ARM FLUOROSCOPY.

FIGURE 7-28 Sample operative report using indents and hanging indents.

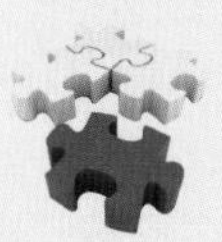

When setting up templates or boilerplates, you can leave paragraph marks (with or without text) in places where you will be transcribing information as the doctor dictates. You can set specific character formatting for a particular spot in the report by setting the insertion point and pressing **CTRL+D**. This will bring up the **Font** dialog box where you can select the appropriate font formatting (eg, the doctor may want allergies typed in bold and all caps). You can do the same thing by applying paragraph formatting to the paragraph mark (press **ALT, O, P** to open the **Paragraph** dialog box). With formatting predefined in your boilerplate or template, you can transcribe an entire report without having to stop to make format changes. See also Chapter 11 for ideas on creating "jumps" to quickly navigate through templates.

Remove Formatting

Every paragraph carries a style definition, even if you don't actually apply a style yourself. By default, Word starts new documents with one paragraph mark carrying the Normal style, and this style is carried throughout the document as you press Enter. Typically, people just add formatting commands on top of the Normal style definition (as opposed to changing formatting by applying a different style). In this case, paragraphs may appear to have different formatting, *but the underlying style is still Normal.* Formatting that is not part of the paragraph's style definition is called **direct formatting**. CTRL+Q will remove any formatting associated with a paragraph that is not part of the paragraph's style definition. CTRL+Spacebar will remove character formatting and return the font to the underlying style of the paragraph.

If you apply the Normal style (CTRL+Shift+N) to a paragraph in your document and the font changes, then you are not working in the default font. Also, if you remove formatting using the shortcut keys described above and the font changes, that's another clue you are not working in the default font. It's always best practice to set the default font to match the primary font to be used in your document. Refer back to page 196 for an explanation of Normal style and the default font.

Troubleshooting Formatting Problems

If you are having problems with formatting, place the insertion point anywhere within the problem text and examine the Horizontal Ruler and the Formatting toolbar/ribbon to see what formatting has been applied. If the toolbars/ribbons and ruler do not reveal enough information, try these tips for diagnosing and fixing formatting problems:

- Press Shift+F1 to display the **Reveal Formatting task pane** (Figure 7-29). Examine the details of the formatting. Click the blue links in the task pane to open the corresponding dialog to adjust the formatting.

- Try removing direct formatting using the shortcut keys CTRL+Q for paragraph formatting and CTRL+Spacebar for character formatting. Click *Distinguish style source* at the bottom of the **Reveal Formatting** task pane to see if direct formatting has been applied.

- Look carefully at the Spacing section of the **Reveal Formatting** task pane. Spacing problems can be created by the *Space after* and *Space before* options. The *Keep with next* option or *Start new page* option can create large white spaces at the bottom of a page (because these commands force text to the next page).

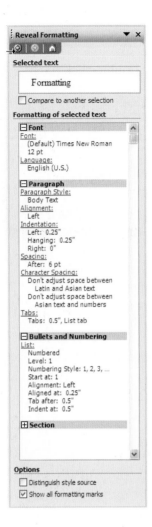

FIGURE 7-29 Use the Reveal Formatting task pane to see all formatting commands applied and to diagnose formatting problems.

- Examine the formatting attributes of the paragraph before and after the problematic paragraph. Spacing commands can make it appear that the problem is in one paragraph when the command is actually originating from the paragraph above or below it.

- Apply the Normal style. Sometimes the easiest fix is to start over by applying the Normal style (**CTRL+Shift+N**) and then reapplying any other formatting commands needed.

- Use Undo. If Word makes an automatic formatting change that you don't want, press **CTRL+Z** as soon as the change occurs to reverse the action.

Page Margins

For a simple one-time change to the page margins, simply drag the edge of the shaded area at each end of the <u>Horizontal</u> and <u>Vertical Ruler</u> to adjust the page margins. You can also set page margins using the **Page Setup** dialog. Follow these steps:

1. Open the **Page Setup** dialog box.
2. Click on Margins (Figure 7-30).

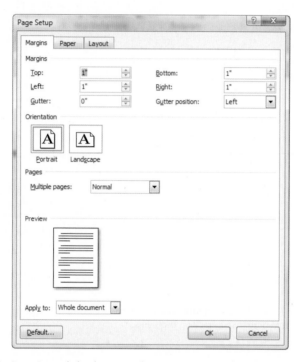

FIGURE 7-30 Use the Page Setup dialog box to set the page margins and to designate default page margins.

3. Type in the margin settings.
4. To make these changes permanent, click the Default button in the lower left corner. Answer Yes to the confirmation box to change all future documents based on the Normal template. If you do not set these as the default values, new documents will revert back to the previous margin settings.
5. To set more than one margin size in a single document, insert a section break and set the margins for each section within the document. Learn more about section breaks below.
6. After inserting a new section, place the cursor in the *new* section and open the **Page Setup** dialog box.

Headers and Footers

Headers are useful for patient reports that exceed one page. The most common use is to place the letterhead in the first-page header and patient demographic information in the header space of subsequent pages. The **header and footer** are treated as separate areas of the document, and text added to the "body" of the

---

Page Setup Dialog Box

Double-click ruler

File > Page Setup
(**ALT, F, U**)

Page Layout >

<u>Page Setup</u>

document does not affect the placement of the text within the header and footer space. Headers contribute to efficiency because patient demographic information at the top of the second (and subsequent) page does not have to be repositioned as the document is transcribed and edited.

When documents are displayed in Print Layout, the header and footer areas appear dimmed. In Normal view or when white space is hidden (see page 127), headers and footers are not displayed at all. Use any of these methods to access the header and footer area:

- Click **ALT, V, H**.
- If the header/footer area is displayed but dimmed, double-click at the very top or bottom of the page to "open" the header and footer. The body of the document will now appear dimmed.
- Use the menu/ribbon. In Word 2003, go to View > Header and Footer. In Word 2007, go to **Insert** > Header and Footer > **Header** > Edit.
- Close the header and footer area by double-clicking in the body of the document, click the **Close** command on the toolbar/ribbon, or repeat the shortcut key **ALT, V, H**.

Once the header and footer area is displayed, Word will display tools for managing the content. Word 2003 displays the Header and Footer toolbar and Word 2007 displays the **Design** tab with **Header and Footer Tools**.

Word 2007 users go to page 227.

Create Different Headers within a Document

By default, a new document has only one header and footer—whatever is typed into the header space will appear on *every page* in the document. To create a report with a different header on the *first* page (eg, the first page has the letterhead and the second page has the patient's name, date of report, and account number), follow these steps:

1. Open the header space.
2. Click the **Page Setup** icon on the Header and Footer toolbar (or click **ALT, F, U**). Figure 7-31 shows a header area displayed along with the Header and Footer toolbar.

(Continued)

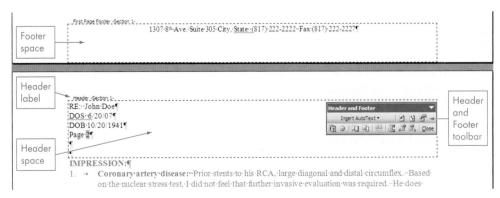

FIGURE 7-31 A sample header and footer with the Header and Footer toolbar floating in the document space.

WORD 2003

3. On the ⎡**Layout**⎤ tab, select *Different first page*. This will tell Word *not* to copy the contents of the first-page header to the second-page header. *This command will apply to the footer as well.*

4. Type the information into the header and footer spaces. Look carefully at the header and footer labels (First Page Header, Header Section 1, First Page Footer, etc) to keep yourself oriented.

5. With *Different First Page* selected, you will need to enter information into both the first-page footer and the second-page footer.

The "first page" refers to the first page of the *document* (if there are no section breaks). The contents of the second-page header will be copied to the remaining headers in the document.

If section breaks are inserted, Word will automatically copy the header information from the first section to all subsequent sections in the same file. The "first-page header" now becomes the first-page header of each *section*. If you do not want to repeat this same header setup in all the sections, click ⎡**Link to Previous**⎤ on the <u>Header and Footer</u> toolbar. The comment "Same as Previous" will disappear from the upper right corner of the header. You will need to repeat this for each section.

Select *Different first page* and ⎡**Same as Previous**⎤ *before* entering text or graphics into the header or footer area. If you add the first-page header and *then* click *Different first page*, the content you just entered in the first-page header will be deleted. Also, removing the Same as Previous designation sometimes deletes content within the header in the previous section. Be sure to double-check all sections using Print Preview (**CTRL+F2**) before printing or returning the report to the client.

Hover the mouse pointer over the Header and Footer toolbar icons to see a ToolTip describing each icon.

Page Numbers and Dates

Simply typing a page number in the header area will copy that same number to the next page header, making all the pages in the document display the same number. You will need to use page number *fields* in a header. Set the insertion point in the header where you would like the page number to appear. Headers and footers automatically have a center and right-aligned tab that are useful for placing page number fields.

Click the Page Number icon (the # sign) to insert a page-number field. To display total pages within the section or the document, click the icon with two plus signs. To format the page numbers (font, number style, etc), select the page number field and then click the third icon.

To insert a preformatted page number into the header space, set the insertion point in the header and open the AutoText drop-down list located on the <u>Header and Footer</u> toolbar. Select an AutoText entry from the list.

Although the Header and Footer tools include fields for inserting the date, date fields are not a good idea in the context of medical transcription. See discussion and warnings for date fields on page 307.

Fields in the header and footer space do not automatically update. If you change information in a header or footer that includes fields, open the header, press **CTRL+A** to select all and press **F9** to force the fields to update.

Word 2003 users to go page 229.

Create Different Headers within a Document

By default, a new document has only one header and footer—whatever is typed into the header space will appear on *every page* of the document. To create a report with a different header on the *first* page (eg, the first page has the clinic letterhead and the second page has the patient's name, date of report, and account number), follow these steps:

1. Open the header space. Click **ALT, V, H** or $\boxed{\text{Insert}}$ > <u>Header and Footer</u> > $\boxed{\text{Header}}$ > Edit. Once the header space is displayed, the ribbon will display the $\boxed{\text{Design}}$ tab with $\boxed{\text{Header and Footer Tools}}$ (see Figure 7-32).

(*Continued*)

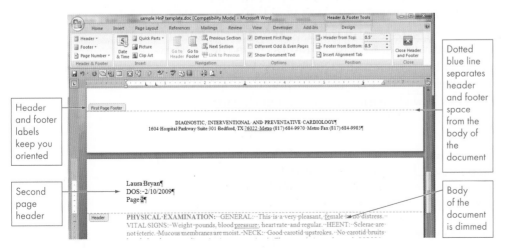

FIGURE 7-32 A sample header and footer space with the Header and Footer Tools displayed.

WORD 2007

2. In the Options group, click Different First Page. This will tell Word *not* to copy the contents of the first-page header to the second-page header. *This command will apply to the footer as well.*

3. Type the information into the header and footer spaces. Look carefully at the header and footer labels (First Page Header, Header Section 1, First Page Footer, etc) to keep yourself oriented.

4. When Different First Page is selected, you will need to enter information into both the first-page footer and the second-page footer.

The "first page" refers to the first page of the *document* (if there are no section breaks). The contents of the second-page header will be copied to the remaining headers in the document.

If section breaks are inserted, Word will automatically copy the header from the first section to all subsequent sections in the same file. The "first-page header" now becomes the first-page header of each *section*. If you do not want to repeat this same header in all the sections, click **Link to Previous** in the Navigation group. The comment "Same as Previous" will disappear from the upper right corner of the header. You will need to repeat this step for each section.

Select Different first page and **Same as Previous** *before* entering text or graphics into the header or footer area. If you add the first-page header and *then* click Different first page the content you just entered in the first-page header will be deleted. Also, removing the Same as Previous designation deletes content within the header in the previous section. Be sure to double-check all sections using Print Preview (**CTRL+F2**) before printing or returning the report to the client.

Page Numbers and Dates

Simply typing a page number in the header area will copy that same number to the next page header, making all the pages in the document the same number. You will need to use page number *fields* in a header. With the header/footer area displayed, click **Page Number** in the Header and Footer group. A drop-down menu of options will appear. Choose an option from the gallery. You may also choose a page number format using Quick Parts. Within the Insert group, click **Quick Parts** > Building Blocks Organizer. Choose an option from the *Page Category* and click **Insert**. Learn more about Quick Parts in Chapter 10.

Although the Header and Footer Tools include fields for inserting the date, date fields are not a good idea in the context of medical transcription. See discussion and warnings for date fields on page 307.

Tips for Working with Headers and Footers (all versions)

To remove all of the text and graphics contained in the header or footer space, place the insertion point in the header or footer and press CTRL+A (select all), Delete. This will not select the entire document—only the contents of the header or footer.

Use Text boxes inside the header/footer space to manage content that is not laid out as straight lines of text. Also, use text boxes to manage content that needs to go outside the boundaries of the header/footer space. Text boxes can actually be placed anywhere on the page, but if placed while the header space is open, the text box will be treated separately from the document content. For example, to create letterhead stationery with a list of names (eg, providers within the same practice) along the side of the document without interfering with page margins, open the header space, insert a text box along the edge of the document and place the names in the text box. Even though the text box is located along the edge of the page, it will be considered part of the header/footer space if it is inserted *while the header is open*. This prevents the text box from interfering with page and paragraph margins. Watch the video on the accompanying CD to learn how to work with text boxes.

If you work with headers and footers extensively, consider assigning shortcut keys to the header and footer commands listed below. See Assigning Shortcut keys on page 394 (Word 2003) and 403 (Word 2007). See also the special project for setting up headers on page 459.

> GoToHeaderFooter
>
> CloseViewHeaderFooter
>
> NormalViewHeaderArea (Opens the header while in Normal view)
>
> ToggleHeaderFooterLink (Removes "Same as previous")
>
> ShowPrevHeaderFooter
>
> ShowNextHeaderFooter
>
> ViewHeader
>
> ViewFooter

Section Breaks

Section breaks allow for different margins, headers, footers, page sizes, and orientations within the same file. Without sections, a page margin setting will apply to every page within the file. Also, without designating sections, the header and footer will appear the same throughout the file. Word offers four types of section breaks:

> *Next page*: This break starts a new section on the next page of the document. It will leave white space on the previous page in order to start the section on a new page.
>
> *Continuous*: This inserts a break on the same page immediately above the insertion point. Continuous breaks are helpful for formatting columns that only take up part of the page, or for changing the margin settings in the middle of a page.

Odd and Even: These breaks begin sections on the following page—odd or even—and may insert a blank page if necessary to start the section on the corresponding odd or even page. Odd page breaks are typically used when formatting books so that a new chapter will always begin on the right-hand page.

Breaks can be viewed on screen by displaying formatting marks. They appear as a horizontal dotted line. Just as paragraph information is stored in the paragraph mark at the end of a paragraph, *section formatting is stored in the section break.* Breaks contain information pertaining to page margins, page size, page orientation (portrait or landscape) as well as header and footer information. Be very careful when deleting section breaks because this will delete the formatting information for the pages *above* the section break.

To insert a section break, open the **Break** dialog box. Select the type of break to be inserted (Figure 7-33). In the context of medical documents, the most likely section break would be a next-page section break. To delete a section break, display formatting marks and set the insertion point above or to the left of the break and press **Delete**.

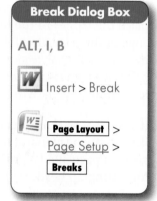

Break Dialog Box

ALT, I, B

Insert > Break

Page Layout >
Page Setup >
Breaks

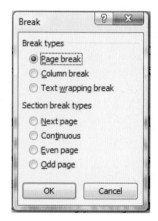

FIGURE 7-33 Select the type of break to insert using the Break dialog box.

  Every document—whether or not a section break has been inserted—has an "invisible" section break stored in the very last paragraph mark, so that means the last paragraph mark in a document contains that paragraph's information as well as information pertaining to the entire document. If a document becomes corrupt, you can sometimes salvage the text by copying the text to a new document, but *omitting the last paragraph mark when selecting the text.* You may have to reformat margins and headers, but at least you will not have to retype the text.

Critical Thinking Questions

1. Explain why an understanding of the paragraph mark is critical to understanding formatting and editing in MS Word. How does Word define a paragraph?

_____

_____

2. What are styles? How do they affect formatting in MS Word? In the context of transcription, what do you need to know about styles?

_____

_____

3. Define the default font and explain how to change it.

_____

_____

4. Describe alignment and indention. Can a paragraph have both an indent and a hanging indent?

_____

_____

5. Describe the most common paragraph formats used in healthcare reports and give their corresponding shortcut keys.

_____

_____

6. What is the difference between line spacing and spacing before and after?

_____

_____

7. Format the following:

 a. H_2O

 b. CO_2

 c. hemoglobin A_{1c}

 d. FEV_1

 e. Lead aV_R

 f. ^{123}I

 g. cm^2

8. Type the following paragraph using nonbreaking spaces between titles and surnames and also within the medication dose to keep dose and form together (ie, 30 mg). Use a nonbreaking hyphen between the hyphenated surnames. After typing, insert enough spaces or dummy text to test your nonbreaking punctuation.

Dr. Smith ordered the following medications for Mrs. Jones-Harvey: Prevacid 30 mg, ibuprofen 200 mg. Mr. Harvey will help Mrs. Jones-Harvey return to the clinic next week for a followup appointment.

9. Turn off Automatic numbered lists and disable Set left and first indent with tabs and backspaces. Format the following report section using shortcut keys to properly format the indents and hanging indents.

Axis I:
1. Adjustment disorder with mixed anxiety and depressed mood (309.28), chronic.
2. Psychosocial factors having an adverse affect on ability to respond to medical treatment.

Axis II: No Diagnosis

Axis III: Obtained from medical record:
1. Lumbar radiculopathy, chronic, status post lumbar interbody fusion at L4-L5.
2. Lumbar facet syndrome, chronic, status post steroid injections X2.

Axis IV: No diagnosis.

Axis V: Current GAF = 60. Highest GAF in the Past Year = 65.

10. Turn off Automatic numbered lists and disable Set left and first indent with tabs and backspaces. Format the following SOAP note using shortcut keys to properly format the indents and hanging indents.

S: The patient returns today for further evaluation of fatigue, nausea, vomiting and general malaise. Since her last visit, she has improved only slightly with the use of Phenergan.

O: Today she is in no acute distress. Blood pressure is 130/80, pulse 80, respirations 16, temperature 99.0°. No abdominal masses. Right upper quadrant tenderness unchanged since last visit.

A:
1. Gastroenteritis following recent travel outside the country. Suspect viral etiology.
2. Peptic ulcer disease.
3. Hypertension, controlled on current medication.

P:
1. Continue to push fluids with strict bed rest. RICE diet for 3 days and then advance as tolerated.
2. Phenergan p.r.n.
3. Return to clinic in 1 week.

CHAPTER 8

Templates

OBJECTIVES

▶ Recognize the role of the Normal.dot file.

▶ Create and use document templates to streamline routine work.

▶ Modify a document template.

▶ Modify the Normal.dot file.

▶ Use the Organizer to copy items between templates (Word 2003).

KEYWORDS

Organizer

global templates

document templates

standard text

Templates folder

Normal.dot

Introduction to Templates

As you learned in Chapter 2, applications use program data files to store information required to run the program. These program data files also supply information about how you prefer to use the program. MS Word has several of these files, the most important of which is the **Normal.dot**. Every time you open Word, you also open a copy of the Normal.dot file—it happens automatically and invisibly. The information in the Normal.dot file is so vital that Word cannot function without it.

You may have already noticed that your documents always open with the same font and margins—no matter how many times you reset them. This is because Word is using the default settings stored in the Normal.dot. The Normal.dot file stores the default font setting, the default paragraph style (Normal style), the default page margin settings, customized toolbars and shortcut keys, and many other preferences. When you open a new document in Word, it always looks the same as the last new document you created because Word is using the information stored in the Normal.dot file to determine how the document appears.

There are quite a few templates already loaded on your computer, as you will see when you open the Template dialog box. They are sorted into categories such as General, Letters, Faxes, and Memos. To see document templates in action, select File > New. Choose On my computer and double-click an icon. Open several templates and see how each file opens with different standard text, graphics, margins, etc.

There are quite a few templates already loaded on your computer, as you will see when you open the New Document dialog box. To see document templates in action, click **Office** > New. Double-click one of the template icons. Open several templates and see how each file opens with different standard text, graphics, margins, etc.

Every time you make a choice about how to use a program (eg, click an option in a dialog box), the computer has to store that information somewhere on your computer. It just so happens that a lot of that information for MS Word is stored in the Normal.dot file.

The Normal.dot file also works as a template file, and is referred to as a global template. **Global templates** supply information to Word all the time and contribute information to *every* document you create. In addition to the global template (Normal.dot), Word can also use **document templates**. These files store information to help create a specific type of document. For example, you can have a template file for creating a fax cover sheet, a letter using company stationery, or a particular type of report. The document template will store information about the font, paragraph styles, page margins, etc, *for that specific type of document*. In the context of transcription, you can create a document template for each type of report (or work type) you routinely create.

In addition to saving specific settings like the font and margins for a given document type, templates can also contain standard text—that is, text that appears in most or all documents of that type. When a document is opened using a template file, the standard text is already contained within the document, ready to be edited as needed. Templates can also store AutoText entries, macros, and even customized toolbars and shortcut keys that are only used when that particular template file is active.

If you type for several doctors or facilities and they each prefer a different font, page margin, and other settings, you do not have to change these settings back and forth each time you "switch gears." You simply open a document based on the doctor's template, and his preferences, headings, and report layout are automatically loaded.

It is common practice among MTs to create a document with margins, report headings, subheadings, and standard text already set so that transcribing is similar to filling in a form. This "base" document is used as a starter for all new reports of that type. Using this approach, you open the document and immediately use Save As to rename the file, so that your base document is preserved and you have a new document with a different name in which to transcribe the report. The biggest drawback to this approach, as veteran MTs will attest, is it is easy to accidentally transcribe new patient information into the base document and click Save instead of Save As. This essentially "contaminates" your base document.

Template files in Word use the same concept of creating a base document as a starter for all new documents of that type, but document templates (dot files) cannot be accidentally changed. When you create a new document *based on a template file*, the information in the template is essentially *copied* to the new document, so the template itself is protected from inadvertent changes to the standard text. Text in the new document can be edited or even completely deleted without affecting the text within the template file. There are many more advantages to using template files that will come to light as you work through this chapter.

The Normal Template

The Normal.dot is *always* active. Simply opening Word starts a new document based on the information saved in the Normal.dot file. Document templates are only used when you specifically open a document based on that template. When you use a document template, the Normal.dot and the document template are both providing instructions to Word, but if the instructions differ between the two, the document template overrides the Normal. For example, if your Normal.dot has a default font of Times New Roman but you open a document based on a template with Arial as the default font, Word will use Arial.

Templates (dot files) store:

- Page setup: Paper size, orientation, and margins
- **Standard text**: Text that appears in most/all documents of that type
- AutoText: Shortcuts for inserting text that is unique to that type of document (eg, common phrases, paragraphs, or sections such as the review of systems or physical exam)
- Default font settings and Styles: Type and size specific to that report type (eg, a specific provider or facility)
- Toolbars and menus: Custom toolbars and instructions for displaying them
- Key assignments: Custom key commands/shortcut keys
- Macro project items: Macros for tasks specific to that type of document

Unless you specify, the above items are automatically stored in the Normal.dot and are available to all documents. If you are working with a document template, any of these items can be stored in that particular template file and those settings will apply only when that template is being used. As you work through this chapter and the remainder of the book, you will learn how to designate a template for storing each of the above items.

Templates can also be found online on the Microsoft Templates website. This site contains templates for use in all the Office applications (PowerPoint and Excel use their own version of template files). Some are created by Microsoft and some are uploaded by individuals willing to share their work. These templates are helpful for creating brochures, flyers, basic contracts, calendars, and other business-related documents.

Safeguarding the Normal Template

Anytime a file is open on your computer, it is liable to become corrupt, especially if there is a power failure or power surge. Since the Normal.dot opens every time Word opens, it is always at a slight risk of becoming damaged. Unfortunately, a damaged Normal.dot file can cause Word to behave strangely. Some features may not work correctly or a command may produce unexpected results. It is important to keep a backup of the Normal.dot and other template files you create in case your hard drive crashes or for some reason the files become corrupt. Follow instructions for backing up this file on page 98. See file locations for each version of Word on pages 71-72.

Word always keeps a "native" copy of the Normal.dot so if for any reason it cannot find the Normal.dot in the exact location specified in the **File Locations** dialog (see page 150 in Word 2003 and page 174 in Word 2007), it will build another Normal.dot to replace the file it cannot find. By default, the Normal.dot and other user templates are stored in the **Templates folder**. Preloaded templates supplied by Microsoft are located in a different folder (depending on the version of Word).

An easy way to access the Templates folder is to type %AppData% in the Address bar of Windows Explorer. This will take you directly to the **Application Data** folder where you will find the Microsoft folder which contains the **Templates** subfolder.

Keep your Normal.dot file backed up routinely! This simply cannot be overstressed. The Normal.dot file will become corrupt—it's not a matter of *if* but *when*. With a recent backup, you will be able to reload your Normal.dot file and be back up and running in a matter of minutes instead of hours or even days.

If Word suddenly changes behavior, and a function or feature is not acting the same as it always has, there is a good chance the Normal.dot has become corrupt. You may never know what caused the Normal.dot to become damaged, and it can be as sudden as "fine this morning, broken after lunch."

Create a Document Template

Creating templates is very easy and will save you a tremendous amount of time and even frustration. One of the most important reasons for creating a template is to use a different font than the one assigned to the Normal.dot. Creating a new template with its own default font will save you a lot of headaches when it comes to formatting. Of course, you can change the default font for the Normal.dot at any time, but if you use two or three different fonts routinely, you might as well create templates for each font. Word was designed to be used with templates, so many of the features and a lot of Word's functionality work best when template files are used. Follow these steps to create a new document template:

1. Start with a blank document or open a document that already contains standard text that you want to appear in your new template.

2. Press **F12** to open the **Save As** dialog box (Figure 8-1).

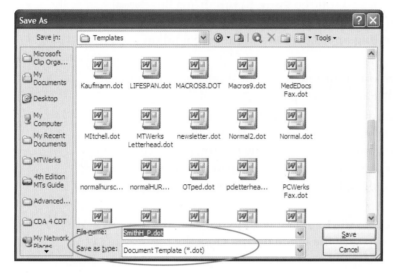

FIGURE 8-1 To create a document template, change the Save as type to Document Template (*.dot).

3. In the *Save as type* box, choose *Document Template (*.dot)*. In the *File name* box, type a name for the new template and then click **Save**. Use whatever file name will help you remember the template's purpose.

4. When you select *Document Template* in the **Save As** dialog box, the folder in the **Save in** box will change to the **Templates** folder. It is important that you save your template in this folder (or a subfolder of the **Templates** folder) so Word will display this template's icon in the **Templates** dialog box.

Now that you have created a new template file, it's time to memorize specifications related to this type of document. This template file will look just like a document and you can edit it just like a document. But remember, it is a template file (note the file name on the <u>Title</u> bar). Make the following changes to the template file:

1. Set the margin settings and click **Default** in the **Page Setup** dialog box (**ALT, F, U** or double-click the margin area of the ruler to open **Page Setup**). Word will confirm that you want to make this a default setting for all new documents based on the current template. Answer **Yes**.

2. Set the font face and size (**CTRL+D**) and be sure to click **Default** in the bottom left corner of the **Font** dialog box. Word will confirm that you want to make this a default setting for all new documents based on the current template. Answer **Yes**.

(Continued)

WORD 2003

3. Add the standard text that you want to appear in all new documents based on this template. Be sure to apply as much paragraph formatting as you possibly can so you won't have to format paragraphs while transcribing.

4. Set up the headers and footers in the template file. If the report type is likely to go to the second page, insert a (temporary) page break (**CTRL+Enter**) in order to view the second-page header. Open the header space (**ALT, V, H**).

5. If there will be different headers on the first page compared to subsequent pages, click *Different first page* on the **Page Setup** dialog box `Layout` tab. Insert the letterhead, if applicable, in the first page header space. (Detailed information on setting up headers and footers is found on page 222.)

6. Insert page number fields or other information that should appear in the header and footer on the first and second pages.

7. After establishing the first and second page headers and footers, delete the temporary page break. Even though you have deleted the page break from the template file, Word will "remember" how to format the second page if the actual transcribed document exceeds the first page. Learn how to automatically update demographic information in the second-page header on page 460.

8. After you have made changes to the template settings and added the standard text, press **CTRL+S** to save the template and close the file (**CTRL+W**).

In the future, to make changes to the standard text contained in the template file, you will need to open the actual template file itself (see below). You can make changes to template settings (as in the case of styles, AutoText, macros, toolbars, and shortcuts) while working on a document based on the template. This will be explained in the chapters related to these topics.

Page 30 explains how you can display file extensions for known file types. With this option selected, the file extension will be displayed with the file name in the <u>Title</u> bar. Displaying file extensions will help you distinguish between documents and templates, especially when you first start using template (dot) files.

Create a document template for each report type you use. Each template can contain standard headings, header and footer information, the signature line, etc. It will also establish the font and margins, and memorize specific AutoText entries for words, phrases, or "normals" that are unique to that doctor as well as any macros that might be needed for that report type. If there is more than one transcriptionist working on the same account, distribute this document template to each MT. This will create consistency for all reports of this type and increase overall efficiency.

If you type multiple reports in a single file, place enough copies of the boilerplate into your template file, one after the other, until you have enough copies for a typical day of dictation. When you open a document based on this template, you will have all your reports set up and ready to type. For example, if the doctor typically dictates ten history and physical reports each day, place ten copies of the history and physical boilerplate into your template. Keep a copy of the boilerplate saved as an AutoText entry just in case you need to insert additional copies on days when more than the usual number of reports is dictated.

Create a Document Based on a Template

To create a document based on a particular template, begin by opening Word. By default, Word will open with a document based on the Normal template. You can close this blank document using **CTRL+F4** or **CTRL+W**. Follow these steps:

1. Open the **New Document** task pane (**ALT, F, N** or File > New). See Figure 8-2.

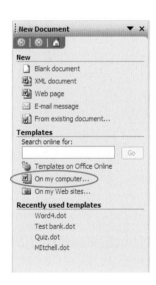

FIGURE 8-2 The New Document task pane allows you to choose templates on your computer or from other locations.

2. On the **New Document** task pane, under *Templates*, select *On my computer*. This will open the **Templates** dialog box as shown in Figure 8-3.

3. If necessary, switch to a different tab (representing a different category of templates) on the **Templates** dialog box.

4. Double-click the template icon or press the first character of the template name to jump directly to that template and press **Enter**.

5. Word will open a new document using the information that is stored in that template (note the Title bar will say Document).

6. Press **CTRL+S** or File > Save and name your document as you normally would.

(Continued)

WORD 2003

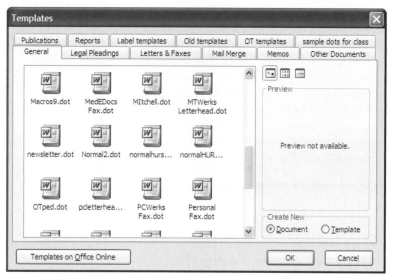

FIGURE 8-3 The Templates dialog box displays an icon for each template available on your computer.

The **New Document** task pane, as shown in Figure 8-2, can be helpful when you are first learning to use Word, but once you know your way around, it can be just one more step to go through. To bypass the task pane and go straight to the **New** dialog box, add the New Dialog command to the File menu, a toolbar, or assign a shortcut key. The command name is FileNewDialog and is found under *All Commands* in the **Customize** dialog box. See Chapter 15 for detailed instructions.

Creating a new document based on a template is fairly quick once you get the hang of it, but if you create many documents a day, these extra keystrokes can add up. To make it faster to start a new document based on a specific template, record a macro to do it for you. Assign the macro to a shortcut key or to a button on the toolbar. See Chapter 12 for specific instructions on recording macros.

Modify Document Templates

To modify the standard text, the document view, or the zoom setting within a template, you need to open the actual template file. Follow these steps to modify the standard text, zoom, or document view:

1. Using the **Open** dialog box (CTRL+O), navigate to the folder containing your templates. Follow the tip below under Putting It Together for easily locating the **Templates** folder.

WORD 2003

2. Choose the template name and click **Open**. Word's Title bar should display the name of your template—*not* Document.

3. Make changes to the standard text, the zoom setting, or the document view. If you change the zoom setting or the document view, you must also make one other change to the file such as typing a word and then deleting that same word—anything that causes Word to detect an actual change to the file.

4. Press **CTRL+S** and close the template file (**CTRL+W**).

Now you can open a document based on that template and see the modified text, and/or the new zoom setting. If you changed the document view (eg, from Normal to Page Layout), documents based on that template will now open in the new document view. The content of *existing* documents is *not affected* by changes you make to the templates on which they are based. Other types of changes, such as changes to the default font, default page margins, AutoText entries, macros, etc, can be made while working with documents that have been opened using the template.

The **Templates** folder can be tedious to locate using the **Open** dialog box. To make it easier, try this: Open the **Save As** dialog box and change the *Files of type* to *Document templates (*.dot)*. This will automatically place the **Template** folder in the *Look in* box. Click Tools > Add to 'My Places'. This will place a link to the **Templates** folder on the Places bar that runs along the left-hand side of the **Open** and **Save As** dialog boxes. Now, whenever you need to access files in the **Templates** folder, simply click the button on the Places bar and the **Templates** folder will be selected in the *Look in* or *Save in* box.

Remember, the *Templates dialog box* will not open a template—only a document *based* on a template. You cannot use the **Template** dialog box to open or back up your template files; you must open the template using the **Open** dialog box.

Modify the Normal Template

If you would prefer that all new documents (not otherwise based on a document template) open with the zoom setting higher or lower than the current setting, you need to modify the Normal.dot itself. Follow these steps (but be very, very careful when making changes to the Normal.dot file in this way):

1. Close Word.

2. Using Windows Explorer, open the **Templates** folder (`%AppData%`, **Microsoft > Templates**).

3. *Right-click* on the Normal.dot file to open the shortcut menu and choose Open (do not double-click the Normal.dot file, as this will open a

(*Continued*)

WORD 2003

document, not the actual Normal.dot). Word will open and the <u>Title</u> bar should read Normal.dot.

4. Change the zoom setting and change the document view if you prefer.

5. Carefully type one word and then delete that one word. Word must detect some change in the file in order to save changes to the zoom and view settings. Be careful not to leave any text remaining in the template file; otherwise, every new document will open with that text.

6. Click **CTRL+S** to save the changes and close the template. Close and reopen Word as you normally do.

> You can change any of your templates (not just the Normal.dot) using the above method of accessing templates directly through the **Template** folder. Place a shortcut to your **Templates** folder on your Desktop (see page 103) to make it easier to access all your templates.

Manage Templates with the Organizer

Macros, AutoText entries, styles, and custom toolbars are stored in templates. You will learn how to save these items into separate templates in the corresponding chapters. To back up these elements, back up your template file. If you have created any one of these elements and want to make it available in another template, or even delete it altogether, you can copy and delete elements using the **Organizer** dialog box (Figure 8-4).

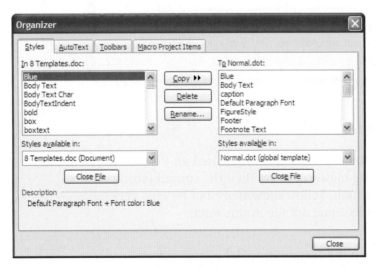

FIGURE 8-4 Use the Organizer to copy or delete specific elements such as AutoText, styles, and custom toolbars between two template files.

To copy elements between templates, follow these steps:

1. To access the Organizer, press **ALT+F8** and click `Organizer`. The **Organizer** consists of tabs for each of the features that are stored in templates: `Styles`, `Macro Project Items`, `Toolbars`, and `AutoText` entries. On each tab, there are two panes. The panes list the individual entries for each category contained within the template file currently displayed in the *Available in* box directly below it.

2. To move items between templates, each template needs to be displayed in one of the panes in the **Organizer**. To change the template displayed in the *Available in* box, use the `Close File` button. The `Close File` buttons are actually toggle buttons. Click once to change the button to `Open File`. Click `Open File` to bring up the **Open** dialog box and select the template name that you want to appear in the *Available in* box.

3. With each template displayed in one of the panes, select an item to copy. Once an item is selected, the `Copy` button will be available (between the two panes) and the copy arrows will point in the direction of the other template (ie, the direction the item will move). Hold down **CTRL** while selecting nonconsecutive entries or hold down **Shift** while clicking the first and last entries to select a range of entries to be copied at once.

4. Use this dialog to copy or delete Styles, AutoText entries, or Toolbars. Learn more about copying Macro Project Items in Chapter 12.

Attach a Template to a Document

Even if you do not start a document based on a specific template, you can still "attach" any template to a document after you have already created the document. This can be helpful if you have a template that contains a macro or a set of styles that you want to use within the current document. You can also attach templates to files that were created by someone else, so you can access some of your favorite tools while working in that file. To attach any template to a document, follow these steps:

1. With the document open, go to Tools > Templates and Add-Ins (**ALT, T, I**).

2. Under *Document Template*, click `Attach` (see Figure 8-5). The **Open** dialog box will appear.

3. Select the template name from the **Open** dialog box and click `Open`.

4. If the template you are attaching contains style definitions that you want available in the current document, click *Automatically update document styles* (see warning below).

5. Click `OK` to close the box.

You can only attach one template file at a time, but you can add and remove template files as needed. To remove a template file, simply open the **Templates and Add-ins** dialog box and delete the template name and the path from the box.

WORD 2003

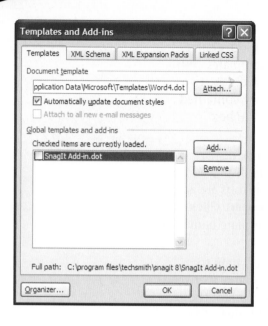

FIGURE 8-5 The Templates and Add-ins dialog allows you to attach a different template file to the current document, giving you access to macros, styles, and other customizations stored in the template file.

Automatically Update Styles

Styles have the ability to update based on the current definition of the style. This means you can open a document created on a different computer or with a different template and the formatting can be updated using the *current definitions* of the styles. If the document you are working on has style definitions that are different than the template you are attaching *and* the styles have the same name (eg, the Normal style in the current document is Times New Roman and the Normal style in the attached template is Arial), the document can be reformatted using the definition of the styles in the *attached* template. To update styles, check *Automatically update template styles* in the **Templates and Add-ins** dialog box. In previous versions of Word, this setting was active (by default), and it caused a tremendous amount of grief because documents created on another computer would be reformatted automatically when opened on a different computer.

If you open a document with the option to automatically update styles (whether it is already checked or you make that selection after opening the document), and the entire document reformats with a different font, immediately remove the check mark from the **Templates and Add-ins** dialog, close the dialog and then press **CTRL+Z** (Edit > Undo). The font will return to the original style definitions.

If you are using Word 2003 and receive documents created in Word 2007, you may encounter problems with the different style definitions used in the two versions of Word. Unless the user has changed the definition, the Normal style in Word 2007 uses the font Callibri and sets the line spacing at 1.15 with a space after of 10 points. To quickly and easily update these documents to reflect the Normal style used in Word 2003 (Times New Roman, single spacing with no space after), open the **Templates and Add-ins** dialog box and click *Automatically update document styles*. The document will be transformed to match the definition of the Normal style on your computer.

Global Templates

It is possible to have more than one global template. Of course, the Normal.dot must always be running, but it is possible to have additional global templates. You can attach a global template using the **Templates and Add-ins** dialog box. Click the Add button and select the template to be used as a global template. This template will remain available to all documents until you specifically remove it using the **Templates and Add-ins** dialog box.

You can also place templates in the Word Startup folder (in the Microsoft folder under **Word / Startup**), which will cause the template to be treated as a global template and will automatically be used every time Word is opened. Global templates are typically used to supply macros, styles, customized toolbars, menus, or other functionality that might be required to work with a specific company's software. In addition, some programs that are designed to work in conjunction with Word may add functionality to Word using a global template. Examples include third-party dictionaries, references, and utilities. If a program has added functionality (eg, a toolbar) that you no longer need, look in the **Templates and Add-ins** dialog to see if there is a global template added. If so, navigate to the **Startup** folder for Word and move the template out of that folder (select the template name in the *Global templates and add-ins* box and look for the path at the bottom of the **Templates and Add-ins** dialog box).

Tips for Using Templates

Templates can actually be stored anywhere on your computer, but only templates in the **Templates** folder will appear in the **Templates** dialog box. To use a template stored in a different location, open the folder containing the template file and double-click the file. A new *document* will open based on that template.

Templates stored outside the **Templates** folder may not automatically load macros contained in the template. Depending on your security settings (see page 148), the macros may be automatically disabled, or you may be presented with the option to enable them at the time you open a document based on that template. To avoid this problem, store the template in the **Templates** folder, where macros are assumed to be safe.

If you use a lot of templates, you may choose to sort the templates into various categories. To create new tabs on the **Templates** dialog box, create new folders within the **Templates** folder. Using Windows Explorer, browse to the **Templates** folder (type `%AppData%` in the <u>Address</u> bar and choose **Microsoft / Templates**). Create new subfolders and drag template files into these folders to sort. The folder name will become the tab name in the **Templates** dialog box.

If someone sends you a template file as an attachment to email, and you know the file to be safe, then save the file to the Templates folder without opening. Do not open the file and use the Save As command to move the file to the **Templates** folder.

WORD 2003

Troubleshoot Templates

Below are common questions related to templates.

Q: Why does Word ask me to save changes to the Normal.dot and how do I answer?

A: Upon closing Word, you may be asked to save changes to the Normal.dot file, and you may be confused about how to answer this question. Since the Normal.dot is used to save various elements (eg, AutoText, formatted AutoCorrect entries, macros, style definitions, custom toolbars and menus, as well as some options) the file changes when any of the above elements have been changed. If you have knowingly made changes to any of these elements, you will want to save these changes when you close the Word session. When presented with the message, as in Figure 8-6, answer Yes. If you are not aware of having made changes to your template, you might consider answering No, as the "change" may actually result in a corrupted Normal.dot file.

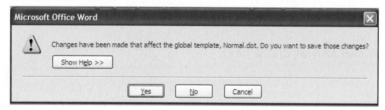

FIGURE 8-6 When changes have been made to the Normal.dot file, Word will ask if you want to save changes.

Q: Why do I get the message "File in Use by Another User"?

A: When you open a file, the computer moves many files into RAM. Word requires many program data files to open in order to function (eg, reference files called DLLs, the Normal.dot, the AutoCorrect list). When you close Word, the information is moved from RAM back to the hard disk. If Word closes abruptly due to an error or improper shutdown, some files may remain in RAM. Files in RAM are considered to be "in use" as far as Windows is concerned. For MS Word, the Normal.dot file and the current file are the most likely files to be left in RAM after an improper shutdown, and they are also the most likely files to become corrupt.

If your computer is having problems that cause Word to shut down (techies call this "ab-end" for abnormal end), Word probably left copies of the current file and the Normal.dot in RAM. When you try to access the file you were working on (when Word shutdown), Word tells you the file is "in use" by another user, as shown in Figure 8-7.

If you are encountering the above problem, then it is likely you are also having problems saving AutoText entries, AutoCorrect entries, macros, and shortcuts stored in the Normal.dot file. When Normal.dot is left open in RAM due to an improper shutdown, Word creates another copy of the Normal.dot when Word

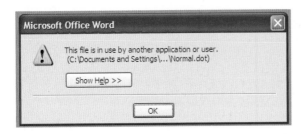

FIGURE 8-7 When more than one copy of the Normal.dot or any other file is still in RAM, Word will present this error message.

is re-opened. After restarting and later closing Word (following an abnormal shutdown), you may be asked to save the Normal.dot using a different file name. As you have probably discovered, Windows will not allow you to save it as "Normal.dot" because the original Normal.dot is still "open" in RAM from the first ab-end. Here's the rub: if you rename the Normal.dot at this point, then Word no longer recognizes the file as *the* Normal.dot, so this file will not be used the next time you open Word. If you bail out of the **Save As** dialog box and do not save this second copy of the Normal.dot, the changes are not saved at all. In either case, any newly created macros, AutoText entries, and other shortcuts are "missing" the next time you open Word.

If you find yourself in that endless loop when Word asks you if you want to save the Normal.dot and the only way out is to type a new file name in the **Save As** dialog box, rename the Normal by appending a number to it (eg, Normal1.dot). To recover any shortcuts or macros created in the Normalx.dot that was just renamed, use the **Organizer** to copy the items from the renamed Normal to the original Normal. You can also recreate the entries, whichever is easier.

There is a way to avoid the above situation. When Word shuts down abnormally, before re-opening Word, check the Task Manager. Press **CTRL+ALT+Del** and choose **Task Manager**. Switch to the **Processes** tab and look for WINWORD on the list of processes (Figure 8-8). If listed (yet Word is closed), select WINWORD and then click **End Task**. Confirm that you do want to end the program (Windows will warn you that you may lose unsaved information, but if Word is "supposedly" closed, there's no information to lose). Press **Esc** to close the dialog box and then re-open Word. See also information on recovering documents on page 75.

Q: When saving my work, I can't change the file type from Document template to Word document.

A: If you are working with the actual template file open (not a document based on a template), you do not want to change the file type to a document. This is the point of using a template file—to protect information in the file. If you attempt to change a template file type to a document file type, you will receive the message displayed in Figure 8-9. This message is meant to remind you that the file will no longer be a template file and will not contain customizations that were stored in the template file, since documents cannot store certain types of customizations the way templates can. Close the template and open a document based on the template. If you would like to duplicate the template file, use Save As and keep the template file type and give the duplicate template a new file name.

WORD 2003

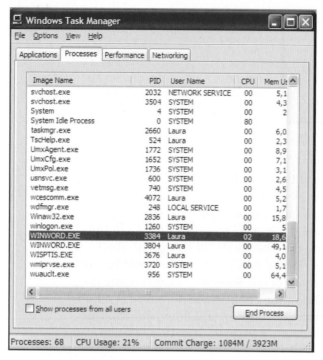

FIGURE 8-8 The Processes tab of the Task Manager showing multiple copies of Winword (Word).

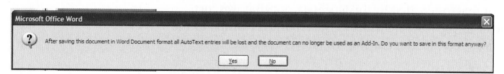

FIGURE 8-9 Word will warn you before changing a template file to a document.

WORD 2007

Q: Can I use templates from earlier versions of Word?

A: Yes, templates are compatible across all versions of Word. If you upgrade Word on the same computer that ran a previous version, the previous templates are moved to a folder named "Old Office Templates" and the templates that installed with previous versions of Word are stored there. Templates *that you have created yourself* will remain in the **Templates** folder and will be available in the **Templates** dialog box as before.

Word 2007 Templates

Word 2007 has slightly modified the template file extensions in the same way the document extensions have been changed. A document template in Word 2007 that has macros enabled will have the extension `dotm`. Templates without macros enabled will have the extension `dotx`. The Normal template in Word 2007 is actually named Normal.dotm. The designation is designed to distinguish templates that have active macros. Word 2007 is still capable of using templates from previous versions of Word and can even open templates with the dot extension, but not all the features in Word 2007 will be functional. When you open a document based on a template created in Word 97 through 2003, Compatibility Mode will be displayed in the <u>Title</u> bar. (See information on converting your templates from previous versions of Word to Word 2007 format on page 477.)

When you first use Word 2007, you will not find a Normal.dotm file. Each time you open the program, Word will build a Normal.dotm file that is functional during that session of Word. When you close Word, that Normal.dotm file is discarded. The file does not persist until you make an actual change to your Normal.dotm file. Examples of changes might include a new AutoText entry saved to the Normal.dotm, a change to an existing style definition, or a change to the default font, paragraph, or page margin settings. When you make one of these types of changes and close Word, the Normal.dotm is saved and will be stored in the **Templates** folder. If you are prompted to save changes to the Normal.dotm file, answer **Yes**.

Create a Document Template

Creating templates is very easy and will save you a tremendous amount of time and even frustration. One of the most important reasons for creating a template is to use a different font than the one assigned to the Normal.dotm. Creating a new template with its own default font will save you a lot of headaches when it comes to formatting. Of course, you can change the default font for the Normal.dotm at any time, but if you use two or three different fonts routinely, you might as well create templates for each font. Word was designed to be used with templates, so many of the features and a lot of Word's functionality work best when template files are used. Follow these steps to create a new document template:

1. Start with a blank document or open a document that already contains standard text that you want to appear in your new template.

2. Press **F12** to open the **Save As** dialog box.

3. In the *Save as type* box, choose *Document Template (*.dotm)*.

4. Make sure the folder location in the **Save As** dialog box reads **Templates**. In Windows XP, click **Trusted Templates** in the <u>Places</u> bar. In Windows Vista, you will need to click the link to the **Templates** folder located under Favorite Links in the **Office Save As** dialog box (see Figure 8-10).

5. In the *File name* box, type a name for the new template. Name the template using the name of the clinic, report type, or the dictator's name—whatever name helps you remember the file's purpose.

WORD 2007

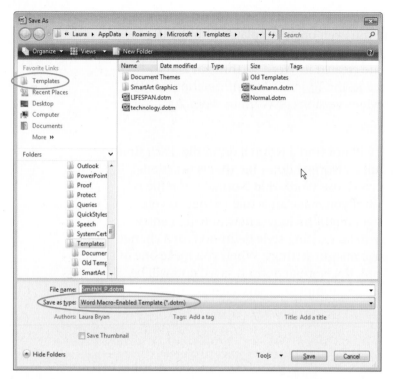

FIGURE 8-10 To create a template file, save a document with the file type *.dotm and store the file in the Templates folder.

Now that you have created a new template file, it's time to memorize specifications related to this type of document. This template file will look just like a document and you can edit it just like a document. But remember, it is a template file (note the file name on the <u>Title</u> bar). Make the following changes to the template file:

1. Set the margin settings and click **Default** in the **Page Setup** dialog box (double-click the margin area of the ruler to open **Page Setup**). Word will confirm that you want to make this a default setting for all new documents based on the current template. Answer **Yes**.

2. Set the font face and size (**CTRL+D**) and be sure to click **Default** in the bottom left corner of the **Font** dialog box. Word will confirm that you want to make this a default setting for all new documents based on the current template. Answer **Yes**.

3. Add the standard text that you want to appear in all new documents based on this template. Be sure to apply as much paragraph formatting as you possibly can so you won't have to format paragraphs while transcribing.

4. Set up the headers and footers in the template file. If the report type is likely to go to the second page, insert a (temporary) page break (**CTRL+Enter**) in order to view the second-page header. Open the header space (**ALT, V, H** or double-click within the header space).

5. If there will be different headers on the first page compared to subsequent pages, click *Different first page*. Insert the letterhead, if applicable, in the first-page header space.

6. Insert page-number fields or other information that should appear in the header and footer on the first and second pages.

7. After establishing the first- and second-page headers and footers, delete the temporary page break. Even though you have deleted the page break from the template file, Word will "remember" how to format the second page if the actual transcribed document exceeds the first page. Learn how to automatically update demographic information in the second-page header on page 460.

8. After you have made changes to the template settings and added the standard text, press **CTRL+S** to save the template and close the file (**CTRL+W**).

In the future, to make changes to the standard text contained in the template file, you will need to open the actual template file itself (see page 253). You can make changes to template settings (as in the case of AutoText, macros, and shortcuts) while working on a document based on the template. This will be explained in the chapters related to these topics.

Page 30 explains how you can display file extensions for known file types. With this option selected, the file extension will be displayed with the file name in the <u>Title</u> bar. Displaying file types will help you distinguish between documents and templates, especially when you first start using template (*.dotm) files.

Create a document template for each report type you use. Each template can contain standard headings, header and footer information, the signature line, etc. It will also establish the font and margins, and memorize specific AutoText entries for words, phrases, or "normals" that are unique to that doctor as well as any macros that might be needed for that report type. If there is more than one transcriptionist working on the same account, distribute this document template to each MT. This will create consistency for all reports of this type and increase overall efficiency.

If you type multiple reports in a single file, place enough copies of the boilerplate into your template file, one after the other, until you have enough copies for a typical day of dictation. When you open a document based on this template, you will have all your reports set up and ready to type. For example, if the doctor typically dictates 10 history and physical reports each day, place ten copies of the history and physical boilerplate into your template. Keep a copy of the boilerplate saved as an AutoText entry just in case you need to insert additional copies on days when more than the usual number of reports is dictated.

WORD 2007

Create a Document Based on a Template

To create a document based on a template you have created, begin by opening Word. By default, Word will open with a document based on the Normal template. You can close this blank document using **CTRL+F4** or **CTRL+W**. Follow these steps:

1. Open the **Template** dialog box (**ALT, F, N** or **Office** > New) as shown in Figure 8-11.

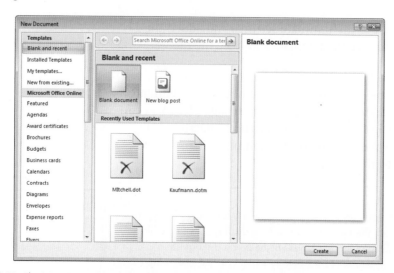

FIGURE 8-11 The New Document dialog box displays various categories of templates that are available on your computer or on Office Online.

2. Choose *My Templates*. Word will open a second dialog box, as shown in Figure 8-12, with your personal templates listed. Double-click the template's icon or click the alpha character to select a template and press **Enter**.

3. Word will open a new document using the information that is stored in that template (note: the <u>Title</u> bar will say Document).

4. Press **CTRL+S** or **Office** > Save and name your document as you normally would. Now you are ready to transcribe.

The **New Document** dialog box as shown in Figure 8-11 may be helpful when you are first learning to use Word, but once you know your way around, it can be just one more step to go through. To bypass the dialog box and go straight to the **New** dialog box (shown in Figure 8-12), assign a shortcut key to the command *FileNewDialog* under *All Commands* in the **Customize** dialog box. See Chapter 15 for detailed instructions.

Creating a new document based on a template is fairly quick once you get the hang of it, but if you create many documents a day, these extra keystrokes can add up. To make it faster to start a new document based on a specific template, record a macro to do it for you. Assign the macro to a shortcut key or to a button on the toolbar. See Chapter 12 for specific instructions on recording macros.

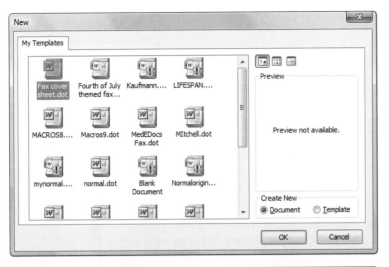

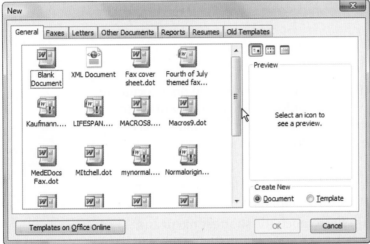

FIGURE 8-12 Two versions of the New dialog box displaying your personal templates. The second dialog box (as shown above) will open with the FileNewDialog command as explained in the Put It Together box on the previous page.

Modify a Document Template

To modify the standard text within a template, you need to open the actual template file and edit the text. Follow these steps to modify the standard text, zoom, or document view:

1. Access the **Open** dialog box (CTRL+O).

2. Make sure the **Templates** folder is displayed in the *Save in* box/Address bar. To access the **Templates** folder in Windows Vista, click Templates under Favorite Links, and in XP, click Trusted Templates in the Places bar. Open the template to be changed. The Title bar should display the name of your template—*not* Document.

3. Make changes to the standard text, the zoom setting, or the document view. If you change the zoom setting or the document view, you must also make one other change to the file such as typing a word and then

(Continued)

WORD 2007

deleting that same word—anything that causes Word to detect an actual change to the file.

4. Press **CTRL+S** and close the template file (**CTRL+W**).

Now you can open a document based on that template and see the modified text, and/or the new zoom setting. If you changed the document view (eg, from Draft to Page Layout), documents based on that template will now open in the new document view. The content of *existing* documents is *not affected* by changes you make to the templates on which they are based.

> Remember, the *New dialog box* will not open a template—only a document *based* on a template. You cannot use the **New** dialog box to open or back up your template files; you must open the template using the **Open** dialog box.

Modify the Normal Template

If you would prefer that all new documents (not otherwise based on a document template) open with the zoom setting higher or lower than the current setting, you need to modify the Normal.dotm itself. Follow these steps (but be very, very careful when making changes to the Normal.dotm file in this way):

1. Close Word.

2. Using Windows Explorer, open the **Templates** folder (type `%AppData%` in the <u>Address</u> bar and choose **Microsoft/Templates**).

3. *Right-click* on the Normal.dotm file to open the shortcut menu and choose Open (do not double-click the Normal.dotm file, as this will open a document, not the actual Normal.dotm). Word will open and the <u>Title</u> bar should read Normal.dotm.

4. Change the zoom setting and change the document view if you prefer.

5. Carefully type one word and then delete that one word. Word must detect some change in the file in order to save changes to the zoom and view settings. Be careful not to leave any text remaining in the template file; otherwise, every new document will open with that text.

6. Click **CTRL+S** to save the changes and close the template. Close and reopen Word as you normally do.

> You can change any of your templates (not just the Normal.dotm) using the above method of accessing templates directly through the **Templates** folder. Place a shortcut to your **Templates** folder on your Desktop to make it easier to access all your templates. Right-click on a template and choose Open on the shortcut menu instead of navigating through the folder tree using the **Open** dialog box.

Manage Templates with the Organizer

Word stores macros and styles in template files, and these items can be copied between template files using the **Organizer**. If you have created one of these elements and want to make it available in another template, use the **Organizer** dialog box to copy from one template to another. To access the Organizer, press **ALT+F8** and click Organizer. Follow the directions under Word 2003 on page 242 for moving styles between template files. Instructions for managing macros will be given in Chapter 12. Note: The Organizer in Word 2003 includes tools for moving macros, styles, AutoText entries, and custom toolbars; Word 2007's **Organizer** only includes macros and styles. In Word 2007, AutoText entries are managed using the **Building Blocks Organizer** (see Chapter 10). Word 2007 does not use custom toolbars, so this feature is not available in Word 2007's Organizer.

Attach a Template to a Document

Even if you do not start a document based on a specific template, you can still "attach" any template to a document after you have already created the document. This can be helpful if you have a template that contains a macro or a set of styles that you want to use within the current document. You can also attach templates to files that were created by someone else, so you can access some of your favorite tools while working in that file. To attach any template to a document, follow these steps:

1. With the document open, go to Developer > Templates > Document Template or press **ALT, T, I**. (If the Developer tab is not displayed, go to Office > Word Options > *Display Developer tab in Ribbon*.)

2. Under *Document Template* click Attach (see Figure 8-13). The **Open** dialog box will appear.

(Continued)

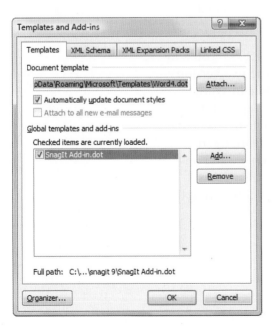

FIGURE 8-13 The Templates and Add-ins dialog allows you to attach template files to your document.

3. Select the template name from the **Open** dialog box and click `Open`.

4. If the template you are attaching contains style definitions that you want available in the current document, click *Automatically update document styles* (see warning below).

5. Click `OK` to close the box.

You can only attach one template file at a time, but you can add and remove template files as needed. To remove a template file, simply open the **Templates and Add-ins** dialog box and delete the template name and the path from the box.

Automatically Update Styles

Styles have the ability to update based on the current definition of the style. This means you can open a document created on a different computer or with a different template attached and the formatting can be updated using the *current definitions* of the styles. If the document you are working on has style definitions that are different than the template you are attaching *and* the styles have the same name (eg, the Normal style in the current document is Times New Roman and the Normal style in the attached template is Arial), the document can be reformatted using the definition of the styles in the *attached* template. To update styles, check *Automatically update template styles* in the **Templates and Add-ins** dialog box. In previous versions of Word, this setting was active (by default) and it caused a tremendous amount of grief, because documents created on one computer would be reformatted automatically when opened on a different computer.

If you open a document with the option to automatically update styles (whether it is already checked or you make that selection after opening the document), and the entire document reformats with a different font, immediately remove the check mark from the **Templates and Add-ins** dialog, close the dialog, and then press CTRL+Z. The font will return to the original style definitions.

If you are using Word 2007 and send documents to users in Word 2003, you may encounter problems with the different style definitions used in the two versions of Word. Unless you have changed the definition, the Normal style in Word 2007 uses the font Callibri and sets the line spacing at 1.15 with a space after setting of 10 points. Word 2003 uses Times New Roman with single line spacing and no space after. If you receive a complaint from another user working in Word 2003, have them open the **Templates and Add-ins** dialog box (found on the Tools menu in Word 2003) and place a check mark at *Automatically update document styles*. The document will be transformed to match the definition of the Normal style on *their* computer.

Global Templates

It is possible to have more than one global template. Of course, the Normal.dotm must always be running, but it is possible to have additional

WORD 2007

global templates. You can add a global template using the **Templates and Add-ins** dialog box. Click the **Add** button and select the template to be used as a global template. This template will remain available to all documents until you specifically remove it using the **Templates and Add-ins** dialog box.

You can also place templates in the Word **Startup** folder (in the Microsoft folder under **Word / Startup**), which will cause the template to be treated as a global template and will automatically be used every time Word is opened. Global templates are typically used to supply macros, styles, customized toolbars, menus, or other functionality that might be required to work with a specific company or that company's software. In addition, some programs that are designed to work in conjunction with Word may add functionality to Word using a global template. Examples include third-party dictionaries, references, and utilities. If a program has added functionality (eg, a toolbar) that you no longer need, look in the **Templates and Add-ins** dialog to see if there is a global template added. If so, navigate to the **Startup** folder and move the template out of that folder (select the template name in the *Global templates and add-ins* box and look for the path at the bottom of the **Templates and Add-ins** dialog box).

Tips for Using Templates

Templates can actually be stored anywhere on your computer, but only templates in the Templates folder will appear in the **New** dialog box. To use a template stored in a different location, open the folder containing the template file and double-click the file. A new document will open based on that template.

If you use a lot of templates, you may choose to sort the templates into various categories. To create new tabs on the **New** dialog box, create new folders within the **Templates** folder. Using Windows Explorer, browse to the **Templates** folder. Create new subfolders and drag templates into these folders to sort. The folder name will become the tab name in the **New** dialog box.

Troubleshoot Templates

Q: Why does Word ask me to save changes to the Normal.dotm and how do I answer?

A: Since the Normal.dotm is used to save various elements (eg, AutoText, formatted AutoCorrect entries, macros, style definitions, as well as some options), the file changes when any of the above elements have been changed. If you have knowingly made changes to any of these elements, you should save these changes when you close the Word session. In this case, answer **Yes** when asked. If you are not aware of having made changes to your template, you might consider answering **No**, as the "change" may actually result in a corrupted Normal.dotm file. You may also be prompted to save changes to the Building Blocks.dotx file as shown in Figure 8-14.

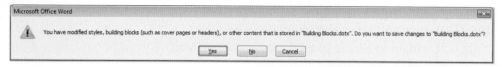

FIGURE 8-14 Word will prompt you to save or discard changes to template files.

Q: Can I use templates from earlier versions of Word?

A: Yes, templates are compatible across all versions of Word. If you upgrade Word on the same computer that ran a previous version, the previous Normal.dot file will be renamed Normal11.dot and stored in the **Templates** folder. Templates *that you have created yourself* will remain in the **Templates** folder and will be available in the **New** dialog box as before. See page 477 to learn more about upgrading to Word 2007 as well as setting up Word 2007 on a new computer using template files from previous versions.

Critical Thinking Questions

1. Explain the difference between a document template and a global template.

   _____

   _____

2. Explain why templates are a better choice for creating new documents compared to using a regular document and the Save As command.

   _____

   _____

3. Why is it important to back up the Normal.dot/Normal.dotm file?

   _____

   _____

4. Why would renaming the Normal.dot/Normal.dotm file help diagnose a corrupt Normal?

   _____

   _____

5. What happens if you use the Save As command to change a dot file to a doc file?

   _____

   _____

6. Explain why displaying file extensions is helpful when learning to use template files.

   _____

   _____

7. Explain how to back up template files.

   _____

   _____

8. Create a new template file and name it Sample.dot. Follow these specifications:

   a. Set the default page margins at 1 inch top and bottom and 1.25 inches left and right.

   b. Set the default font as Times New Roman 12 point.

   c. Type the headings and the standard text as shown in the sample report on page 423.

   d. Set font formatting so that the patient's name inserts in bold and uppercase.

e. Format the header space so that the patient's name, date of service, and page number appear on the second page (but not the first).

f. Save the changes and close the template file.

g. Create a document based on this template and name it Exercise D. doc (Word 2003) or Exercise D.docx (Word 2007).

CHAPTER 9

AutoCorrect

OBJECTIVES

▸ Recognize how each AutoCorrect option affects what you type.

▸ Add, remove, and modify AutoCorrect entries.

▸ Create AutoCorrect entries to efficiently format abbreviations and insert symbols and special characters.

▸ Create AutoCorrect entries to correct misspelled words and habitual typos.

▸ Control AutoCorrect changes using Undo and the AutoCorrect Options button.

▸ Back up AutoCorrect entries, restore entries after a computer problem, and move entries to another computer.

KEYWORDS

short form

third-party text expander

text expander

With text

Replace text

Introduction to AutoCorrect

The AutoCorrect feature built into Word was designed to "automatically correct" errors. Since it is designed to correct errors, it is always "on," meaning anytime the "error" is typed, it will be corrected without you having to think about it (compare this to AutoText, which only makes changes when you specifically instruct Word to do so). AutoCorrect has many uses, only one of which is to correct errors. You can use the AutoCorrect feature to automatically correct typos and misspelled words, change capitalization, format text, expand shortcuts into longer words and phrases, insert symbols, and flag potential errors.

You may have already seen AutoCorrect at work since Word installs with over a thousand entries to correct common typos, misspelled words, and misused phrases. Examples of corrections already included in the AutoCorrect list include:

- Common typos —teh changes to the
- Common spelling errors —judgement changes to judgment, alot changes to a lot

- Misplaced or dropped spaces — `saidthat` changes to `said that` or `againstt he` changes to `against the`
- Phrase errors —`should of been` changes to `should have been` or `their are` changes to `there are`
- Misplaced or missing apostrophes —`wouldnt` changes to `wouldn't`

Although Word installs with many entries to get you started, you are in complete control of the list. You can examine the list, add to the list, and delete items from the list. To see the list of entries, display the **AutoCorrect** dialog box and scroll through the list. To remove an entry, select the entry and click <u>**Delete**</u>.

To use AutoCorrect, simply type the "incorrect" form (also called the *Replace* text) and press the *Spacebar* or *any* punctuation key. The incorrect form will be replaced with the correct form instantly.

AutoCorrect Options

The **AutoCorrect** dialog box offers six different options that can be turned on or off. Most of the features are very helpful and there is no particular reason to disable any of the features. Open the **AutoCorrect** dialog box (Figure 9-1) and examine the options listed in the upper half of the **AutoCorrect** dialog box. Learn more about these options on page 153 (Word 2003) and 178 (Word 2007).

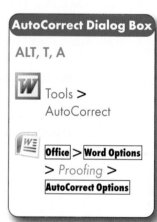

AutoCorrect Dialog Box

ALT, T, A

Tools >
AutoCorrect

Office > **Word Options**
> *Proofing* >
AutoCorrect Options

AutoCorrect includes many options for correcting text automatically as you type

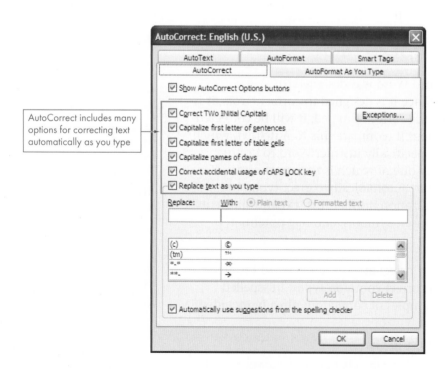

FIGURE 9-1 The AutoCorrect dialog box.

The option to *Capitalize first letter of sentences* will not cap the first word of a sentence following a sentence that ends in a digit or an abbreviation such as b.i.d. See page 454 for instructions on writing a macro to capitalize missed caps.

Ideas for Using AutoCorrect

Once you begin using AutoCorrect, you will discover many ways to take advantage of its power and convenience. The following are a few ideas for using AutoCorrect:

- Correct common misspellings (eg, change recieve to receive)
- Correct typos (eg, change apin to pain)
- Quickly format subscripts and superscripts (eg, CO_2)
- Change Latin words to italic (eg, *in situ*)
- Insert symbols (eg, the degree symbol ° or Greek letters ά, β, and γ)
- Convert abbreviations to all caps (eg, change cabg to CABG)
- Format awkward formats (eg, HER-2/*neu*, hemoglobin A_{1c})
- Format Latin abbreviations (eg, change tid to t.i.d., bid to b.i.d.)
- Change the function of a key (eg, avoid using the **Shift** key by changing brackets [ ] to parentheses ( ) or = to +)
- Correct accidental use of the **Shift** key (eg, change **Shift+period**, which inserts the greater-than sign, to a period)
- To conform to style guidelines (eg, to change q4h to q.4 h. with the correct spacing and period placement)
- To avoid using abbreviations on the Joint Commission's *Do Not Use* list (eg, change qd to daily)

As powerful as it can be, AutoCorrect can also unwittingly create problems if you are not careful. Since the correction/change happens as soon as you press the **Spacebar** or *any punctuation key*, you effectively cannot avoid inserting the replacement text. For this reason, AutoCorrect entries should be reserved for corrections, changes, and shortcuts that you want to insert *every time you type the incorrect text.*

Transcription typically involves typing the same words and phrases many times a day. Creating shortcuts to reduce the number of keystrokes required to insert long words, phrases, paragraphs, and even boilerplates can increase productivity and increase accuracy tremendously. A utility that allows you to type **short forms** (abbreviations for words, phrases, and boilerplate text) to insert text is referred to as a **text expander**. AutoCorrect can be used as a text expander utility, and many transcriptionists use AutoCorrect extensively in this manner. If you decide to take this approach to increasing your productivity, you should be aware of the caveats.

A significant disadvantage of using AutoCorrect as a text-expansion tool is the lack of flexibility. Many two- and three-letter combinations are logical shortcuts for more than one phrase (eg, CVA can mean costovertebral angle and cerebrovascular accident), but AutoCorrect allows only one expansion per short form. You cannot work around this limitation by creating lists for each physician or medical specialty because Word only allows one AutoCorrect list per user. In addition, AutoCorrect entries are limited to 255 non-formatted characters, which may not be enough to accommodate a standard paragraph such as a review of systems or a physical exam.

Also, be aware that it is easy to unwittingly create a short form using an actual word (eg, eat for evaluation and treatment), a short patient name (eg, ed could be a patient or doctor's name as well as a short form for erectile dysfunction and emergency department), or a common abbreviation (eg, mi could be the short form of myocardial infarction, myocardial ischemia, and the abbreviation for Michigan). You will also be surprised at how easy it is insert the wrong expansion without noticing, especially since *any* punctuation mark will invoke AutoCorrect. If you use AutoCorrect as a text expander, devise a method to distinguish short forms from actual words and abbreviations (eg, append an x to each short form). It is important to implement a systematic approach to creating text expansions *before* you have created and memorized hundreds of short forms, because eventually you will be trying to memorize and use thousands of short forms! A good reference for learning how to create shortcuts is *Saving Keystrokes* by Diana Rolland.

Using AutoCorrect extensively requires careful proofing for inadvertent insertions, which, ironically, defeats the purpose of using AutoCorrect in the first place.

A **third-party text expander** is a separate software program that runs in conjunction with your word processor. These programs store short forms and then insert the corresponding word or phrase directly into the document when the short form is typed. They are very reliable, simple to use, offer more flexibility than AutoCorrect, and are worth every penny. Many MTs use AutoCorrect to expand hundreds, if not thousands, of short forms into words and phrases, and if your circumstances do not allow for a third-party expansion program, then by all means take advantage of AutoCorrect to increase your efficiency. But if you have a choice and can use a text expander program, you will increase your options for creating shortcuts and improve overall accuracy and efficiency. In Chapter 10, you will also learn about AutoText, a feature in MS Word that can be used to insert text.

Third-party expander programs are typically more portable than AutoCorrect. Generally speaking, it is easier to move between various transcription platforms using a third-party expander program rather than relying solely on AutoCorrect. Some platforms that do use Word disable the AutoCorrect feature in favor of their own built-in expansion tool. Examples of third-party text expansion programs include Instant Text and SpeedType.

I use a combination of AutoCorrect, AutoText, and Instant Text (my personal favorite program for expanding text). I use the semicolon key (not the Spacebar or other punctuation) with Instant Text to expand phrases so I am deliberate in my decision to expand. I use AutoCorrect to insert "universal" shortcuts that I want to insert every time I type the incorrect text or the short form. Most of my AutoCorrect entries insert format or capitalization changes or spelling corrections. I never use AutoCorrect to expand a short form into a longer word or phrase.

Create New Entries

In addition to the extensive list of entries already included with Word, you can create your own entries quickly and easily. There are several approaches, depending on the type of entry you want to create. Follow the steps below for each type of AutoCorrect entry.

Correct Typing Errors

To create a new entry that will correct a common typo, follow these steps:

1. Open the **AutoCorrect** dialog box (**ALT, T, A**).
2. In the *Replace* box, type a word or phrase that you often mistype or misspell. For example, type `usaly`.
3. In the *With* box, type the correct spelling of the word `usually` (see Figure 9-2).
4. Press **Enter** to create the new entry or click ⬚**Add**⬚. The dialog box will remain open so you can create a new entry. Click ⬚**OK**⬚ or **Esc** to close the dialog box when you are finished.

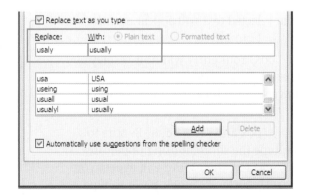

FIGURE 9-2 To create an AutoCorrect entry to correct a common misspelling or typo, type the incorrect word in the Replace box and the correct word in the With box.

Use this same method to insert punctuation or change capitalization (eg, `tid` to `t.i.d.` or `cabg` to `CABG`). You can also create an entry by typing the *With* text directly into the document and selecting that text before opening the **AutoCorrect** dialog box. The selected text will appear in the *With* box, so you can type the incorrect form in the *Replace* box.

Carefully select the text within your document when creating a new Auto-Correct entry. If you pick up a leading or trailing space in your selection, those spaces will become part of your AutoCorrect entry and you will insert extra spaces into your document when you insert the entry. If you pick up a paragraph mark, your new entry will insert a paragraph break when it is inserted into your document. To be sure that you select exactly what you intend, display formatting marks (see page 197) before selecting text.

Create Formatted Entries

AutoCorrect is a terrific tool for applying formatting, especially when the formatting is awkward to apply, as in chemical names with superscripts and subscripts. These entries have to be created and formatted within the document itself since there are no formatting commands available within the **AutoCorrect** dialog box. To create an entry that contains formatting such as bold, italic, subscript, or superscript, follow these steps:

1. Make sure paragraph marks are displayed (**CTRL+Shift+8**).

2. Type the text into the document and apply formatting.

3. If the final character is a subscript or superscript character (eg, CO_2), make sure the space following the last character is normal type. Otherwise, when the entry is inserted while transcribing, the next text you type following the insertion will insert as superscript or subscript. Even though you do not actually include the trailing space in your AutoCorrect entry, Word "remembers" that the space following should be normal type.

4. Carefully select the text without picking up leading or trailing spaces or the paragraph mark (unless of course you really do want to add spaces as part of the entry).

5. Open the **AutoCorrect** dialog box. Your selected text will appear as unformatted text in the *With* box.

6. Click *Formatted text* just above the *With* box. Your entry will now display as formatted text within the *Replace* box (see Figure 9-3). The *Formatted text* option will only be available if you have selected formatted text before opening the dialog.

7. Type the shortcut (eg, co2) in the *Replace* box and press **Enter**. Be sure to type your shortcut in lowercase. If you type the shortcut using uppercase letters (eg, CO2) when *Formatted text* is selected, then Word will expect you to type your shortcut in uppercase too. Of course, it's much easier to type lowercase.

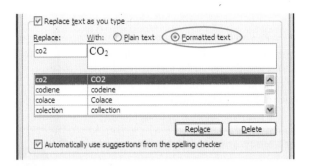

FIGURE 9-3 Click the Formatted text button to save formatting information with the AutoCorrect entry.

Pay close attention to the formatting of spaces following formatted entries such as **HISTORY OF PRESENT ILLNESS**. Be sure to remove bold formatting from the space immediately following the last character of the heading before selecting and creating your AutoCorrect shortcut. Otherwise, each time you use the shortcut, the text that you type immediately after the formatted entry will continue with the formatting. You will be quite annoyed by the need to adjust formatting while transcribing.

Create a shortcut in AutoCorrect to make it easier to type the patient's age using the hyphenated phrase −year-old. Instead of having to create a shortcut for every possible age, you can create a single shortcut that works with any number (age). This shortcut works well because it closes up the space between the number and the hyphen. To make this work, you must start your *Replace* text with a punctuation mark. Choose a shortcut that is easy to type, such as ; y, and type this into the *Replace* box of the **AutoCorrect** dialog box. In the *With* box, type −year-old. To use, type the patient's age followed by the **Spacebar**. Then type ; y **Spacebar**. The punctuation mark at the beginning of the *Replace* text will cause Word to jump backward and close up the space between the number and the hyphen

Normally, Word changes the first c in the abbreviation for courtesy copy to uppercase (Cc:) because Word interprets it as the first word in a sentence. Create a shortcut to insert cc: at the end of a document so that the first c is not capitalized. When creating the AutoCorrect entry, click the formatted text button and Word will retain the formatting (cc:).

Normally, AutoCorrect inserts entries in whatever font is currently in use. If you create a formatted entry, it will not only preserve the subscript or superscript formatting information, but it will also retain the font size and style. This may present problems if you transcribe documents in different fonts or font sizes. If you need to create a formatted shortcut that will adjust to the current font, use AutoText instead. Learn about AutoText in Chapter 10.

Insert Symbols

AutoCorrect is a terrific tool for quickly inserting symbols into your document. Several symbols are already included in AutoCorrect and are listed at the beginning of the list in the **AutoCorrect** dialog box. Follow these steps to add other symbols to your list:

1. Open the **Symbol** dialog box (Figure 9-4).
2. Locate the symbol within the grid and click to select. You may need to change the *Font* or the *Subset* to find the symbol you need (scrolling through the symbol grid will also change the *Subset*).
3. Click **AutoCorrect**, which will open the **AutoCorrect** dialog box. The selected symbol will appear in the *With* box. Type a shortcut in the *Replace* box. To create a single-key shortcut for common symbols such as the degree symbol, use keys on the "outer edges" of your keyboard that you rarely use anyway such as the **Accent** key (to the left of the **1**) or the **Backslash** key (above **Enter**).

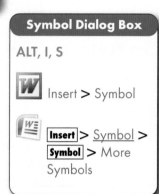

Symbol Dialog Box

ALT, I, S

Insert > Symbol

Insert > Symbol > **Symbol** > More Symbols

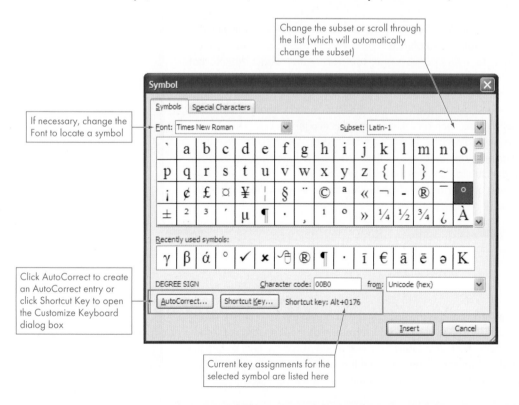

FIGURE 9-4 Locate a symbol in the Symbol dialog box to create an AutoCorrect entry for inserting that symbol.

Notice that the **Symbols** dialog box also displays a shortcut key (bottom center) for some of the symbols as well as a [Shortcut Key] button that opens the **Customize Keyboard** dialog box. The difference between an AutoCorrect shortcut and a shortcut key is shortcut keys use modifier keys (**ALT**, **CTRL**, **Shift**) and AutoCorrect entries do not.

AutoCorrect works well for easily inserting a degree symbol. One clever way to do this is to use the **Accent** key (the key to the left of the 1 and above the **Tab**). This key is not used in transcription, so it can be used as the shortcut for inserting the degree symbol. Locate the degree symbol in the **Symbol** dialog box as described above and click [AutoCorrect]. In the *With* box, type **Accent**. To use, type a number followed by the **Accent** key (eg, 98.6`) and it will automatically convert to a degree symbol.

Brackets are easy keys to reach but are rarely used in transcription, so they are good keys to use with AutoCorrect to insert a symbol or to substitute for parentheses (the bracket is easier to type than **Shift+9** and **Shift+0**). To change the function of the **Bracket**, simply type a **Bracket** in the *Replace* box and a **Parenthesis** in the *With* box.

Combine AutoCorrect with Spell Checking

If you find that you misspell a word consistently, you can add this word to the AutoCorrect list during a spell check. Instead of correcting the word, choose [AutoCorrect] from the **Spelling and Grammar** dialog box or the Spelling and Grammar right-click menu. Choose the correct spelling from the list of suggested words (Figure 9-5). Word will create an AutoCorrect entry based on the incorrect-correct spelling pair. The next time you type the incorrect spelling, AutoCorrect will correct it for you. Learn more about the spelling and grammar feature in Chapter 14.

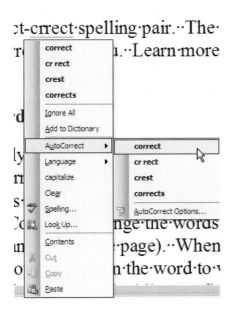

FIGURE 9-5 Use the Spelling and Grammar right-click menu to create a new AutoCorrect entry for words you habitually misspell.

Flag Incorrect Words

Some typos can easily go undetected because the mistyped word is actually another word. Examples include `form` and `from`, `please` and `pleas`, `her` and `here`. Only very careful proofreading will catch these types of errors, but AutoCorrect can help. For words that you habitually mistype, use AutoCorrect to change the words to bold text (or any other format that will cause the word to stand out on the page). When the formatted word inserts into your document, pause to confirm the word was spelled correctly and then press **CTRL+Z** (see explanation below) or confirm and remove formatting during proofreading.

Use the Spell Checker with AutoCorrect

At the bottom of the AutoCorrect dialog box you will see the option to *Automatically use suggestions from the spelling checker*. When this option is enabled, Word will automatically correct the spelling of a word, even if the misspelled word is not included in the AutoCorrect list, but only when the spell checker determines there is only one possible correction. Since Word's spelling and grammar feature normally offers suggestions for correcting the spelling of a word, this setting simply bypasses the need to select the correct word when there is only one possible correct word. Learn more about Word's spelling and grammar feature in Chapter 14.

I was initially skeptical of Word's ability to automatically correct words using the spell checker, but I have used this setting for several years, and the feature has proved to be reliable. This feature will correct many words when letters are simply transposed (eg, `iwll` instead of `will`). I have never seen Word change a medical term to the incorrect medical term. I have also found that it will automatically correct the capitalization of brand-name drugs. To take advantage of this, I type all drug names in lowercase; the generic names remain lowercase and brand-name drugs are automatically capitalized. If the drug name is misspelled *and* the capitalization is incorrect, Word will mark the word as incorrectly spelled and not make any automatic changes.

Reverse an AutoCorrect Change

The AutoCorrect feature is a tremendous tool for ensuring accuracy and increasing speed, but occasionally it introduces a problem. For example, when typing `cc` (courtesy copy) at the end of a report, AutoCorrect changes it to `Cc` because of the setting *Capitalize the first letter of sentences*. An easy fix is to simply click Undo (**CTRL+Z**) immediately after Word makes the change. A similar problem arises if you have an entry to convert `bid` to `b.i.d.` You may have occasion to actually type the word `bid` (as in an auction). Again, type `bid`, strike the **Spacebar** and then press **CTRL+Z**. The automatic correction will be reversed and you can continue transcribing.

You will also notice that any time AutoCorrect makes a change in your document, a blue line will underscore the character that was changed (Figure 9-6). Move the cursor next to the character to display the underscore or hover over the area with the mouse to display the $\boxed{\text{AutoCorrect Options}}$ button (see Figure 9-7). Click the button to display a drop-down menu of options for controlling the corresponding AutoCorrect action. You can also display the drop-down menu by pressing **ALT+Shift+F10** while the blue line is displayed.

Cc:···John·Smith,·MD¶

FIGURE 9-6 A blue line will appear under a character that has been affected by one of the AutoCorrect features.

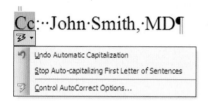

FIGURE 9-7 The AutoCorrect Options button opens a drop-down menu for controlling the AutoCorrect feature.

The first option on the AutoCorrect Options menu (eg, Undo Automatic Capitalization) has the same result as **CTRL+Z**—it reverses the action this one time. The second option on the menu removes the check mark in the **AutoCorrect** dialog box that controls that particular AutoCorrect feature (eg, Capitalize first letter of sentences). The third option will open the **AutoCorrect** dialog box so you can make changes as necessary. The AutoCorrect Options menu will change depending on the type of automatic correction that was made.

Modify an AutoCorrect Entry

You can modify any AutoCorrect entry—those you created or those that installed with Word. To change an AutoCorrect entry stored as plain text, open the **AutoCorrect** dialog box. Select the entry from the AutoCorrect list (scroll through the list or type the Replace text to quickly bring that entry to the top of the list). Change the entry in the *With* box. Click $\boxed{\text{Replace}}$.

If you want to change an AutoCorrect entry that contains a long passage of text, a graphic, or formatting, you have to make the changes in the document, not in the **AutoCorrect** dialog box.

Follow these steps:

1. Start by inserting the (old) entry into your document.

2. Make the changes to the entry within the document and then select the revised entry.

3. Open the **AutoCorrect** dialog box and type the AutoCorrect entry's shortcut in the *Replace* box and click Replace.

The **AutoCorrect** dialog box is easy enough to use for a few simple corrections now and then, but it can be tedious to use if you need to make a lot of changes or want to delete a large number of your entries. To make extensive changes to your AutoCorrect list, see instructions for using the AutoCorrect utility on page 474.

AutoCorrect Exceptions

It is possible to create an "exceptions list" that specifies corrections you do not want AutoCorrect to make. Open the **AutoCorrect** dialog box and click Exceptions to display the **Exceptions** dialog box (Figure 9-8). Word has three categories of exceptions that correspond to the AutoCorrect options *Capitalize first letter of sentences*, *Correct two initial capitals*, and *Automatically use suggestions from the spelling checker*.

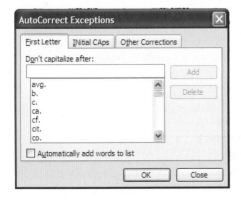

FIGURE 9-8 The AutoCorrect Exceptions dialog box.

To prevent Word from capitalizing the word following an abbreviation that ends with a period (eg, Inc.), click the First letter tab and then type the abbreviation (including the period) in the *Don't capitalize after* box. Click Add.

I haven't found any abbreviations that are commonly used in medical transcription that need to be added to the Exceptions list. Most medical abbreviations that have periods are the Latin abbreviations such as p.r.n. and t.i.d. Even though these particular abbreviations end with a period, Word does not interpret them as the end of a sentence because there are multiple periods separated by individual letters. These Latin abbreviations do not need to be added to the Exceptions list.

To prevent Word from correcting a word that contains mixed uppercase and lowercase letters such as MTips, select the INitial Caps tab and type the word in the *Don't correct* box. Click Add.

If you enable *Automatically use suggestions from the spelling checker* (as described above), you may have a reason to create an exception to this automatic behavior (remember, these are AutoCorrect actions that do not have a correct/incorrect word pair saved in the AutoCorrect list). If there is a particular word that you do not want Word to automatically correct, add the word to the Other Corrections tab of the **AutoCorrect Exceptions** dialog box.

Notice at the bottom of the **Exceptions** dialog box there is an option to *Automatically add words to list*. If you use the **Backspace** key or the **Left** arrow key to back up and correct a word that was just changed by the AutoCorrect feature, Word assumes you want to create an exception to the rule and automatically adds the word to your exception list. You may actually be making a change to your document based on the dictation—not because you are reversing an AutoCorrect action—and therefore not realize you are creating an exception to the rule. Automatically adding words to the exception list has the potential to create confusion, because exceptions added inadvertently will cause the capitalization rules to appear random (ie, Word won't make capitalization changes when you might otherwise expect it to). This feature is enabled by default, but most likely you will want to remove the check mark (disable it) on all three tabs of the **AutoCorrect Exceptions** dialog box.

 If automatic capitalization appears to behave erratically, it may be that Word has added exceptions to your AutoCorrect list without you realizing it. Before giving up on the capitalization feature and disabling it, check the exceptions list. Remove words from the list and see if Word behaves more predictably.

Back Up AutoCorrect

No doubt a lot of work goes into building an AutoCorrect list, so it is important to keep this data backed up. You will lose precious time rebuilding a list that has been lost due to a hard drive crash, not to mention the frustration of working without your "fix-it list." Entries that contain any type of formatting (eg, bold, italic, or a paragraph mark) are stored in the Normal.dot/Normal.dotm file. Plain-text AutoCorrect entries are stored in the AutoCorrect file named MSO1033.acl. (MSO stands for Microsoft Office; 1033 is the language identification number for US English; and acl stands for AutoCorrect list). Therefore, two files are required to fully back up all your AutoCorrect entries. Likewise, if you need to restore your entries to the same computer (after a crash) or to a new computer, you will need both files. Refer to page 70 for instructions on locating and backing up the Normal.dot and the AutoCorrect list.

If disaster strikes and you must restore your AutoCorrect data, copy the Normal.dot/Normal.dotm from your backup disk to its appropriate folder and copy the MSO1033.acl file to the Office folder (as above). Word must be closed while you restore the files. Remember, you must use the copy and paste commands to place these files in their respective folders. Do not try to open these files.

Microsoft also offers an AutoCorrect utility which creates a document listing all AutoCorrect entries. This document can be used to view, edit, move, and restore the AutoCorrect list. See page 474 for instructions on using this utility.

Critical Thinking Questions

1. Explain why you cannot use AutoCorrect to create a shortcut for inserting a title (such as Dr.) followed by a nonbreaking space (ie, the shortcut to include both the title and the nonbreaking space).

   _____

   _____

2. Why is it important to reveal formatting marks before selecting text when creating a new AutoCorrect entry?

   _____

   _____

3. Even though the AutoCorrect entry does not include the space immediately following it, why is it important to remove the formatting from the space immediately following a formatted character?

   _____

   _____

4. What is the difference between a shortcut key and an AutoCorrect entry?

   _____

   _____

5. Make a list of words you habitually misspell or mis-key. Type these words into a document. Right-click each misspelled word and create an AutoCorrect entry to correct them.

   _____

   _____

6. Create an AutoCorrect entry for each of the following:

   a. t.i.d.

   b. q.i.d.

   c. cbc to CBC

   d. H_2O

   e. CO_2

   f. aV_R

   g. ^{123}I

   h. -year-old

   i. HISTORY OF PRESENT ILLNESS:

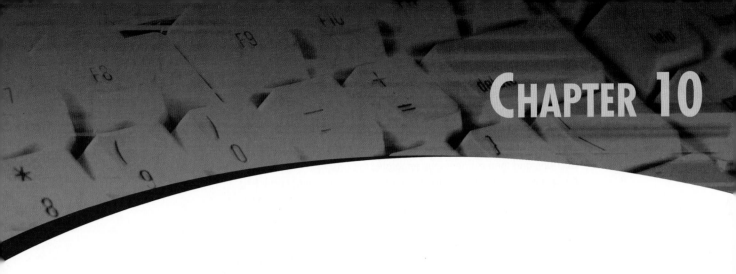

CHAPTER 10

AutoText

OBJECTIVES

- Differentiate AutoText and AutoCorrect and describe the best application of each feature.
- Use AutoText to store boilerplate text and other shortcuts.
- Troubleshoot AutoText formatting problems.
- Manage AutoText entries using the Organizer (Word 2003).
- Manage AutoText entries using the Building Blocks Organizer (Word 2007).
- Back up AutoText entries.

AutoText offers a way to store and quickly insert text, graphics, fields, tables, bookmarks, and other items that you use frequently. AutoText is useful for inserting boilerplate text and "normals" so you do not have to retype the same text over and over. AutoText entries can be as long as you like and can include fields, formatting, graphics, tables—almost anything. AutoText entries can be stored in the Normal.dot, where they will be available to all your documents, or they can be stored in document templates so they are available only when working on a document based on that template. For example, the phrase "right upper sternal border" is a common phrase, so it could be stored in the Normal.dot. A specific phrase like "fundus height measures" would most likely be limited to an obstetrician, so you could save that phrase in a template for obstetrics.

You will want to keep your AutoText entries separated into template files as much as possible to make them easier to manage. By storing entries in separate templates, you do not have to clean out a list of shortcuts for accounts you no longer type—simply stop using the template and the shortcuts will never be in your way. Yet another advantage to sorting your list into templates is the ability to duplicate shortcut names. For example, the short form CVA can insert the phrase `costovertebral angle` in one template and `cerebrovascular accident` in another.

KEYWORDS

Normal template
Default font
Building Blocks (Word 2007)

Shortcut keys
F3
ALT+F3

Managers and business owners can create templates that contain Auto-Text entries for common phrases and normals used by a given physician or account, and then distribute the templates to transcriptionists that work on the given account. This approach creates consistency among all MTs working on the same account and gives them immediate access to common phrases and normals needed to accurately transcribe the account. It also lessens the MT's training time for the given account.

Word has many AutoText entries already built in, including entries for inserting page-number fields, document properties, and salutations. Word 2007 has greatly expanded the number of built-in entries and has incorporated AutoText into the Building Blocks feature.

AutoText vs AutoCorrect

AutoText and AutoCorrect use different methods to insert entries; AutoText is "optional" and AutoCorrect is "automatic." After setting up an AutoText entry, you can choose whether or not to insert the text into your document. By contrast, when you use AutoCorrect to automatically change the text as you type, Word will always insert the change. AutoText entries can be stored in different templates so that you can make them available only when needed, whereas AutoCorrect entries are always available. Also, AutoText entries will maintain formatting and capitalization and will not be changed by any of the AutoCorrect features (eg, automatic capitalization). The advantages and disadvantages of each method of creating shortcuts will become more apparent as you work through this chapter.

Create an AutoText Entry

To create a new AutoText entry, type, format, and select the text, table, field, or graphic that you want to store as an AutoText entry and then press **ALT+F3**. This will bring up the small window as in Figure 10-1. Type a name at *Please name your AutoText entry* or accept the default name (the first few letters or words of the entry) and press **Enter**. The AutoText name is also the shortcut that you will use to insert the text into your document.

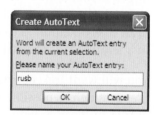

FIGURE 10-1 The Create AutoText box allows you to quickly create a new AutoText entry.

Use the **Create AutoText** box if you do not need to designate a particular template to store the AutoText entry. By default, entries will be added to the Normal.dot (or the template already designated in the **AutoText** dialog box—see next paragraph). If you select a graphic or any other non-text element, the graphic itself will not appear in the *Name* box, but instead you will see an asterisk. Replace the asterisk with a name (shortcut) for your graphic.

Word includes a full-function dialog box as well as an <u>AutoText</u> toolbar for creating and managing AutoText entries (Figure 10-2). To display the toolbar (Figure 10-3), choose View > Toolbars > AutoText. On the toolbar, click the left icon to open the full dialog box and the New button to open the **Create AutoText** quick-entry box (Figure 10-1).

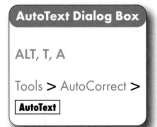

AutoText Dialog Box

ALT, T, A

Tools > AutoCorrect > **AutoText**

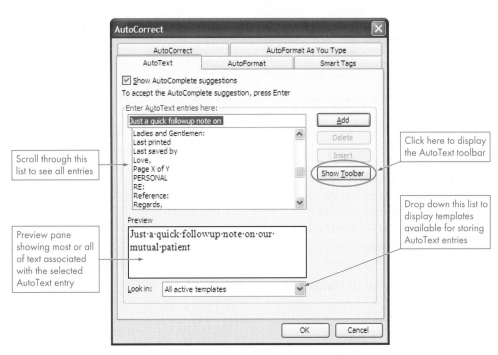

FIGURE 10-2 The AutoText dialog box helps you manage all your AutoText entries.

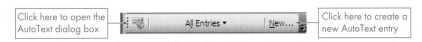

Click here to open the AutoText dialog box

Click here to create a new AutoText entry

FIGURE 10-3 The AutoText toolbar can be displayed while you work to help you manage your AutoText entries.

If you are working with a document based on a template, and the text to be stored as an AutoText entry is unique to that template (ie, you will only use the text when transcribing a report based on that template), you may choose to store your AutoText entry in that particular template.

WORD 2003

To designate a template to store your new AutoText entry, follow these steps:

1. Open the **AutoText** dialog box.

2. Open the *Look in* drop-down box and select the current template. Your choices will be *All active templates*, the current template, or the *Normal template* as shown in Figure 10-4. (You don't have to make any change to the *Look in* box if you want to store your entry in the Normal template.)

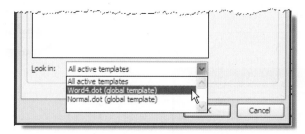

FIGURE 10-4 To separate your AutoText entries into separate templates, select a template name from the Look in box on the AutoText dialog box.

3. Click **OK** to close the dialog box.

4. Select the text within the document that will be the new AutoText entry. Oddly enough, if you select text and *then* change the template, the suggested name for the new entry is removed from *Enter AutoText entries here* box and you have to return to the document and select the text again. The template designation in the *Look in* box will remain selected until you specifically change it back to *All active templates*.

5. Open the **AutoText** dialog box and accept the suggested name or type a different name for your entry.

6. Press **Enter** to save and close the box.

Once you have changed the template designation, you can create additional entries to be saved in that template using the **Create AutoText** box (ie, select text and press **ALT+F3**).

The *Look in* box tells Word "where to look" for AutoText entries, so when you have finished adding your AutoText entries, be sure to change the *Look in* box back to *All active templates*. Otherwise, when you resume transcribing, Word will not look for entries stored in the Normal.dot and it will appear as if your entries are missing.

Formatted AutoText Entries

If you apply font characteristics such as bold or italic, this information will be saved with the AutoText entry, and it will always insert with these characteristics. It is also important to note that AutoText will preserve the capitalization exactly as it is saved. If you save an AutoText entry without capitalizing the first word and then insert it at the beginning of a sentence, AutoCorrect's automatic capitalization feature will not override the formatting—the first word of the sentence will remain lowercase.

AutoText entries saved with a paragraph mark will insert with the paragraph formatting carried by that paragraph mark (ie, centered, justified, align right or left), as well as a hard return. Decide whether you want this information included with your AutoText entry. Be sure to reveal paragraph marks (**CTRL+Shift+8**) before selecting the text to be memorized as an AutoText entry so you are certain whether the mark is included in the selection or not. Also take note of leading or trailing spaces so you don't create spacing problems when you insert the entry into your text.

AutoText works really well for creating shortcuts for titles (eg, Dr., Mrs., Mr.) followed by a nonbreaking space, because the AutoText entry will insert without inserting an additional space or punctuation mark. The cursor remains at the point of insertion (unlike an AutoCorrect entry that always includes a space or punctuation mark at the end of the insertion). For example, you can create a shortcut for inserting Dr. followed by a nonbreaking space so you can immediately type the surname without having to backup and remove a regular space before typing the surname. Remember, using a nonbreaking space will prevent Dr. and the surname from separating across a line break. To create, type the title and a non-breaking space (**CTRL+Shift+Spacebar**). Select the characters, including the nonbreaking space, and press **ALT+F3**. Name the entry with a simple name such as d or dr and insert using **F3**.

Assign Fonts to New Entries

If you use AutoText entries and you transcribe in more than one font (eg, Dr. Smith uses Arial and Central Clinic uses Times New Roman), it is especially important that you use template files and assign the default font to match the font used in the template. When AutoText entries are created, Word memorizes the *status of the font relative to the current default font*. If the AutoText entry is created in the same font as the default font, then Word remembers to insert the entry in the default font—whatever the current default font is. If the entry is created in a font that *differs* from the default font, Word remembers that the entry is an *exception* to the default and assumes that you always want to insert the text exactly as typed regardless of the surrounding text. Using AutoText entries in documents with mismatched font settings will cause what appear to be random (and very irritating) font changes.

This concept may be difficult to grasp at first, and may even seem convoluted, but it actually makes sense when you think about the way the majority of companies use Word. Companies often require all company correspondence to adhere to a given style, including a specific font. If you worked for a company that used Tahoma for all its correspondence but used a decorative script for the company's slogan, you would want that slogan to always insert in the decorative font—otherwise you would be reformatting the entry each time it was used, and that takes away from AutoText's usefulness. Almost all of Word's features are built around the concepts of templates and styles, and its functionality assumes that template files and default fonts are being used.

The issue of the font becomes a problem in transcription when you type in more than one font yet you use the same AutoText entries across all document types. The solution is to use template files and designate default fonts (remember, simply changing the font using the toolbar or the dialog box does not change the underlying font associated with the document). Review templates in Chapter 8 and font formatting on page 203. If your employment situation does not allow for the use of template files (dot files), then you can change the default font before transcribing each document. In other words, if you *must* type a document in another font, don't just change the font, designate that font as the default and do this each time you create a new document with a different font. You could create a macro with a shortcut key to accomplish this in a single keystroke, which would be somewhat of a nuisance to remember, but not nearly as aggravating as correcting font changes in the middle of your document.

 After creating or changing entries to AutoText, you may be prompted to save changes to the Normal.dot or the document template. Be sure to answer **Yes** or your changes will be discarded.

Insert AutoText Entries

You have two options for inserting an entry into your document using the keyboard—the Enter key or **F3**. When you type the fourth character of the AutoText name, a yellow ToolTip will appear just above the current line of text. Press Enter as long as the suggestion is displayed and the AutoText entry will insert. If you do not want to insert the entry, simply continue typing and the ToolTip will disappear. If you need to clear the ToolTip from the display so you can press the Enter key (without inserting the AutoText entry), press Esc. AutoText entries with a name (shortcut) of three characters or less can be inserted using F3.

The two methods of inserting an AutoText entry give you choices about naming your AutoText entry. AutoText entries can be named with a single character or using an actual word (eg, eat for evaluation and treatment), since there is less danger of expanding a shortcut unintentionally as can easily happen with AutoCorrect. Since the Enter key will insert an AutoText entry, you may occasionally find that an entry inserts at the end of a line when you didn't really intend to insert it. If this happens, press CTRL+Z to reverse the insertion.

If you type for several doctors who each have a different physical exam section, you can save the boilerplate text in AutoText and name each of them "PE". The trick is to store them in each doctor's template file. This way, the correct AutoText entry will only be available to you when you open a document based on that doctor's template. Even though you have several entries named PE, you will always insert the correct PE format. This keeps your abbreviation system simple and consistent, and that means fewer items to remember!

In the same way, create AutoText entries for phrases that are unique to that dictator and save them in his/her template file. Save them using the first few words of the phrase and the suggestion box will appear on the screen when you begin to type the phrase, reminding you that you have a shortcut available. When you change work assignments, you can simply delete the template file(s), and your system will not be "cluttered" with shortcuts you no longer use.

The AutoText Toolbar

As described above, the AutoText toolbar can be displayed, giving you quick access to the dialog boxes used to create and manage your entries. The **New** button (see Figure 10-3) will only be available if you have selected content in your document first. The icon on the left side of the toolbar opens the **AutoText** dialog box. The center button opens a drop-down menu of AutoText entries.

When you create a new AutoText entry, Word notes the style associated with the entry at the time it was created. Word uses styles to sort the AutoText entries into categories, and these categories are displayed on the toolbar button's drop-down menu and also on the AutoText menu (on the Insert menu). You will also notice that the center button on the toolbar will change from **All Entries** to a particular style name based on the style at the current location of the cursor. When a style name is listed on the toolbar, only the entries associated with that style will display on the drop-down menu. If the toolbar displays **All Entries**, the drop-down menu will display all AutoText entries as well as style names that have more than one AutoText entry associated with them; AutoText entries associated with a style will be on the style's submenu.

As a transcriptionist, you are not likely to use a lot of different styles, so the sort-by-style feature may be of little value. But it is important to note how entries are displayed on the toolbar so you will know how to locate entries when needed. For a transcriptionist, the real advantage of AutoText is to be able to type a shortcut and insert text with a few keystrokes *without perusing a long list of entries or clicking a menu item with the mouse*. So the bottom line is you may rarely use the toolbar to insert your entries. Occasionally you may forget the name of an entry, and in that case you can scan the menu for the entry's name. You can also use the **AutoText** dialog box to scan the list to locate an entry.

WORD 2003

Some of the built-in AutoText entries contain fields associated with document properties, including fields for dates. Review Chapter 11 on using fields before inserting date fields into a medical report.

An AutoText entry can contain fields but it cannot contain commands. Macros, on the other hand, can contain commands. Combining macros, fields, and AutoText entries works well for inserting boilerplate text that will be subsequently edited. For example, you may need to insert a physical exam boilerplate and then add the vital signs. Record a macro that inserts the AutoText entry and then moves the cursor up to the first vital sign entry. Learn how to use fields in Chapter 11 and macros in Chapter 12.

Manage AutoText Entries

Individual entries can be deleted by simply opening the **AutoText** dialog box, selecting the entry from the list, and clicking **Delete**. To delete multiple AutoText entries, it may be easier to delete them using the **Organizer** dialog box. To use the **Organizer**, follow these steps:

1. To open the **Organizer**, press **ALT+F8** and click **Organizer** in the bottom right corner.

2. Change the tab to **AutoText**. The entries for the current template should appear in one pane and the entries stored in the Normal.dot will appear in the other pane (see Figure 10-5).

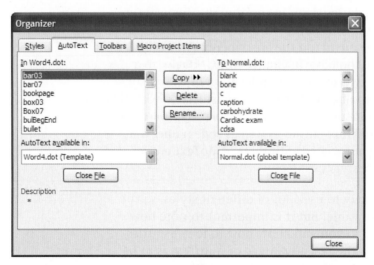

FIGURE 10-5 Use the Organizer to delete AutoText entries.

3. Select nonconsecutive entries by holding down **CTRL** while clicking on individual entries with the left mouse button. To select a range of entries (consecutive entries), select the first entry, hold down **Shift** and click the last entry. This will select all entries between the first and last selection.

4. With entries selected, click **Delete** in the middle of the dialog box.

WORD 2003

You can also copy AutoText entries to another template using the **Organizer** dialog box. Click `Close File` then `Open File` to select a template to be displayed in one of the panes. With each template displayed in one of the panes, select the entries to be moved and click `Copy`. See more detailed information on using the **Organizer** on page 242.

Print AutoText Entries

To print AutoText entries, open a document based on a template that contains the AutoText entries you want to print. Press CTRL+P to open the **Print** dialog box.

In the *Print what* box, select *AutoText entries* as in Figure 10-6. This will print AutoText entries contained in the Normal.dot as well as the currently active template (if applicable).

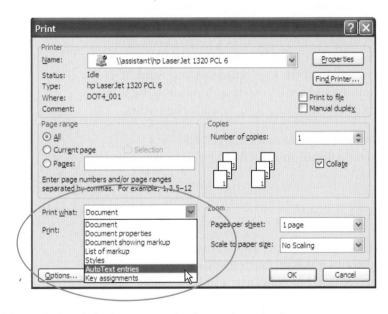

FIGURE 10-6 Use the Print dialog box to print a hard copy of your AutoText entries.

Back Up and Share AutoText Entries

Since AutoText entries are stored in templates, you back them up by backing up your template files. Custom document templates are saved in the same folder as the Normal.dot. See page 71 for paths to the **Templates** folder.

To share your AutoText entries (and only AutoText entries) with another person, place the appropriate template file on removable media. Insert the removable media into the other computer and open Word. Use the **Organizer**, as explained above and on page 242, to copy the AutoText entries from one template to another.

To access AutoText entries stored in another template, you can also attach the template to the current document using the **Templates and Add-ins** dialog box. This will give you access to AutoText entries without copying the entries from one template file to another. See page 324 for instructions on attaching templates.

Troubleshoot AutoText

The following are frequently asked questions related to AutoText.

The suggestion box does not appear or entry does not insert

The name of your AutoText entry is also the shortcut for inserting the entry. AutoText entries stored in the same template need to have unique names. For example, if you have four sentences that start with "The patient. . ." and you accept the default name (The patient) for each of these AutoText entries, these entries will not have unique names. If you type the patient, AutoText will not give you a suggestion box, because it will not know which of the four sentences you want. If you are not getting a ToolTip, check your list and see if you have duplicated the first seven or eight characters of another AutoText entry, and if so, rename the entries.

Also, if you have added entries to another template and changed the *Look in* location, entries in the Normal template will not insert. Change the *Look in* box back to *All active templates*.

Why do my entries insert with a different font?

Many transcriptionists have experienced the mysterious "font change" when inserting an AutoText entry. You will encounter this problem if you change fonts between documents (eg, Dr. A prefers Times New Roman and Dr. B wants Courier New) and do not assign the default font. Not only will this create problems when memorizing AutoText entries, but you will be very frustrated with the constant need to change the font. Review the information on page 281 related to assigning fonts.

Building Blocks

At first glance, it would appear that AutoText has been removed from Word 2007, but actually it still exists and can be used in much the same way as in previous versions of Word. AutoText has been incorporated into a larger feature called Building Blocks. Word 2007 has many building blocks that can be used to insert more than just text. A building block can include a cover page, fully formatted header and footer, fields, tables, table of contents, text boxes, and watermarks. Many of these features will have limited application in the context of routine medical documentation, but may be helpful for business owners who need to create business correspondence, reports, or marketing materials. On a day-to-day basis, transcriptionists will find the most value in being able to insert phrases and boilerplate text quickly and easily by typing a shortcut and then pressing **F3**.

Word 2007 has added an additional template specifically for storing building blocks called Building Blocks.dotx. In previous versions, AutoText entries were stored in the Normal template by default, but now you have another global template from which to choose. Building Blocks.dotx is a global template, so entries stored in this template will be available at all times. You can still separate your entries into your custom document templates, and for account-specific shortcuts, that is your best option.

Until you use building blocks extensively, you may have a hard time deciding whether to store entries in the Building Blocks template or the Normal.dotm. Personally, I have retained my entries in the Normal.dotm. I made this decision partly because they were already in the Normal.dot when I migrated my files to Word 2007. It is possible to move entries to another template, so you can start out using the Normal and later change your mind if you find a compelling reason to use the Building Blocks template. I still separate entries that are unique to a dictator or account into their respective document templates.

Building blocks are accessible through galleries that drop down from command buttons on the ribbon. Each building block is assigned to a gallery and a category and then further divided into templates. The gallery, category, and template settings are referred to as properties. Figure 10-7 shows the Alphabet building block assigned to the *Headers* gallery (in the **Building Blocks Organizer**) and its corresponding entry in the *Header* gallery that drops down from the Header button.

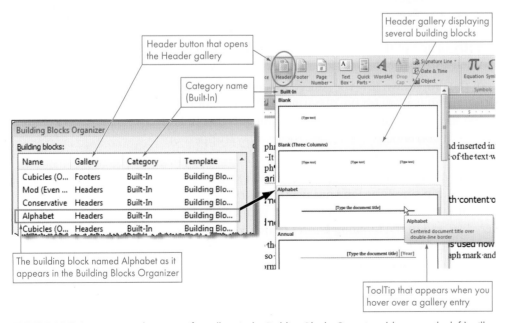

FIGURE 10-7 Items assigned to a specific gallery in the Building Blocks Organizer (shown on the left) will display on the corresponding drop-down gallery on the ribbon.

If you have used AutoText in previous versions of Word, you may find the new terminology in Word 2007 confusing. From a practical standpoint, AutoText entries and building blocks are the same thing and function the same way. In Word 2007, an AutoText entry is a *type* of building block that appears in the AutoText gallery. The gallery setting determines where the entry appears on the ribbon, but does not affect the way the entry functions. In the context of medical transcription, it still makes sense to refer to entries as AutoText entries, as the types of entries that you will most likely use can logically be saved in the AutoText gallery (as opposed to one of the other galleries such as Header, Footer, Cover Pages, Page Numbers, Tables, Tables of Contents, Text Boxes).

Create an AutoText Entry

Follow these steps to create a new building block in the AutoText gallery:

1. Type and select the text, table, or graphic that you want to store.

2. Press **ALT+F3** or choose Insert > Quick Parts > Save Selection to Quick Part Gallery. This will open the **Create New Building Block** dialog as in Figure 10-8.

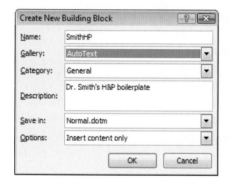

FIGURE 10-8 The Create New Building Block dialog box allows you to create a new AutoText entry.

3. Type a name for the entry or accept the default name (the first few letters of the entry). The *Name* will also be the shortcut for inserting the entry.

4. Choose a *Gallery* from the drop-down list. The gallery selection will determine which drop-down menu (gallery on the ribbon) will display your new entry. If this is a routine shortcut to be used while transcribing, I recommend using the *AutoText* gallery. If you choose *Quick Parts*, the entry will appear on the drop-down menu under Insert > Text > **Quick Parts**.

5. Select a *Category*. You can create your own categories such as exams, boilerplates, normals, etc, or you can simply assign your new entry to *General*. One advantage of assigning a category is to be able to sort your entries on the drop-down gallery lists and in the **Building Blocks Organizer** (see Figure 10-11). To create a new category, open the category drop-down list and choose *Create new category*. Type a new category name of your choosing.

6. Type a *Description* if you would like, but this is optional. The description will appear as a ToolTip when you hover over the entry in a drop-down gallery (see Figure 10-7).

7. Next, choose the *Template* that will store your new entry. If the entry is specific to one type of report and you have created a template for that report, save the entry in that specific template. (Of course, you must be working in that template currently for it to be listed.) The new entry will default to the Building Blocks template if you don't choose otherwise.

8. Last, choose how you want the entry to insert. Most likely, you will want to choose *Insert content only*. Other options include *Insert content in its own paragraph* and *Insert contents in its own page*. *Insert content in its own paragraph* will break the paragraph at the current insertion point and then create another paragraph after the entry. *Insert contents in its own page* will insert page breaks above and below the entry when the entry is inserted.

To quickly move through the **Create New Building Block** dialog, press **Tab**. Tap the first letter of the option in each drop-down box to quickly select an option. For example, type a name, press **Tab**, tap the **A** (to select *AutoText* gallery), press **Tab**, tap the **G** for *General* category, etc. Press **Enter** when finished.

At first, you may find all the options somewhat confusing, but the good news is all these options are easily changed. Create your entries however you feel best suits your needs, and if you learn that you made a poor choice or that your entry doesn't work optimally, change the entry's properties (see below). Experience, in this case, will be your best guide.

In the context of transcription, by far the majority of my Building Blocks (AutoText entries) is made up of phrases, paragraphs, and boilerplates that are unique to a dictator or an account. I don't usually create building blocks for headers and footers, because I set up these elements (only once) in my template file and never have to add these elements during routine transcription. Since I use the AutoText feature to insert text as I am transcribing, I want to be able to insert text quickly and efficiently without picking up the mouse or navigating through the ribbon and drop-down menus. For this reason, the gallery option is technically of little significance. The category option is helpful for sorting and locating entries using the **Organizer**, but there's no harm if you choose not to use these categories.

Name AutoText Entries

The name of your AutoText entry is also the shortcut for inserting the entry using the keyboard. AutoText entries saved in the Normal template or within the same document template should have unique names if you want to be able to insert them by typing the shortcut name. For example, if you save four sentences

WORD 2007

that start with "The patient. . ." and you accept the name suggested by Word (ie, The patient), these entries will not have unique names. When you type the shortcut name (ie, the patient) Word will not know which of the four sentences you want and will not insert any text. A warning will appear on the <u>Status Bar</u> (as in Figure 10-9) to let you know the name is not unique.

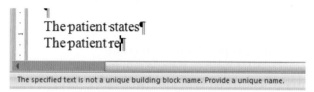

The·patient·states¶
The·patient·re¶

The specified text is not a unique building block name. Provide a unique name.

FIGURE 10-9 A message appears on the Status Bar when an AutoText name has been duplicated and Word is unable to insert the entry.

Word allows duplicate or near-duplicate names for AutoText entries because you can get around duplicates by inserting entries using the drop-down menus—duplicate names only come into play when you use the shortcut name to insert the entry. AutoText entries stored in separate document templates *can* have the same name.

The real advantage of AutoText is to be able to insert a block of text *without picking up the mouse to peruse a long list of entries*. If your entry doesn't insert, rename your AutoText entry so it has a more unique name. The less unique the name, the more characters you have to type before Word can distinguish one entry from another with the same beginning characters. You can also use single letters and even numbers as an AutoText shortcut.

Also be aware that Word 2007 has many building blocks built in and the chances of duplicating names or having shortcut names collide is more likely than in previous versions of Word. If you accidentally insert the wrong text, simply press CTRL+Z to remove the unintentional insertion and then rename one of the entries or delete the offending building block (see instructions below).

If you type for several doctors who each have a different physical exam section, you can save the boilerplate text in AutoText and name each of them "PE." The trick is to store them in each doctor's personal template file. This way, the correct AutoText entry will only be available to you when you open a document based on that doctor's template. Even though you have several entries named PE, you will always insert the correct PE format. This keeps your abbreviation system simple and consistent, and that means fewer shortcuts to remember!

In the same way, create AutoText entries for phrases that are unique to that dictator and save them in his/her template file. When you change work assignments, you can simply delete the template file(s), and your system will not be "cluttered" with shortcuts you no longer use.

AutoText works really well for creating shortcuts for titles (eg, Dr., Mrs., Mr.) followed by a nonbreaking space, because the AutoText entry will insert without inserting an additional space or punctuation mark. The cursor remains at the point of insertion (unlike an AutoCorrect entry that always includes a space or punctuation mark at the end of the insertion). For example, you can create a shortcut for inserting Dr. followed by a nonbreaking space so you can immediately type the surname without having to backup and remove a regular space before typing the surname. Remember, using a nonbreaking space will prevent Dr. and the surname from separating across a line break. To create, type the title and a nonbreaking space (**CTRL+Shift+Spacebar**). Select the characters, including the nonbreaking space, and press **ALT+F3**. Name the entry with a simple name such as d or dr and insert using **F3**.

After creating or changing entries to Building Blocks, you may be prompted to save changes to the Normal.dotm, the Building Blocks.dotx, or the document template. Be sure to answer Yes.

Formatted AutoText Entries

If you apply font characteristics such as bold or italic, this information will be saved with the AutoText entry, and it will always insert with these characteristics. It is also important to note that AutoText will preserve the capitalization exactly as it is saved. If you save an AutoText entry without capitalizing the first word and then insert it at the beginning of a sentence, AutoCorrect's automatic capitalization feature will not override the formatting, and the first word of the sentence will remain lowercase.

AutoText entries saved with a paragraph mark will insert with that paragraph formatting (ie, centered, justified, align right or left), as well as a paragraph break, even if you select *Insert content only* (the paragraph mark will be considered part of the content). Decide whether you want this information included with your AutoText entry. Be sure to reveal paragraph marks (**CTRL+Shift+8**) before selecting the text to be memorized as an AutoText entry so you know whether the paragraph mark is included in the selection. Also take note of leading or trailing spaces so you don't create spacing problems when you insert the entry into your text.

Assign Fonts to New Entries

If you use AutoText entries and you transcribe in more than one font (eg, Dr. Smith uses Arial and Central Clinic uses Times New Roman), it is especially important that you use templates and assign the default font to match the font used in the template. When AutoText entries are created, Word memorizes the *status of the font used relative to the current default font*. If the AutoText entry is created in the same font as the default font, then Word remembers to insert the entry in the default font—whatever the current default font is. If the entry is created in a font that *differs* from the default font, Word remembers that the entry is an *exception* to the default and assumes that you always want to insert the text exactly as typed regardless of the surrounding text. Using AutoText entries in documents with mismatched font settings will cause what appear to be random (and very irritating) font changes.

This concept may be difficult to grasp at first, and may even seem convoluted, but it actually makes sense when you think about the way the majority of companies use Word. Companies often require all company correspondence to adhere to a given style, including a specific font. If you worked for a company that used Tahoma for all its correspondence but used a decorative script for the company's slogan, you would want that slogan to always insert in the decorative font—otherwise you would be reformatting the entry each time it was used, and that takes away from AutoText's usefulness. Almost all of Word's features are built around the concepts of templates and styles, and its functionality assumes that templates and default fonts are being used.

The issue of the font becomes a problem in transcription when you type in more than one font yet you use the same AutoText entries across all document types. The solution is to use template files and designate default fonts (remember, simply changing the font using the toolbar or the dialog box does not change the underlying font associated with the document). Review templates in Chapter 8 and font formatting on page 203. If your employment situation does not allow for the use of template files (dotm or dotx files), then you can change the default font before transcribing each document. In other words, if you *must* type a document in another font, don't just change the font, designate that font as the default and do this each time you create a new document with a different font. You could create a macro with a shortcut key to accomplish this in a single keystroke, which would be somewhat of a nuisance to remember, but not nearly as aggravating as correcting font changes in the middle of your document.

Insert an AutoText Entry

To use an AutoText entry, simply type the shortcut (the AutoText name) and press **F3**. The entry will insert at the insertion point. You may not have to type the entire AutoText name before pressing **F3**, but you do have to type enough characters for Word to distinguish it from any others that start with the same characters.

If you forget the name of your building block, you can use the corresponding gallery or the **Building Blocks Organizer** to insert your entry. For example, items saved to the Quick Parts gallery will appear on the Quick Parts drop-down menu.

Go to |Insert| > <u>Text</u> > |**Quick Parts**| (see Figure 10-10) and choose from the menu (gallery). If you saved your entry to the AutoText gallery, or if you cannot locate the correct gallery, go to |Insert| > <u>Text</u> > |**Quick Parts**| > Building Blocks Organizer. Select the entry and click |Insert|.

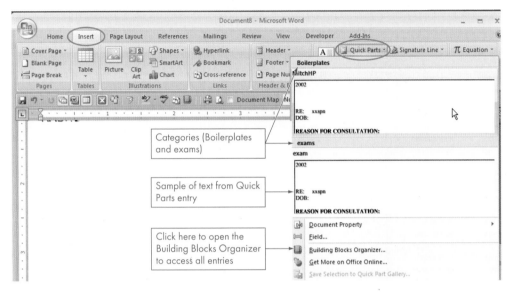

FIGURE 10-10 Entries saved under Quick Parts will display in the Quick Parts gallery and will sort by category if applicable. Click an entry to insert into your document.

 You can add an AutoText drop-down menu to the <u>Quick Access</u> toolbar for easy access to the items saved in the AutoText gallery. See instructions on page 400 for adding commands to the <u>Quick Access</u> toolbar. The AutoText drop-down menu is found under *All Commands* > *AutoText*.

 Many of the built-in building blocks contain fields associated with document properties, including fields for dates. Review Chapter 11 on using fields before inserting date fields into a medical report.

 An AutoText entry can contain fields but it cannot contain commands. Combining macros, fields, and AutoText entries works well for placing paragraphs to be edited. Create a macro that inserts an AutoText entry and then moves the cursor to the first position within that paragraph to continue transcribing. For example, you may need to insert a physical exam boilerplate and then edit the vital signs. Record a macro that inserts the AutoText entry and then moves the cursor up to the first vital sign entry. Learn how to use fields in Chapter 11 and macros in Chapter 12.

Manage AutoText Entries

Word includes the **Building Blocks Organizer** for managing all your building blocks (Figure 10-11). To open the organizer, click `Insert` > Quick Parts > Building Blocks Organizer.

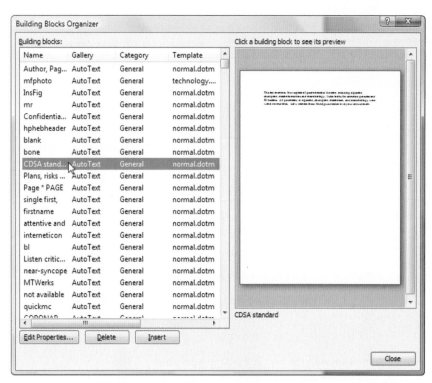

FIGURE 10-11 Use the Building Blocks Organizer to manage all your entries.

Here are a few tips for managing your entries:

- The **Organizer** lists entries in tabular form. Click any of the column headers to sort the building blocks alphabetically by that column.
- The list is quite long, so move through the list quicker by tapping the first letter of an item's name.
- To delete an entry, simply select it from the list and click `Delete`.
- To change one of the entry's properties (eg, move to a different gallery), select the item and click `Edit Properties`. The **Modify Building Block** dialog box opens, which looks exactly like the **Create New Building Block** dialog (see Figure 10-7). Choose a different gallery from the drop-down list.

To copy/move an entry to a different template file, follow these steps:

1. Open a document based on the template that contains the AutoText entry, or if the item is stored in the Normal.dotm or Building Blocks.dotx, open a document based on a template that you want to contain the AutoText entry.
2. Open the **Building Blocks Organizer** and select the item to be moved.

3. Click **Edit Properties**. The **Modify Building Block** dialog box opens, which looks exactly like the **Create New Building Block** dialog (see Figure 10-8).

4. Choose a template from the *Save in* drop-down list.

5. After making changes, confirm that you want to redefine the entry. Any change will prompt the message to "redefine" the entry.

Modify an Entry

You cannot modify the contents of a building block using the **Building Blocks Organizer**. To edit the text of an entry, you will need to insert the entry into your document and make your edits in the document. Once you have made the changes, select the entry again and re-save it. If you duplicate the name and all the properties exactly, Word will ask if you want to replace the previous entry. If you do not recreate the name and all the properties exactly as before, Word will create another entry. This duplication can cause problems when inserting (and you may inadvertently insert the wrong text). It may be easier to delete the first entry (after inserting it into your document) and then save the newly edited entry as if it was a brand new entry.

To make it easier to access the **Building Blocks Organizer**, place an icon on the <u>Quick Launch</u> toolbar. Right-click the menu item for the Building Blocks Organizer (Figure 10-12) and choose Add to Quick Access Toolbar. A small green book will appear on the <u>Quick Access</u> toolbar.

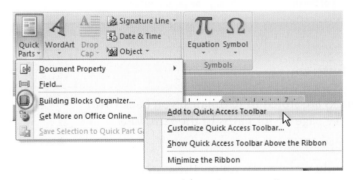

FIGURE 10-12 Add the Building Blocks Organizer to the Quick Access toolbar.

Print AutoText Entries

To print AutoText entries, open a document based on a template that contains the AutoText entries you want to print. Press **CTRL+P** to open the **Print** dialog box.

In the *Print what* box, select *Building Blocks entries* as in Figure 10-13. This will print AutoText entries contained in the Normal.dotm and the currently active template. Since Word 2007 installs with so many building blocks already, this print job will be extremely large (possibly over 100 pages).

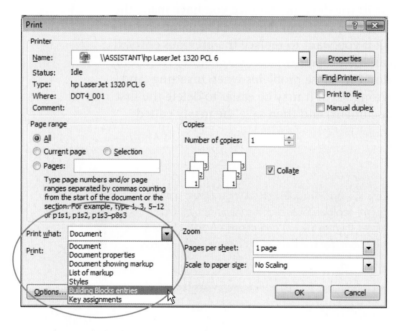

FIGURE 10-13 Use the Print dialog box to print a list of building blocks, although be prepared for this to print as many as 100 or more pages.

Back Up and Share AutoText Entries

Since AutoText and other building blocks are stored in templates, you back them up by backing up your template files. See page 71 for paths to the **Template** folder and the Building Blocks.dotx.

To share your AutoText entries with another computer, follow these steps:

1. Copy the template file containing the building blocks and place on removable media.

2. If the entries are stored in the Normal template or the Building Blocks template, rename the template slightly before copying to the receiving computer.

3. Place the template on the computer that you want to receive the new entries.

4. Open a document based on this template (see page 252).

5. Open the **Building Blocks Organizer** and click the column header to sort by template.

6. Select an entry to be moved and click to open the **Modify Building Block** dialog box.

7. In the *Save in* box, change the template name to Normal.dotm or Building Blocks.dotx.

 To access AutoText entries stored in another template, you can also attach the template to the current document using the **Templates and Add-ins** dialog box. This will give you access to AutoText entries without copying the entries from one template file to another. See page 324 for instructions on attaching templates.

Troubleshoot AutoText

Many transcriptionists have experienced the mysterious "font change" when inserting an AutoText entry. You will encounter this problem if you change fonts between documents and do not assign the default font. Not only will this create problems when memorizing AutoText entries, but you will be very frustrated with the constant need to change the font. Review the information above on Assigning Fonts to a New Entry on page 291.

Critical Thinking Questions

1. Compare and contrast AutoCorrect and AutoText. Give three examples of how you can use each feature.

   _____

   _____

2. List three advantages to storing AutoText entries in document templates.

   _____

   _____

3. Describe the relationship between the formatting associated with an Auto-Text entry and the default font.

   _____

   _____

4. Consider this scenario: Template A has a default font of Times New Roman. Template B has a default font of Arial 10 point. An AutoText entry is created in Template A using Arial 12 point font and is then inserted into a document based on Template B. How will the entry appear in the document based on Template B?

   _____

   _____

5. Why do you think Word allows AutoText shortcuts to be duplicated but not AutoCorrect shortcuts?

   _____

   _____

6. Word 2007 only: Describe the relationship between Building Blocks and AutoText entries.

   _____

   _____

7. How do you back up AutoText entries?

   _____

   _____

8. Create AutoText entries for the following:

   a. The SOAP note format created in Chapter 7.

   b. Main headings shown in the sample template on page 423.

CHAPTER 11

Fields

OBJECTIVES

▸ Use empty fields to navigate boilerplate text.
▸ Use shortcut keys to manage fields.
▸ Use data fields to insert document information and patient demographics.

Fields are one of the most powerful tools in MS Word. These tiny little workhorses can transform the way you work and save you a tremendous amount of time. This chapter will introduce both empty fields and data fields as well as give examples of how to use both in the context of medical documentation.

KEYWORDS

data field
Document properties
empty field
field code
field results
lock
source
unlinking
update

Shortcut keys
ALT+F9
CTRL+F9
F11

Using Empty Fields

One of the drawbacks of using templates with standard text or even boilerplate text is maneuvering through the text quickly as you are transcribing. Moving the insertion point to the next spot within the text to continue transcribing can be tedious. Placing "jump points" throughout the text solves this problem, making templated reports efficient and easy to use.

The classic "jump" (used by transcriptionists since the days of Word Perfect 5.1) uses characters such as two question marks (??) or an asterisk (*) to mark the spot for the next text insertion. A macro (a series of commands) is then used to search for the characters and set the insertion point. In MS Word, an **empty field** can be used to create these jump points instead of placing symbols. For example, to easily transcribe vital signs, you can set up a sentence in your boilerplate containing an empty field at each data point.

VITAL SIGNS: Blood pressure { }, pulse { }, respirations { }, temperature { }°.

The braces { } represent jump points (empty fields). Once you have set up your boilerplate text with jump points, you simply press **F11** to jump from one position to the next, quickly filling in the data without having to repeatedly tap the arrow keys or pick up the mouse to place the insertion point.

Empty fields have several advantages over the symbol-and-macro approach. Empty fields can be placed anywhere in a document, including tables, headers, and footers. They can even be saved as part of an AutoText entry. Unlike asterisks and other characters, you do not have to worry about deleting unused markers. Empty fields are not like form fields (a different feature in MS Word), so they do not have to be "protected," and you are not limited to the type or amount of text that you can place in the field. Also, you can pre-format an empty field with font characteristics such as bold and all caps.

Here are a few tips for working with empty fields:

- To place an empty field, place your insertion point where you want to set a jump point and then press **CTRL+F9**. A pair of braces will appear with two spaces between them. Use the arrow keys to move the cursor outside the braces without disturbing the spacing between the braces.

- The set of braces will appear when you first place the field, but after you close and reopen the file, the braces will be hidden.

- To display or hide empty fields (ie, the braces), press **ALT+F9** (a toggle command). This shortcut key corresponds to the option *Switch between field code and its result* (see page 135 in Word 2003 and page 172 in Word 2007).

 Shading fields makes them stand out so they are easier to work with. To display field shading, go to Tools > Options > **View** and select *Field shading: Always*.

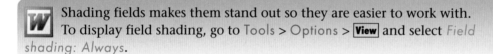 Shading fields makes them stand out so they are easier to work with. To display field shading, go to **Office** > **Word Options** > **Advanced** > **Show Document Content** > *Field Shading: Always*.

 The options to display field codes and field shading are local settings, meaning they do not follow the document. The next person to view the document will not see field codes or field shading unless they have these options set on their own copy of Word.

Each time you press the **F11** key, you will move from one empty field to the next. Word calls this "browsing by fields." Using the **F11** key will change your "browse" settings, which changes the way the **Page up** and **Page down** keys function (see page 125 for a full explanation). **CTRL+Page down** and **CTRL+Page up** will now move to the next field or the previous field (respectively).

You can return the **Page up** and **Page down** keys to their native function if necessary. At the bottom of your Vertical scroll bar, click the small center button (see Figure 11-1) or press **CTRL+ALT+Home** to open the **Browse Object** dialog box. Select the page icon and press **Enter**. Of course, the next time you hit **F11**, **CTRL+Page up** and **CTRL+Page down** will revert back to browsing by field.

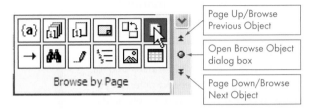

FIGURE 11-1 Use the Browse Object dialog box to restore the function of the Page up and Page down keys.

 If you need **CTRL+Page up** and **CTRL+Page down** to retain their function (ie, move to the top of the previous or next page), reassign the commands BrowsePrev and BrowseNext to a different key combination (other than the **Page up** and **Page down** keys) or remove the key assignments altogether. See Chapter 15 to learn how to reassign shortcut keys.

Formatting Empty Fields

Applying formatting to empty fields makes this template-navigation technique even more useful. When formatting is pre-defined, you can jump to the empty field and continue transcribing without pausing to make formatting changes. To format a field, set the insertion point and then open the **Font** dialog box (**CTRL+D**) and/or the **Paragraph** dialog box (**ALT, O, P**) to make the necessary format selections. Immediately after making the format changes, press **CTRL+F9** to set the empty field.

If the text that immediately *precedes* a field is formatted differently (see example below), set an empty field then select the field along with the space or tab character that immediately precedes the field and then apply the font attributes. This will ensure that the field itself carries the correct formatting.

 The allergy section of a document is a good place to apply special formatting. Often, allergies are to be typed in bold and uppercase. Set a field at this position within the standard text and open the **Font** dialog box. Select *Bold* and *All caps*. When you press **F11** to type the allergies, the characters will insert as bold and all caps (without having to press caps lock).

 If you use the All caps formatting, be sure you press **F11** or an arrow key, not the **Enter** key, to move the insertion point to the next position to continue transcribing. If you press the **Enter** key, the formatting commands will carry forward and you will continue to type in bold and all caps.

Carefully test your formatting before finalizing your template or saving your boilerplate. Press **F11** to jump to each field and examine the toolbars/ribbons for the correct formatting, or type a few characters to make sure they insert correctly. Press **CTRL+Z** (not **Delete**) to remove the text without disturbing the field or formatting. Uses for fields are only limited by your imagination!

It is critically important that you display formatting marks when setting up your standard text containing empty fields. Remember, the spaces and tab characters retain character formatting just like any other character, so you must pay attention to spaces and tabs on either side of your empty fields. If the spaces that immediately precede your empty field carry the bold format, then text inserted at that point will insert in bold (see Figure 11-2). If you do not pay close attention to the formatting when setting up your standard text, using the template will be very frustrating, because you will have to adjust the formatting while you are transcribing.

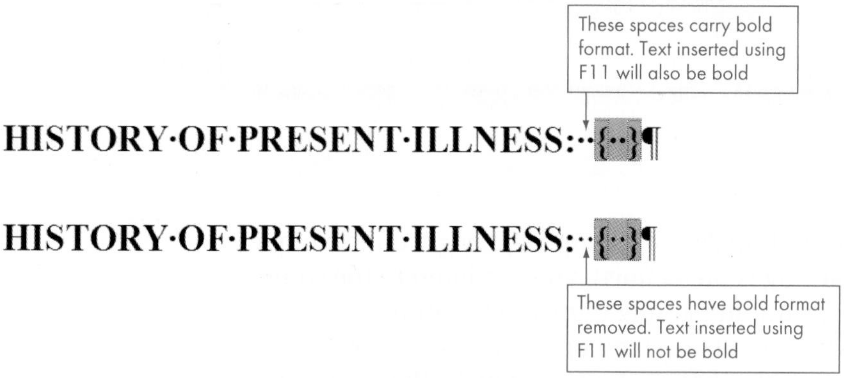

These spaces carry bold format. Text inserted using F11 will also be bold

HISTORY·OF·PRESENT·ILLNESS:··{··}¶

HISTORY·OF·PRESENT·ILLNESS:··{··}¶

These spaces have bold format removed. Text inserted using F11 will not be bold

FIGURE 11-2 Display formatting marks while setting up boilerplate text. Note that spaces and paragraph marks with bold formatting are displayed in heavier type.

As in the example above, empty fields are perfect for typing vital signs and filling in other details of the physical exam. Place empty fields throughout your standard text, so you can go immediately from the patient name to the date of the report to the medical record number, etc. See also sample templates in Chapter 16.

If your doctor has a sentence that he uses often, but it changes only slightly (eg, lab results like a CBC or CMP or standard text for EKG results), you can create an AutoText entry with empty fields placed at points where you will insert each individual result. When needed, insert the AutoText entry, press **Home** or **Up** to move the insertion point above the first empty field, then press **F11** to jump to the first field. You could also record these steps as a macro (see Chapter 12).

I place empty fields throughout standard paragraphs, such as a review of systems, at the beginning of each sentence or at the beginning of commonly changed phrases. I tap the F11 key to follow the dictator through the paragraph, sentence by sentence. If the dictator makes a change to the standard text, my insertion point is already in place to begin editing. I use macros to quickly delete phrases and sentences from the standard to be replaced with the newly dictated text. Learn more about editing techniques in Chapter 14 and macros in Chapter 12.

Hiding or Displaying Fields

You can transcribe with fields displayed or hidden; it's often a matter of personal preference. The F11 key will move to the next empty field whether fields are displayed or not. You can easily toggle the fields "on" and "off" using ALT+F9. I prefer to transcribe with the fields hidden, but you should try it both ways to see how it works best for you. If you work in Word along with a transcription platform or a text-expansion program, you may need to try both ways to see how the different software features interact with each other.

If fields are displayed while transcribing, the F11 key will jump to the field and select the field. When you begin typing, the field will be replaced with the text (ie, typing over selected items replaces the item). One drawback to deleting fields as you transcribe is it will prevent you from being able to "jump backwards" or from using the fields to navigate the document during proofreading. Since empty fields take up four spaces when displayed, they can potentially change page breaks. Be sure to double-check page breaks with fields hidden before delivering the document.

It was not Microsoft's intention to use empty fields for jump points. Empty fields were actually created so that advanced users could create their own data fields. It just so happens that using empty fields as jumps is a clever way to take advantage of a feature that was designed for a very different use. On the job, you may work on a transcription platform that provides you with a document for each new job to be transcribed or edited. These documents may already contain data fields that interact with the transcription platform. These fields may be used to insert the patient name, date of service, dictation system ID, dictation date, or other pertinent data. These data fields will contain actual field codes—not just empty braces. Usually there's no harm in mixing empty fields with data fields; just be aware that displaying empty fields will display the field codes for these other fields as well (see further explanation below). Be sure that you don't delete the data fields inserted by the transcription platform.

Using Fields for Notations

When setting up templates, it can be helpful to leave notes or instructions to guide you while transcribing, especially if the account has a lot of specifications. Leaving embedded instructions is also very helpful for training new MTs on an account, since you can leave notations right where the information is needed. To embed instructions in a template, insert an empty field at the point where the instruction applies. Set the insertion point between the two spaces inside the brackets and type a / (forward slash). Immediately follow the slash with a note or instruction. Examples of notes might include:

```
{/type medications in paragraph form}

{/do not delete this disclaimer}

{/use list format if obstetrical history is dictated}
```

Simply toggle **ATL+F9** to display or hide the notes as necessary. The client will not see these notes unless by some chance they were to turn on field codes (which is not likely). You can type the report with field codes showing or not. Fields with notes displayed will take up space and potentially shift page breaks, so the layout should be checked with field codes hidden before delivering the document.

Be sure to start the note with a slash, otherwise the phrase **Error: Bookmark not found** will be displayed in the document. If not removed from the document, this notation will also print.

Working with Data Fields

A **data field** (not an empty field) can be thought of as a "go fetch" command that can be placed anywhere in a document. In their most basic form, fields contain instructions for retrieving information from another **source** and placing that information within the field. The source can be somewhere within the same document or even outside the current document. Fields are also capable of performing mathematical calculations (eg, retrieving numbers from various locations in a document and displaying the sum) and transforming data from one format to another (eg, changing a date from 1-15-2009 to January 15, 2009). Fields are powerful tools for automating your work, but it is important to understand a little bit about fields before you use them extensively. Fortunately, you don't need to understand how to program fields to take advantage of them; Word has many fields built in and ready to use.

A field consists of the **field code** (instructions) and the **field results** (the information obtained based on the instruction). Figure 11-3 shows a snippet from a document with two fields displayed as field codes and then as field results. Toggle **ALT+F9** to switch between field codes and field results.

¶ I
PATIENT·NAME: → {·DOCPROPERTY·"ReversePatName"·*·MERGEFORMAT·}¶

TYPE·OF·REPORT: → PROCEDURE·NOTE¶

DATE·OF·VISIT: → {·DOCPROPERTY·"ServiceDate"·\@·"MMMM·DD,·yyyy"·*·
MERGEFORMAT·}¶

¶
PATIENT·NAME: → DAYLE·PORTER¶

TYPE·OF·REPORT: → PROCEDURE·NOTE¶

DATE·OF·VISIT: → March·24,·2009¶

FIGURE 11-3 The same fields displayed as field codes (above) and field results (below).

The above figure shows the fields with shading around the field itself. The shading immediately identifies the information as a field and provides a visual reminder that you cannot directly edit the information contained in the shaded area. *If you use fields, turn field shading on!*

 To display field shading, go to Tools > Options > |View|. Under *Field Shading*, choose *Always*.

 To display field shading, go to |Office| > |Word Options| > |Advanced| > |Show Document Content| > *Field shading: Always*.

The biggest advantage to using fields is their ability to automatically adapt to changes. **Update** causes a field to refer back to the source of the information and make necessary changes to the results. Some fields automatically update as the information changes (eg, page-number fields change as soon as you add a new page), while other fields must be forced to update. Many fields are designed to update when the document is closed and reopened. To force a field to update, set the cursor in the field and press **F9**. To force all fields to update, press **CTRL+A, F9**. To update fields inside the header or footer space, display the header and footer (**ALT, V, H**) and press **CTRL+A, F9**.

The most important thing to remember when working with fields is that *you cannot directly edit the results of a field,* you must edit the *source* of the information. For example, if you have a field that retrieves the patient name and places it in a given position in the document and you discover that the name is spelled incorrectly, you cannot correct the patient name in that field—you have to correct the name *at the source*. If you edit the field itself, it may appear to reflect the change, but when you close and reopen the document, the field will update based on the source, and the name will revert to the incorrect spelling.

Fields are very useful for automating your work. You can use them to keep document information current, consistent, complete, and accurate—with little or no effort on your part. Word includes many fields, and some are easily accessible on ribbons, toolbars, and menus. For example, the page number icon accessible when the header and footer space is open is actually the command to insert the page number *field*. Place fields in your template files or boilerplate text and let Word automatically update information for you. See sample projects using fields on pages 456 and 460. Some fields that are useful in medical transcription include:

- Page number
- Date and Time
- User initials
- Document properties (eg, document name, word or character count, author)
- Bookmarks and Cross-references

Inserting Fields

Insert a field by first placing the insertion point where you want the field to appear and then press the shortcut key associated with the field (eg, page number and date fields). If the field does not have a shortcut key assigned, locate the specific field command on the Insert menu (Word 2003) or the **Insert** tab (Word 2007). If you cannot locate the field on a ribbon or toolbar, use the **Field** dialog box (Figure 11-4).

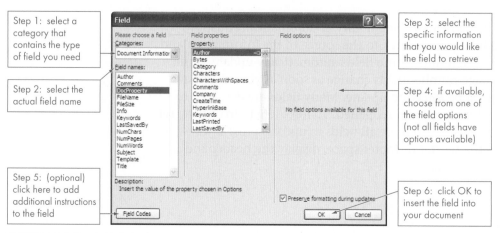

FIGURE 11-4 The Field dialog box.

Figure 11-4 describes how to use the **Field** dialog box. The Field Codes button in the bottom left corner allows you to add more instructions (called switches) to the field, such as how to display a date (eg, in digits or spelled out) or how to format the field results (eg, uppercase, lowercase, or title case).

The following paragraphs describe various fields that you may find useful.

Page numbers: Page-number fields work really well when placed in headers and footers. To insert, click icons available on the Header and Footer toolbar/ribbon or press **ALT+Shift+P**. AutoText (in Word 2003) also includes page number entries in several different formats (eg, Page X and Page X of Y where Y is total number of pages in the document).

Date and Time fields: These fields insert dates and time stamps, which can be helpful, but there are a few words of caution in order. The date field that will insert with the shortcut **ALT+Shift+D** is the *current* date. This field refers to your computer's system date as set by the **Date and Time Properties** box on the Control Panel. This is not an appropriate date field to use as the transcription date, dictation date, or date of service, because it will update when the document is opened on a different day. The Create Date field, on the other hand, inserts the date the document was created and does not update. This field works well for entering the transcription date. Open the **Field** dialog box and choose *Category: Date and Time* then *Field name: CreateDate*. Choose a date format under *Properties*.

User Initials: This particular field can be used to place initials in your report. Place a User initials field at the end of your reports to automatically place your initials or transcriptionist ID. Open the **Field** dialog box and choose *Category: User Information* then *Field name: UserInitials*. This field inserts information based on the **User Information** dialog (see page 146 in Word 2003 and 160 in Word 2007).

Document Properties: Use this field to insert information associated with the **Document Property** dialog box. Fields applicable to transcription might include *Author, FileName, NumChars* (number of characters), and *NumWords* (number of words). Learn more in the next section Using Document Properties. Also, see page 465 under Special Projects for an example of using document-information fields to help build log sheets that include the file name and character count.

Bookmarks and Cross references: These two features work together to take information from one part of the document and copy it to another part of the document. The bookmark acts as a "source" field. The cross-reference field "fetches" the bookmarked information and places that text in the cross-reference field. A good example of their use in transcription would be to automatically transfer the patient name from the primary position in the document (usually at the beginning of the report) to a second-page header or other location within the document.

Cross-reference fields can also be saved using AutoText. Using the patient name as an example, the name can be typed into a bookmarked area of the document and then the AutoText entry that references the bookmark can be inserted "on the fly" wherever the patient name is needed. See page 462 under Special Projects for an explanation of this technique.

If you cannot set a specific place in your template for a field, you can place a field "on the fly" by saving the field itself as an AutoText entry. To do this, insert the field into a document, select the field, and press **ALT+F3**. Type a name for your field in the dialog box. The name will be the shortcut for inserting the field when needed. To insert the field, type the AutoText name and press **F3**. The field will insert and instantly update with the field results. Remember, the field result displayed at the time you create your AutoText entry doesn't matter; it's the field *code* that you are capturing in your AutoText entry. The field results will update based on the information in the document at the time it is placed.

Locking and Unlinking Fields

You may choose to **lock** fields so that they cannot update—even if you try to force an update with the update command (**F9**). To lock a field, place the cursor in the field and press **CTRL+F11**. To lock all fields in a document, press **CTRL+A** to select all and then press **CTRL+F11**. This same key will also unlock fields.

You can also convert field results to regular text by **unlinking** the field from its source. To unlink a field, set the insertion point in the field and press **CTRL+Shift+F9**. A field that has been locked can be unlocked and then updated, but a field that has been unlinked is no longer a field (it's just regular text). An unlinked field cannot be converted back to a field; therefore, it cannot be updated.

It can be useful to lock fields or unlink fields when transferring information away from the source. For example, if you copy field information such as the character count from your document and copy it into a log sheet, you do not want the character count to update—that will give you the character count for the log sheet. In this case you can either lock the field before copying the field to a new document or unlink the field.

Using Document Properties

Every document has document properties, and this information can be leveraged to increase your efficiency. **Document properties** are a form of metadata (data which describes data). Document properties include the document's file name, the author, the title, subject matter, and many other types of information that describe the file. Properties also include statistical information about the document such as the file size, page count, and character count, as well as the date the document was created, last modified, or printed. The **Properties** dialog box can be viewed from inside the document

(File > Properties). You can also access **Properties** from Windows Explorer (right-click file name and choose Properties or press **ALT+Enter**).

To apply these concepts to transcription, use document properties for entering patient demographics (eg, name, date of service, date of birth, medical record number, etc). Place document property fields in your template along with the standard text and then type patient information into the corresponding text box in the **Properties** dialog box. Follow these steps:

1. Choose one of the fields to represent the patient's name (or other demographic data) and insert this field into your document where you want the patient's name to appear. Go to Insert > Field > Document Information > DocProperty and choose a specific Property.
2. If applicable, insert the same field in the second-page header space.
3. To use the fields during the transcription process, display the **Properties** dialog box (File > Properties) and type the patient's name directly into the document **Properties** dialog box. This information will transfer to the corresponding fields in the document itself.

Repeat this process for other types of patient information such as date of birth or medical record number. This approach will save you time by typing the information only once and also will avoid the possibility of typos when retyping the information in other areas of the document. In addition, any subsequent corrections to patient demographics can be made in the **Properties** dialog box (inside or outside of Word) and all related fields in the document will update automatically.

Not all document properties are strictly limited to the labels assigned to them by Microsoft, so several of them can be "repurposed" for patient demographic information. For example, the Keyword field could be used as the date of service. The Subject might actually be used as a date of birth field or the medical record number. You can be creative in the way you use these properties.

If you use this approach, you can have Word open the **Properties** dialog box automatically when you first save the document. Go to Tools > Options > **Save** and place a check mark at Prompt for document properties.

WORD 2003

As a bonus, document properties can be displayed in Windows Explorer. In Details view, some of the document properties can be displayed as a column header (see Figure 11-5). Right-click a column header in Explorer and choose which columns to display based on the document properties you want to see. In this way, Windows Explorer combined with Word's document properties can build a database-type view of all documents in a folder so you can quickly sort and locate reports by patient name, file name, date of service, or similar information.

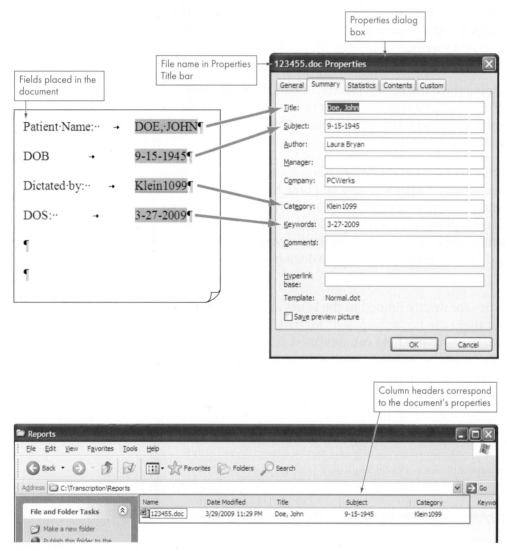

FIGURE 11-5 Document properties can be used as fields in the document itself and displayed as column headers in Windows Explorer.

 A list of helpful shortcut keys for working with fields can be found on page 313.

WORD 2007

Using Document Properties

Every document has document properties, and this information can be leveraged to increase your efficiency. **Document properties** are a form of metadata (data which describes data). Document properties include the document's file name, the author, the title, subject matter, and many other types of information that describe the file. Properties also include statistical information about the document such as the file size, page count, and character count, as well as the date the document was created, last modified, or printed. The **Properties** area can be viewed from inside the document (Office > Prepare > Properties) or from Windows Explorer (right-click file name and choose Properties or press **ALT+Enter**).

To apply these concepts to transcription, use document properties for entering patient demographics (eg, name, date of service, date of birth, medical record number, etc). Place document property fields in your template along with the standard text and then type patient information into the corresponding text box in the **Properties** dialog area. Follow these steps:

1. Choose one of the fields to represent the patient's name (or other demographic data) and insert this field into your document where you want the patient's name to appear. Go to Insert > Quick Parts > Document Property and choose a specific property.

2. If applicable, insert the same field in the second-page header space.

3. To use the fields during the transcription process, display the **Properties** dialog area (Office > Prepare > Properties) and type patient demographic information directly into the **Properties** dialog area. This information will transfer to the corresponding fields in the document itself.

Repeat this process for other types of patient information such as date of birth or medical record number. This approach will save you time by typing the information only once and also will avoid the possibility of typos when retyping the information in other areas of the document. In addition, any subsequent corrections to patient demographics can be made in the **Properties** dialog area (inside or outside of Word) and all related fields in the document will update automatically. Displaying patient demographic information across the top of the document can also provide at-a-glance information about the current file.

Add the Document Properties icon to the Quick Access toolbar (Office menu > Properties) or assign the command (TogglePropertyPanel) to a shortcut key to quickly display/hide the **Document Properties** area (see Chapter 15 for instructions on customizing key assignments and the Quick Access toolbar). Once you display the **Properties** area, it will remain open, even if you create a new document.

Not all document properties are strictly limited to the labels assigned to them by Microsoft, so several of them can be "repurposed" for patient demographic information. For example, the Keyword field could be used as the patient's name or the dictating physician's ID. The Subject might actually be used as a date-of-birth field or the medical record number. You can be creative in the way you use these properties.

As a bonus, document properties can be viewed in Windows Explorer. In Details view, some of the document properties can be displayed as column headers (see Figure 11-6). Right-click a column header in Explorer and choose which columns to display based on the document properties you want to see. In this way, Windows Explorer combined with Word's document properties can build a database-type view of all documents in a folder, allowing you to quickly sort and locate reports by patient name, file name, date of service, or similar information.

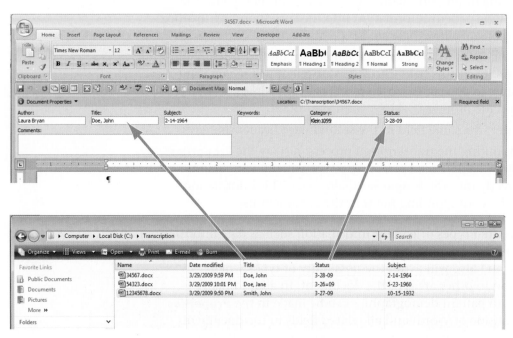

FIGURE 11-6 Document properties correspond to the column headers in Explorer.

Helpful Shortcut Keys

Table 11-1 lists shortcut keys associated with fields.

Table 11-1	Shortcut keys for working with fields.
CTRL+F9	Insert an empty field
F9	Update selected fields (forces the selected field(s) to update). To update all fields in a document, press CTRL+A, F9
ALT+F9	Switch between all field codes and their results—toggles all fields in the document
Shift+F9	Switch between a field code and its result—toggles the selected field only
ALT+Shift+D	Insert a date field (this date WILL automatically update when the document is open—do not use for dictation date, date of service, or transcription date).
ALT+Shift+P	Insert a page number field
ALT+Shift+T	Insert a time field
ALT+CTRL+L	Insert a field for numbering lists (LISTNUM field). This is not the same as the automatic numbering feature described in Chapter 13)
CTRL+Shift+F7	Update linked information in a Word source document
CTRL+Shift+F9	Unlink a field (turns the field results into regular text so it is no longer a field and no longer associated with the field source)
ALT+Shift+F9	Run GOTOBUTTON or MACROBUTTON from the field that displays the field results
F11	Go to the next field
Shift+F11	Go to the previous field
CTRL+F11	Lock a field (prevents the field from updating)
CTRL+Shift+F11	Unlock a field (unlocks a field so it can be updated)

Critical Thinking Questions

1. List at least three advantages of using empty fields as jump points compared to using symbols.

   _____

   _____

2. Explain why you cannot edit a data field directly.

   _____

   _____

3. Why should you display field shading?

   _____

   _____

4. Describe the relationship between document properties and column headers in Windows Explorer.

   _____

   _____

5. Add empty fields to the template you created in Chapter 8 (Sample.dot). Make sure the fields are formatted correctly so you do not have to apply or correct formatting as you transcribe.

6. Using the sample report on page 436 as a guide, create a document template. Add empty fields and make sure the fields are formatted so that jumping to the field automatically formats the text. Use document properties and data fields to place patient demographic information into the document.

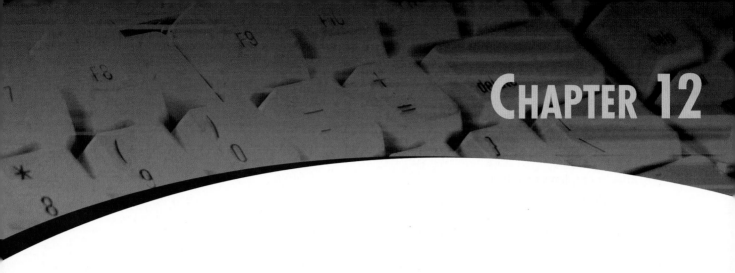

CHAPTER 12

Macros

OBJECTIVES

‣ Identify specific tasks that can be streamlined using a macro.

‣ Create macros using the Macro Recorder.

‣ Identify rules for naming and creating macros.

‣ Manage macros using the Macros dialog box.

‣ Share macros between templates or with other transcriptionists.

KEYWORDS

Macro Recorder

Macros dialog box

modules

Organizer

Run

Visual Basic for Applications

Shortcut keys

ALT+F8

Navigation keys (page 189)

If you perform a task repeatedly in Word, you can automate the task by using a macro. A macro is a series of Word commands that you group together as a single command to accomplish a task quickly and efficiently. Instead of stepping through a series of time-consuming, repetitive actions in Word, memorize the steps as a macro (in effect, a custom command) that accomplishes the task for you. Word includes a feature called the **Macro Recorder** for easily creating macros. Word actually records a macro as a series of Word commands in **Visual Basic for Applications** (VBA). This may sound complicated, but actually, the Macro Recorder creates the actual code for you. The Macro Recorder has some limitations, but is still powerful enough to create very useful macros without any knowledge of programming. After you gain more experience with recording macros, you may choose to use advanced methods of editing the macro code or writing VBA code yourself.

Recording macros is simple. If you can step through the commands and repeat the steps consistently, then you can create the macro by simply stepping through the commands with the Macro Recorder turned on. The recorder captures your steps, memorizes them, and then "plays them back" with lightning speed. Remember, use the Macro Recorder for shortcutting a *series of commands*. Whenever you find yourself repeating the same sequence of commands, especially mouse clicks, record those steps as a macro. You can use macros to:

- speed up routine editing and formatting
- quickly change an option or setting located in a dialog box
- open a new document based on a template
- manage templates and standard text

(Continued)

- navigate a template or boilerplate text when the report is not dictated in the same order as the template
- create log sheets
- attach templates to a document
- add additional templates to documents

Word already has many built-in commands, so before recording a simple macro, review the list of Word commands to see if the function is already available (see page 183). If the command is available, assign a shortcut key instead of recording a macro (see page 394 in Word 2003 and 403 in Word 2007 for instructions on assigning shortcut keys). You will be pleasantly surprised to learn that you will not need a tremendous number of macros. If you use boilerplate text, template files, fields, and Word's built-in commands, there are probably only a few tasks left to be streamlined using macros.

The macro feature in Word is *not* the best tool for saving shortcuts to insert routine phrases and paragraphs. There is a limit to the number of macros you can store in a single template file (up to 150 per template), so using the macro recorder as a text expander is a poor use of resources. AutoText, AutoCorrect, and third-party text expanders are much better choices for saving shortcuts for inserting text. An exception to this would be to create a macro that first inserts an AutoText entry containing standard text and then moves the cursor to a given position in the paragraph to quickly resume transcribing (eg, insert a physical exam paragraph and then move the insertion point to the vital sign section to fill in data). Using AutoText to store the actual text (and then inserting the AutoText entry as part of the macro) gives you more control over the text formatting and also makes it easier to modify the standard text if it changes at some point in the future. If you use templates that already contain the majority of your standard text, you will not need an extensive number of these types of macros.

Any reference to Normal.dot in this chapter also refers to the Normal.dotm file in Word 2007. Remember, only files with the docm and dotm extensions in Word 2007 are capable of storing macros.

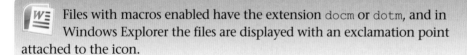

Files with macros enabled have the extension docm or dotm, and in Windows Explorer the files are displayed with an exclamation point attached to the icon.

Recording Tips

Before you record a macro, plan the steps carefully. Macros that include only 2 or 3 steps can be recorded easily without too much planning, but longer macros should be planned out, written down, and practiced before actually recording. Making a change to a macro after it is recorded can be difficult (but it is possible). If you make a mistake, it's probably easier to delete the macro and record it again. If necessary, you can pause during the recording.

When you record a macro, you can use the mouse to click commands and options on toolbars, menus, ribbons, and within dialog boxes and task panes, but the macro recorder does not record mouse movements in *the document space*. For example, you cannot use the mouse to move the insertion point to a specific place in the document, such as the top of the page or the beginning of a paragraph. You also cannot use the mouse to select, copy, or move text by clicking or dragging. You must use shortcut keys for navigating documents and selecting text. Refer to shortcut keys in Chapter 6 for moving the insertion point throughout the document space and study the keyboard editing techniques in Chapter 14. Mapping out the needed shortcut keys should be part of your planning.

To reach a given point in a document, it's often best to move the cursor to the beginning of the document (CTRL+Home) and then map out the path to reach that defined point. This approach creates a consistent and reproducible approach to placing the insertion point in documents with slightly varying content. For example, to select a given heading in the document, go to the beginning of the document and use the Find feature (CTRL+F) to search for and select that heading. Or move to the beginning of the document and count the number of lines (Down) or paragraphs (CTRL+Down) to reach a defined point. Another approach is to tag a position in the document with an asterisk, question mark, or unique combinations of these characters then use Find to locate those characters. Once the point is located, delete the marker characters as part of the macro. Learn more about the Find feature in Chapter 14.

Try to anticipate any messages that Word might display. For example, if your macro includes a command to close a document, be sure to include the Save command as part of the macro so Word will not stop in the middle of the macro to display a message to save changes. Another example applies to the **Find** and **Replace** dialog box. Make sure the Search Options box displays the correct search direction (Up, Down, or All). If the macro searches up or down only, Word will stop the macro when it reaches the beginning or end of the document and display a message asking whether you want to continue searching.

You can use a macro to change an option or setting located in a dialog box, but you cannot end a macro with a dialog box open. When you open a dialog box as part of a macro to change a setting, check *all the settings* in that dialog box to make sure they will apply in all cases. Word will not just record the single setting that you change, but will also record all other current settings within that dialog. A good example is using a macro to make font changes. If you simply want to apply bold as part of your macro, use the toolbar button or the shortcut key, not the **Font** dialog box; otherwise, all the font attributes currently selected in the **Font** dialog box will be recorded as part of your macro—they may or may not be what you want in all cases.

Macros can be used to open specific documents (eg, a reference document that you use routinely), but the file to be opened cannot be renamed or moved to another folder after the macros is recorded. If you move the file or rename the file, the macro will no longer be able to locate the file and you will receive an error when you use the macro.

In order for the macro to apply in all circumstances, make sure that the macro does not depend on any particular information contained in the document that is used to record the macro. If you record a macro that involves naming a file, the file name used to record the macro will become a permanent part of the macro and all documents named using that macro will have the same name. You can modify the VBA code to change the macro's behavior so that it gives each file a unique name (Note: The accompanying CD contains a sample macro for naming a file using information from within the document.). Consult a reference on Visual Basic for Applications to learn more about editing VBA code.

You can pick up on a little bit of Visual Basic by examining the code that is created using the Macro Recorder. After recording a macro, open the **Macros** dialog box (**ALT+F8**), select the macro name, and click **Edit**. Compare each line of the code with the steps you just recorded. If the macro included steps to open a dialog box, note how each command within the dialog box is recorded. Learn more about editing macros in the Special Projects chapter.

Naming Macros

Part of recording a macro will include naming the macro. There are several rules you must follow when naming macros. Keep these items in mind when naming your macro:

- Macro names cannot contain spaces or punctuation
- Macro names *can* contain numbers but they cannot *start* with a number
- Mixed case or underscore characters can be used to make the name more readable (eg, OpenSmithHnP or Delete_Sentence)

If you give your macro an invalid name, upon closing the **Record Macro** dialog, Word will display the error message "Invalid Procedure Name" and you will have to start over.

If you give a new macro the same name as an existing built-in macro, the new macro's actions will be added to the existing actions. For example, the Close command (to close a document) has a macro attached to it called FileClose. If you record a new macro and name it FileClose, it becomes attached to the Close command. When you choose the Close command, Word performs the new actions you recorded. To view a list of built-in macros in Word, press **ALT+F8**. In the *Macros in* list, click *Word Commands* (see directions for printing this list on page 183.)

Recording a Macro

Once you have planned your macro, you are ready to record each of your steps using the Macro Recorder. Follow these steps to record a macro:

1. Open the **Record Macro** dialog box using the menu/ribbon or double-click the `Macro Recorder` button on the <u>Status Bar</u> (see Figure 12-1). The `REC` button is displayed by default in Word 2003. To place the recorder icon on the <u>Status Bar</u> in Word 2007, right-click the <u>Status Bar</u> and place a check mark at Macro Recording.

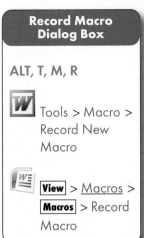

Record Macro Dialog Box

ALT, T, M, R

Tools > Macro > Record New Macro

`View` > <u>Macros</u> > `Macros` > Record Macro

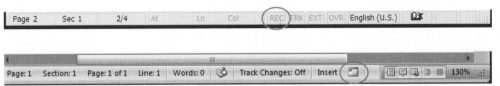

FIGURE 12-1 Macro recorder buttons on the Status Bar in Word 2003 (top) and Word 2007 (bottom).

2. The `Record Macro` button will open the **Record Macro** dialog box (Figure 12-2). In the *Macro name* box, type a name for the macro. By default, Word will suggest Macro*N* (where *N* is the next macro number in the sequence), but it is better to give your macro a specific name that identifies the macro and its purpose. If you happen to forget to name your macro, you can rename it after you complete the macro recording (see page 322).

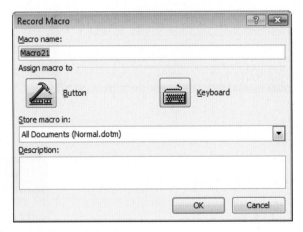

FIGURE 12-2 Use the Record Macro dialog box.

3. In the *Store macro in* box, select the template or document in which you want to store the macro. Store the macro in *All documents (Normal.dot)* in Word 2003 and *All documents (Normal.dotm)* in Word 2007. This will make the macro available at all times. If you plan to store a macro in a particular template, you must have a document based on that template open at the time you record the macro so the document name will be available in the

(Continued)

Store macro in box (template files are covered in Chapter 8). It's not likely that you will store a macro in a document, as it would only be available while working in that *one* document. In Word 2007, you cannot save a macro in a `dotx` or `docx` file (only `dotm` or `docm`).

4.   Type a description for the macro in the *Description* box. A description is optional but can be helpful.

5.   At this point, you may choose to assign your macro to a shortcut key or a button on a toolbar. Click the appropriate button in the middle of the **Record Macro** dialog to open the **Customize** dialog box. See detailed information on using the **Customize** dialog box in Chapter 15. Once you are adept at using the **Customize** dialog box and the macro recorder, you will be able to combine these tasks into the same routine. In the meantime, you can record the macro and assign shortcuts to your macro after you have completed the recording.

6.   After completing the **Record Macro** dialog box, click OK . The dialog will close and the mouse pointer will have a tape icon attached indicating you are recording.

7.   Perform the actions you want to include in your macro. If necessary, you can pause the recording. In Word 2003, click the red dot on the recorder toolbar that appears while recording. In Word 2007, go to View > Macros > Macros > Pause Recording. Remember, you can use the mouse to click commands, but the macro recorder cannot record mouse movements *in the document space*.

8.   To end the macro, click the same button that you used to start the macro. (In Word 2007, the icon on the Status Bar will have changed to a blue box.)

See Special Projects starting on page 443 for more ideas on how to use macros.

Running Macros

The command name for "playing back" a macro is **Run**. To run a macro, follow these steps:

1.   Open the **Macros dialog** box (see Figure 12-3).

2.   Type the macro name or select from the list.

3.   Once selected, click Run .

This approach will always work, but of course these steps will probably negate much of the advantage of using a macro (unless it is a long, complicated macro that you seldom use). For utmost efficiency, place shortcuts for your macros on toolbars and/or menus or assign shortcut keys (or all of these!). You will learn how to create shortcuts for your macros in Chapter 15.

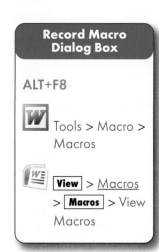

Record Macro Dialog Box

ALT+F8

Tools > Macro > Macros

View > Macros > Macros > View Macros

Managing Macros

To manage your macros, you need to understand a little about how they are stored in Word. Individual macros are stored in **modules**, and modules are stored in templates and documents. A document or a template file can contain more than one module. (Think of one macro as being a pea, and the module as a "can of peas." The template is the "pantry" that can hold more than one can of peas.) By default, Word stores macros in the Normal template unless you designate a different storage file at the time you create the macro. By default, the module within the Normal.dot file is called NewMacros. Technically, the macros you create and store in the Normal template are named Normal.NewMacros. <name> where <name> is the actual name you assign to your macro. Macros stored in other templates are named TemplateProject.NewMacros.<name>. You will see the macro name listed with its full name in the **Customize** dialog box (see page 390 in Word 2003 and page 402 in Word 2007).

Use the **Macros dialog box** (Figure 12-3) to manage your macros. This dialog lists the individual macros using just the last part of the name (the name you assign to the macro). Select a macro from the list and then choose a command button:

- The **Edit** button opens the Visual Basic Editor to make changes to the actual code.
- The **Step Into** button runs the selected macro in "debugging" mode, which is used to find errors in the code when the macro is not programmed correctly. It's not likely you will ever use **Step Into** unless you learn Visual Basic (the programming language).
- **Delete** allows you to remove the selected macro.
- **Organizer** opens the **Organizer** dialog box.

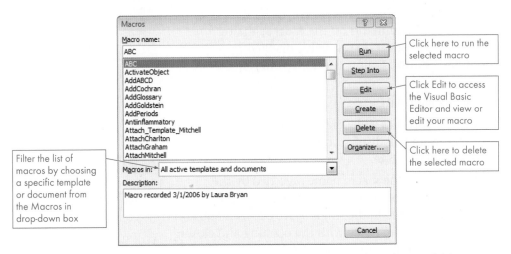

FIGURE 12-3 Use the Macros dialog box to manage individual macros, including editing and deleting.

The **Organizer** dialog box shown in Figure 12-4 lists the *modules* stored in a template and allows you to copy or delete an *entire module*. So, to work with modules (the can of peas), use the **Organizer**. To manage individual macros (the peas), use the **Macros** dialog box. Unless you want to share your macros with another user, you may never actually use the **Organizer** to work with your macros. See page 468 for instructions on copying modules between templates. See page 470 for instructions on copying individual macros to other computers.

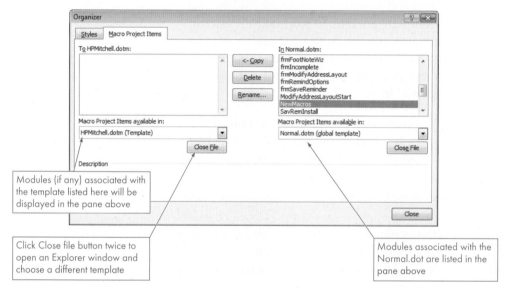

FIGURE 12-4 Use the Organizer to copy macro modules to other templates.

Renaming Macros

Unfortunately, there is not a "rename" command on the **Macros** dialog box. Renaming a macro is not difficult, but it does involve displaying the macro's code in the Visual Basic Editor. Follow these steps to rename a macro:

1. Open the **Macros** dialog box (**ALT+F8**).

2. Select the macro from the list and click **Edit**. The Visual Basic Editor will open (see Figure 12-5). The Editor will display your macros in a continuous list, with each macro separated by a line.

3. The first line of the macro displays the macro name preceded by the word Sub (see Figure 12-6). To edit the name, carefully edit the text following the word Sub. Be sure to retain the single space between Sub and the macro name and follow the macro name with the opening and closing parentheses. Also, don't forget to follow macro naming rules (as discussed on page 318).

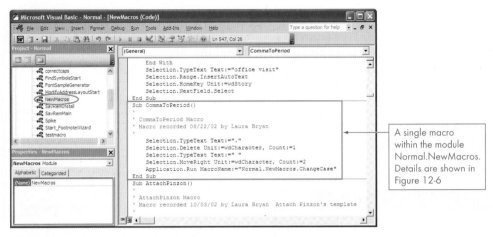

FIGURE 12-5 The Visual Basic Editor displays the programming code used to play back macros.

```
Sub CommaToPeriod()
'
' CommaToPeriod Macro
' Macro recorded 08/22/02 by Laura Bryan
'
    Selection.TypeText Text:="."
    Selection.Delete Unit:=wdCharacter, Count:=1
    Selection.TypeText Text:=" "
    Selection.MoveRight Unit:=wdCharacter, Count:=2
    Application.Run MacroName:="Normal.NewMacros.ChangeCase"
End Sub
```

FIGURE 12-6 Details of a single macro showing the macro's code written in Visual Basic.

4. You can also edit the description of the macro. Any line within the macro that begins with an apostrophe is ignored when the macro runs. You can see that these lines are also displayed in green text. Any green text can be modified without affecting the macro itself.

5. Close the Visual Basic editor. Changes are automatically saved when you close the editor window.

Sharing Macros

You may at times want to use a macro that you have created and stored in another template. To make the macro available, designate the template (that contains the macro you want to use) as a global template. To do this, follow these steps:

1. Open the **Templates and Add-ins** dialog box.
2. Click **Add** (see Figure 12-7).

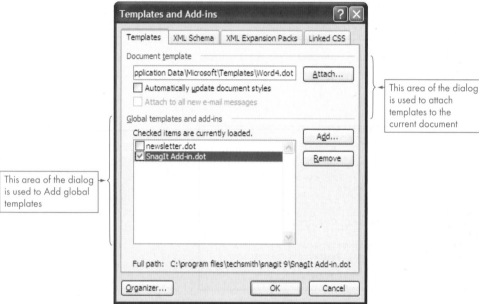

FIGURE 12-7 Use the Templates and Add-ins dialog box to add a global template, making macros stored in the template available to the current document.

3. Select the template containing the macros.
4. Click **OK**.
5. Enable or disable the template as needed by placing or removing the check mark next to the template name.

Transcription service owners can create customized macros and distribute the template file containing the macros. MTs can add the template as a global template using the **Templates and Add-ins** dialog box.

Global templates give you access to macros, AutoText entries, Building Blocks (Word 2007), and custom menus and toolbars that are stored in that template. Formatting information such as styles and margins as well as other settings are ignored. Any template can act as a global template. You can use the same

---

Templates and Add-ins Dialog Box

ALT, T, I

Tools > Templates and Add-ins

Developer > Templates > **Document Template**

(see page 160)

template as a document template in some circumstances and a global template in other circumstances. Global templates will remain active, even if you switch between documents or close Word. To remove the template from the list of available global templates, select the template name in the **Templates and Add-ins** dialog box and click Remove.

Programs that add functionality to Word (or other Office applications) may do so by attaching a global template. You may see templates listed in the Global templates pane even though you did not personally add them. Some brands of transcription software work in tandem with Word and add toolbars, menus, and other customizations to Word using global templates.

You can also make macros available by *attaching* the template file to the current document using the same **Templates and Add-ins** dialog box. *Attaching* a template may affect the formatting of the current document, whereas *adding* a template as a global template will *not* affect formatting. An attached template only affects the current document, whereas an *added* template will remain active across all documents.

You cannot attach more than one template to a document, so if you have already opened a document based on a template, you cannot attach a second template (you can switch the template, but you cannot attach multiple templates). You can *add* more than one global template. See page 243 (Word 2003) and 255 (Word 2007) for more information on attaching templates.

In addition to adding and attaching templates to access macros, you can also copy macros between templates and/or between computers. See the instructions on page 467 for copying macros to another computer.

● ●

Notes

Critical Thinking Questions

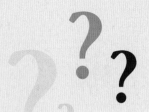

1. Describe the best application of a macro in MS Word.

   _____

   _____

2. List at least two specific ways you can use a macro in Word.

   _____

   _____

3. Why do you think you may only need a few macros to use on a routine basis?

   _____

   _____

4. Explain how you can and cannot use the mouse when recording a macro.

   _____

   _____

5. List the rules for naming a macro.

   _____

   _____

6. Describe how you back up macros.

   _____

   _____

7. Describe three ways to share macros with other users.

   _____

   _____

8. Describe the difference between *attaching* a template and *adding* a template as a global template.

   _____

   _____

9. Record the following macros described in the Special Projects section:

   a. Open a new document based on a template described on page 458.

   b. Move to another position within the document (Jumping Jacks) on page 445.

CHAPTER 13

Numbered Lists and Tables

OBJECTIVES

▸ Differentiate the AutoFormat As You Type *feature* from Automatic numbered list *format*.

▸ Manage automatic numbered lists.

▸ Use tables to manage complex formatting.

▸ Use tables to manage data.

Automatic Numbered Lists

Word has a built-in **automatic numbered list format** which is a defined format that includes the list number (as a number field), an indent and a hanging indent. It is called "automatic" because the numbering is controlled by the formatting commands and each new list number will insert automatically. Of all the features in Word, automatic numbered lists are probably the most frustrating for the medical transcriptionist.

Word has the ability to "detect" the start of a numbered list and automatically apply numbered list formatting (hence the name **AutoFormat As You Type**). You can also apply the automatic number format using the format commands on the toolbar/ribbon. And of course, you can format a list yourself without using the automatic number format at all.

To apply automatic numbered list format, follow these steps:

1. Begin a list of items but do not type the list number or apply formatting. You can type the first item in the list or type the entire list.

2. After you have typed part or all of the list, select the list and click the Numbering button on the Formatting toolbar/**Home** tab

(Continued)

KEYWORDS

AutoFormat As You Type

Automatic numbered list format

promote

demote

sublist

gridlines

Shortcut Keys

ALT+Shift+Num5

CTRL+ALT+U

CTRL+Enter

CTRL+Shift+Enter

Shift+ALT+Right

Shift+Enter

(Figure 13-1). Word will insert list numbers at the beginning of each paragraph and apply an indent and a hanging indent.

3. The automatic numbered list format includes number fields as well as commands for controlling the formatting (these commands are saved in the paragraph mark). To add to a list that is already numbered, set the insertion point at the end of a list item and press **Enter** to carry the formatting forward. A new list item will insert and the numbering will automatically adjust.

4. Press **Enter** twice to end an automatic numbered list.

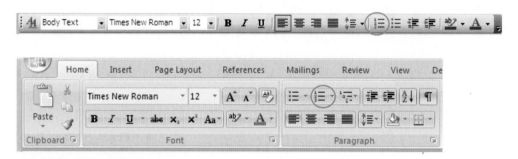

FIGURE 13-1 The numbered list and bulleted list icons on the toolbar in Word 2003 (above) and the ribbon in Word 2007 (below).

 Rules for working with automatic numbered lists also apply to bulleted lists. Use these same instructions for managing bulleted lists. The Bullets icon is next to the Numbering icon.

You can also create a numbered list *automatically as you type* if you have selected this feature in the **AutoFormat As You Type** dialog box (see page 157). Follow these steps:

1. Type **1, Period, Tab** followed by the text for the first list item.

2. When you press **Enter** to add the next list item, Word automatically inserts the next number, indents the list, and applies a hanging indent.

3. To finish the list, press **Enter** twice.

4. Insert new list items within the list by setting the insertion point at the end of a list item and press **Enter**. The numbering will automatically adjust.

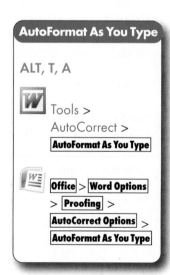

AutoFormat As You Type

ALT, T, A

Tools >
AutoCorrect >
AutoFormat As You Type

Office > **Word Options** > **Proofing** > **AutoCorrect Options** > **AutoFormat As You Type**

Occasionally you may encounter an odd situation where the number is formatted differently than the text associated with it. You can't select the number field to correct the formatting, so the problem becomes quite perplexing. Since the format of the number in the number field is controlled by the formatting information carried in the paragraph mark, the solution is to apply the correct formatting to the *paragraph mark* at the end of the list item. Display formatting marks and you will probably notice that the paragraph mark carries the same mismatched formatting as the number field. Select just the paragraph mark and apply/correct the formatting.

There are two options that determine how Word's numbered lists behave and how Word responds to your keystrokes. It's important to understand how these options affect the automatic numbering behavior so you can determine which options work best under what circumstances. Examine the options in the **AutoFormat As you Type** dialog box as shown in Figure 13-2 (see also page 157). If you do not want Word to detect the start of a numbered list and apply the automatic numbered list format, remove the check mark at *Automatic numbered lists*. If you do not want to use the **Tab** key to set indents and hanging indents, remove the check mark at *Set left-and first-indent with tabs and backspaces*. Learn more about this setting below and review the information on page 217.

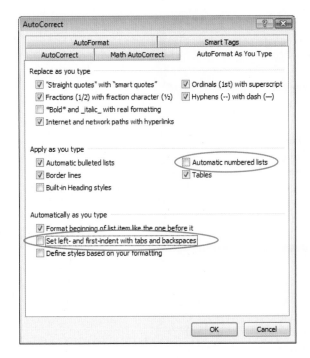

FIGURE 13-2 Options on the AutoFormat As You Type dialog affect the automatic numbered list feature.

The Automatic numbered list format inserts a field—not an actual number. This particular field cannot be selected, and there's the rub—you can't make a direct change to the number field. It is important to understand how to manage automatic numbered lists so you feel like you are in control—not Word. If the options are too frustrating, turn off automatic numbered lists and simply type numbered lists "manually."

AutoFormat vs Numbered List Format

It is important to distinguish the AutoFormat As You Type *feature* from automatic numbered list *format*. Automatic numbered lists is a style that is predefined by Word to include indents and hanging indents. This format also includes the fields and commands for numbering the list. AutoFormat As You Type is a feature that tells Word to *detect* the start of a numbered list based on certain cues (see page 157, option 8) and to automatically apply numbered list formatting. It doesn't really matter how the text attains the automatic numbered list style (by you applying it or Word picking up cues and applying it for you)—automatic numbering becomes a part of the paragraph formatting.

Even with the Automatic numbered lists feature turned off in the **AutoFormat As You Type** dialog box, you can still apply the numbered list format using the toolbar button. Opening a document on a computer with *Automatic numbered lists* disabled will not affect the automatic number formatting that is already applied. The list will continue to automatically insert numbers when you press the Enter key to continue the list.

If Word detects a list and applies list formatting when you do not need it, immediately press CTRL+Z to undo the list formatting.

Using automatic numbered list format uses fields for the item numbers, and these fields do not always translate well if the Word document is subsequently converted to plain text (txt files), rich text format (rtf files), or is imported into electronic record systems. Check with your client or employer to make sure these number fields will convert correctly when the document reaches its final disposition.

Removing Indents

When applying *automatic numbered list format*, Word will automatically indent the numbered list. You cannot permanently change this option to make the list insert flush with the left margin. To work around this, follow these steps:

1. Type the first item in your list.
2. Press Enter. The "2" will appear and the numbered list will indent.
3. Before you type the second item in your list, press Up one time to move the cursor into the paragraph of list item number 1.
4. Press **ALT+Shift+Left**. This will promote the entire list (return the list to the left margin).
5. Press Down to return to the second line item and continue typing.

Although this will return your list to the left margin, it is quite cumbersome to do while the dictator is talking a blue streak! Record these steps as a macro and assign a shortcut key, or better yet, start the numbered list in your template file and format it at the left margin as above. When transcribing, list items 1 and 2 will already be available and correctly formatted. If the list goes beyond list item 2, Word will continue with automatic numbering when you hit the Enter key at the end of list item 2.

To start a list in your template, you have to type a little bit of "dummy" text for Word to actually detect a list. Type a "fake list" that includes the first two items in the list and move the list to the left margin. Once you have the list formatted, carefully delete the dummy text but *do not delete the paragraph marks*. Insert empty fields (CTRL+F9) as jump points (see Chapter 11).

> Indents and hanging indents can be changed once the list is inserted, but you cannot make *permanent* changes to the automatic numbered list format—any format changes you make to the list format in one document will be retained for that document but will be discarded when you start a new document.

Creating Lists within Lists

A potentially frustrating problem you may encounter while working with automatic numbered lists is creating a **sublist**. Each time you press Enter to start a new line, Word interprets this as a new list item and inserts the next number in the list. So the problem is how to create a new line of text that has the sublist format (usually a deeper indent with lowercase letters instead of numbers). There are several approaches to creating a sublist. Your circumstances may determine the best approach for you.

AutoFormat As You Type includes the option to *Set left- and first-indent with tabs and backspaces*. With this setting enabled, creating sublists is not difficult. Follow these steps:

1. In the middle of a list, press Enter to start a new list item then press Tab. Word will **demote** the list (indent it further) and insert a lowercase letter a.

2. Press Enter at the end of each sublist item to continue the sublist.

3. After typing each item in the sublist, press Enter to start a new list item. Press Shift+Tab to **promote** the next list item (ie, decrease the indent) and return to the next number in the sequence.

> If your work involves creating paragraphs that are formatted with both indents and hanging indents, such as the SOAP note or a typical Operative note, the option to *Set left- and first-indent with tabs and backspaces* can cause a lot of frustration (see page 219). Your circumstances will determine whether you should enable or disable this feature.

> If you find the automatic settings to be too difficult to manage, disable *Automatic numbered lists* and/or the option to *Set left- and first-indent with tabs and backspaces*. You may also choose to toggle between these options depending on the type of report you are working on. If you change this setting often, create a macro to toggle these settings. Learn more about creating macros in Chapter 12.

A second option for creating sublists is to use a line break instead of a paragraph break to control sublists. To create a sublist without invoking the next number in the list, use the line break (**Shift+Enter**) instead of the paragraph break (**Enter**). The formatting mark for a line break is a curved arrow, as shown in Figure 13-3. The sublist will line up with the hanging indent. Remember, a line break does not create a new paragraph, so you cannot apply separate paragraph formatting to the sublists.

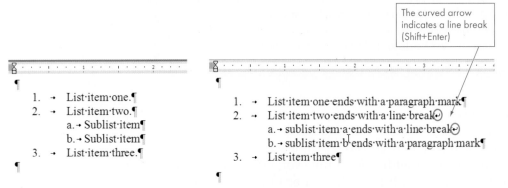

The curved arrow indicates a line break (Shift+Enter)

FIGURE 13-3 Two approaches to creating a sublist. The sublist on the left has been created using the demote command. The sublist on the right has been created using line breaks.

Also, you may be able to use the Demote command to format a sublist. To do this, begin a list in numbered list format. Indent the first item in the sublist by pressing **Shift+ALT+Right**. When you reach the end of the sublist, press **Enter** and then press **Shift+ALT+Left** to promote the list. Word should continue the numbering accordingly.

Breaking a List Across a Page

You have two options for controlling automatic numbered lists when they approach a page break. The first option is to apply the *Keep with next* setting (see page 212) to the list items that you want to "stick together." Assign a shortcut key as explained on page 394 (Word 2003) and page 403 (Word 2007) to the Keep with next command (ParaKeepWithNext) to make it easy to apply "on the fly." This approach works well because you do not have to worry about the list breaking at the wrong point if the text above it is subsequently edited.

The second option is to insert a manual page break at the point where the list should break. This option is initially quick to apply but it can create problems if the document is subsequently edited; you have to double-check the position of the page break (and possibly readjust) if the text above the break is edited. To insert a manual page break, place the insertion point *in front of the first word* of the list item that you want to force to the next page (Figure 13-4) and press **CTRL+Enter**.

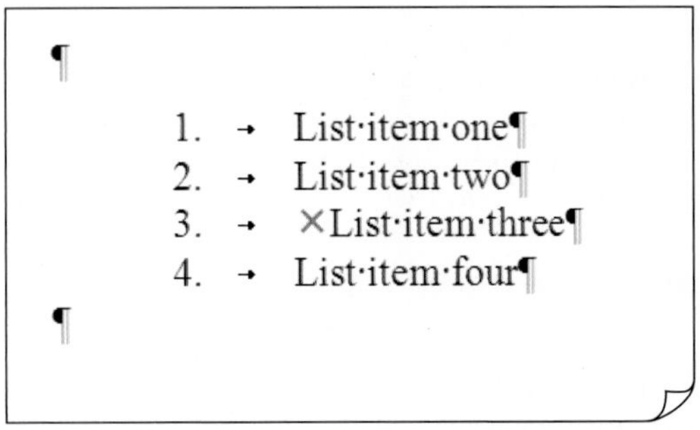

¶

    1. → List·item·one¶
    2. → List·item·two¶
    3. → ✕List·item·three¶
    4. → List·item·four¶

¶

FIGURE 13-4 Place the insertion point at the red X and press CTRL+Enter to force item number 3 to the next page.

Repairing a Numbered List

It is easy to repair an automatic numbered list that has gone "haywire." Continue typing until you finish the list and then select the entire list. Click the numbering icon on the toolbar twice. The first click will strip the number formatting completely and the second click will reapply it correctly. To pull the list back to the left margin, while the list is still selected, press ALT+Shift+Left.

If Word does not begin a list with the number 1 (ie, Word continues the numbering from a previous list), place the insertion point in the first incorrect list item, right-click and choose Restart numbering. By the same token, if you want to continue a list from the previous, set the insertion point in the first list item, right-click, and choose Continue numbering.

Setting the Number Style and Alignment

Using the **Numbering** dialog box, you can fine tune your numbered lists and create a specific format that can be re-used while you are in the current document. This dialog displays a gallery of list styles that can be further customized. Follow these steps to use the **Numbering** dialog box:

1. Once you begin a list, go to Format > Bullets and Numbering or right-click and choose Bullets and Numbering.
2. Click a thumbnail that closely matches the list style you want to use (Figure 13-5).

(Continued)

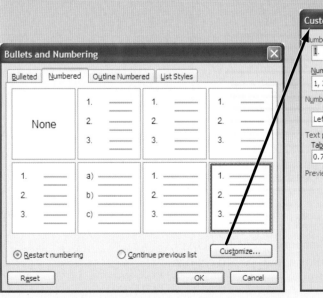

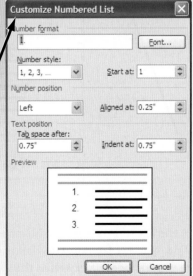

FIGURE 13-5 The Numbered gallery displays various numbering formats to choose from. Click Customize to fine tune your numbered list.

3. To further customize the list style, choose Customize. The **Customize Numbered List** dialog allows you to change the Number format and Number style as well as the Text Position.

Text Position changes the numbers' alignment within the number "column." For example, if the list exceeds 9 items, the number 10 could line up even with the 9 on the right (the zero below the 9) or on the left (the 1 below the 9).

Using the Numbering Library, you can fine tune your numbered lists and create a specific format that can be re-used while you are in the current document. This gallery displays a selection of list styles that can be further customized. Follow these steps to use the Numbering Library:

1. Once you begin a list, click the down arrow next to the `Numbering` button on the `Home` tab, or right-click and choose Numbering.

2. Click a thumbnail that closely matches the list style you want to use (see Figure 13-6).

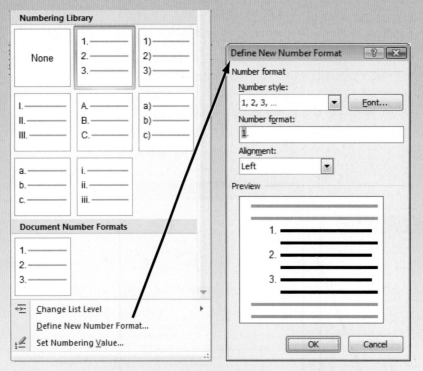

FIGURE 13-6 Tweak numbered lists using the Numbering Library.

3. To further customize the list style, access the Numbering Library as above and choose Define New Number Format. This dialog allows you to change the Number style and Number format as well as the Alignment.

Alignment changes the numbers' position within the number "column." For example, if the list exceeds 9 items, the number 10 could line up even with the 9 on the right (the zero below the 9) or on the left (the 1 below the 9).

Unfortunately, any changes you make to the gallery of numbered and bulleted lists will only "stick" for the current document. As soon as you open a new file, all gallery settings revert back to their native settings and you will need to change the settings again. The gallery is useful for long documents with many lists, but transcriptionists typically work with many short documents, making this feature less useful in the long run.

Tables

Some formats can be difficult to manage, and oddly enough, using a table to control the layout is a viable solution. Traditionally, tables are used to align lists or numbers in columns that can be tabulated and sorted, but you can also use them to place text in a specific format. You can also use a table to set up a complicated letterhead containing text and graphics. Since each cell within a table can be formatted independently of other cells, this approach works well in letterhead formats with numerous provider names, addresses, and departments (see sample report on page 434). Start with a basic table and drag the table borders to create cells of varying sizes to accommodate text and graphics. Tables hold their formatting regardless of how much or how little information is added to them. They can also solve formatting problems when indents and numbering are involved.

Use these tips when working with tables:

- To make tables easier to use, place empty fields in table cells to control the direction of the insertion point (**F11** moves left to right across a row and down through rows).
- Format an entire column or row with bold, all caps, or other font characteristics for quick and flawless typing. As more rows or columns are added "on the fly," the formatting follows.
- Use tables to manage multiple indents and hanging indents as in Figure 13-7.
- Set up tables wherever there will be a list and start with one or two rows as a part of the template. Add more rows as needed "on the fly" by simply pressing **Tab** at the end of the last row.
- Hide border lines so the printed document will not appear to be formatted as a table.
- Display **gridlines** to easily visualize the cells when working with tables that have the borders hidden (see instructions below for displaying grid lines).
- The end of a table cell is marked by a small circle. Even when gridlines are hidden, you will know you are working with a table because you will see the end-of-cell markers.

Formatting can be adjusted as needed by deleting columns or rows that are not needed. For example, in Figure 13-7, the single entry "Bilateral tubal ligation" can be moved to the left by deleting the empty column (where the numbers would be if there was more than one item). Tables also work well for patient demographics as in Figure 13-8. If any of the names are particularly long, they will wrap to the next line within their own cell without distorting the rest of the formatting.

HISTORY¶

SURGICAL:◻	◻	Bilateral·tubal·ligation.◻	◻
¶			
MEDICAL:◻	1.◻	Non-insulin·dependent·diabetes·mellitus.◻	◻
◻	2.◻	Hypertension.◻	◻
◻	3.◻	Congestive·heart·failure.·The·patient·was·hospitalized·for·6·days·in·November·of·2008.◻	◻
¶			
MEDICATIONS:◻	1.◻	Amaryl·4·mg◻	◻
◻	2.◻	Toprol·XL·25·mg·b.i.d.·◻	◻
◻	3.◻	Lasix·40·mg·daily◻	◻

¶

HISTORY

SURGICAL:		Bilateral tubal ligation.
MEDICAL:	1.	Non-insulin dependent diabetes mellitus.
	2.	Hypertension.
	3.	Congestive heart failure. The patient was hospitalized for 6 days in November of 2008.
MEDICATIONS:	1.	Amaryl 4 mg
	2.	Toprol XL 25 mg b.i.d.
	3.	Lasix 40 mg daily

FIGURE 13-7 An example of a table used to format sections of a history and physical report. The lower image shows the same report with no table borders or formatting marks displayed.

Name:··Joseph·Smith-Johnson◻	**Date:**···3/19/09◻	**Chart:**···#3456◻	◻
Physician:···Hamilton◻	**Ref·Physician:**···Montenegro◻	**Tape:**···#345◻	◻

¶

Name: Joseph Smith-Johnson	**Date:** 3/19/09	**Chart:** #3456
Physician: Hamilton	**Ref Physician:** Montenegro	**Tape:** #345

FIGURE 13-8 An example of a table used to format patient demographics. The lower image shows the same report with no table borders or formatting marks displayed.

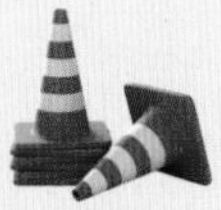

Word counts the lines within *each cell* of a table, so line counts will be higher than if the text was not placed in a table. Using Figure 13-7 as an example, starting at HISTORY and ending at Lasix, Word calculates 25 lines. Character counts are not affected by tables.

Creating Tables

To create a simple table, follow these steps:

1. Set the insertion point where you want to insert a table.
2. Click the Insert table button on the Standard toolbar (Figure 13-9). A grid will appear.

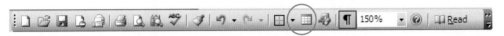

FIGURE 13-9 Click the Insert Table icon to create a new table.

3. Move the mouse over the grid to select the number of columns and rows you need and click the left mouse button to insert the table. If there are not enough columns or rows on the grid, select them all, then insert more rows and columns directly into the table once it is placed.
4. You can also go to Table > Insert > Table and fill in the dialog box to create a new table.

If you use a table occasionally but not in every report, create a table and store it in AutoText to quickly insert when needed.

Working with Tables

When formatting tables, you must specify exactly what part of the table you want to format. Here are tips for working with tables:

- To select rows with the mouse, double-click just to the left of the row and the entire row will backlight.
- To select an entire column, hover the mouse just over the top border/gridline until you see a down-pointing arrow and then click.
- You can also select the table, a column, or a row using Table > Select and then choosing Table, Column or Row.
- To select cells within a table using the keyboard, hold down the **Shift** key and press **Left/Right** or **Up/Down**.
- You may find it useful to display the Tables and Borders toolbar (Figure 13-10) for creating and formatting tables (right-click in the toolbar area and choose Tables and Borders).

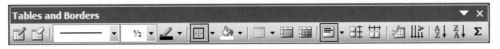

FIGURE 13-10 The Tables and Borders toolbar contains command buttons for managing tables.

WORD 2003

When working with tables, the "select" commands will select the table's *contents*, not the table itself. Applying commands to the selection will affect the contents only.

If you will be working with tables often, assign shortcut keys to the commands: TableSelectRow and TableSelectColumn (see Chapter 15). Table Select is already assigned to **ALT+Shift+Num5** (also written **ALT+Clear**).

Applying Paragraph and Font Formatting

You can preset the font and paragraph format within individual cells, rows, or columns. For example, if you format a column with bold and all caps, you will not have to press **Caps Lock** or **CTRL+B** when you type text in that column, even if you add more rows. Select the applicable row or column and press the shortcut key to apply the font format.

Paragraphs within cells can be formatted in the same way as paragraphs outside of a table. To change the horizontal alignment (justified, left, right, centered), use the same paragraph alignment shortcut keys (**CTRL+J, CTRL+L, CTRL+R, CTRL+E**).

Cells can also be formatted with automatic numbering. Select the column or row and click the numbering icon on the <u>Formatting</u> toolbar. As each new column or row is inserted, the numbers will increment.

To count the number of rows (items) in a long table, select a column and apply numbering to that column. Each cell in the column will be numbered, so you can easily determine the number of rows.

The AutoCorrect feature includes the option to automatically cap the first word in a table cell. This option is turned on by default, but if you prefer to start table cells with a lowercase word, remove the check mark. Go to Tools > AutoCorrect > *Capitalize first letter of table cells*.

Aligning Text Vertically

Text within a table can be aligned vertically at the top, center, or bottom of the cell. By default, Word aligns text in a table to the upper left of a cell. To set the vertical alignment within a cell, click the down arrow next to the Alignment icon ⊟▾ on the <u>Tables and Borders</u> toolbar, or right-click, choose Cell alignment, and then select the icon corresponding to your desired format.

Formatting Borders

By default, tables have a black, ½ pt, single, solid-line border that will print. Here are tips for managing table borders:

- To manage table borders, click the down arrow next to the corresponding icon on the <u>Tables and Borders</u> toolbar. You can also use the **Borders and Shading** dialog box as shown in Figure 13-11. To open the dialog, go to Format > Borders and Shading, or right-click within a table cell and choose Borders and Shading.

Choose a Setting to apply to the entire table. Use the buttons on the right to customize borders

Click the border icons representing the sides of table cells to place or remove borders

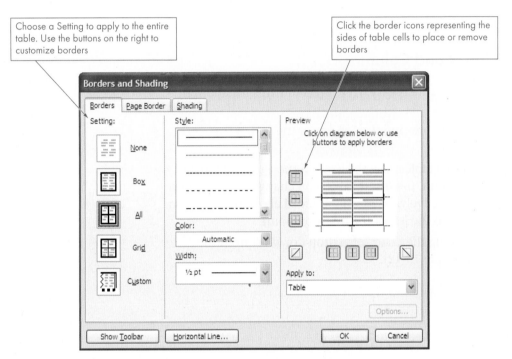

FIGURE 13-11 Use the Borders and Shading dialog to control the lines around and within a table.

- Remove all table borders by pressing **CTRL+ALT+U**.
- Apply borders to individual cells, a row, or the entire table. Use the grid in the **Borders and Shading** dialog box to apply borders to the *selected cells*.
- Even with borders removed, Word will show you light gray gridlines to define the table cells. If you do not want to see these gridlines on your screen, you can hide them by selecting Gridlines on the Table menu (**ALT, A, G**). This command toggles on/off.

With gridlines displayed, tables can sometimes appear differently than when viewed without gridlines. Check your table layout using Print Preview (**CTRL+F2**) before finalizing the document.

Adjusting Cell Height and Width

To set the width and height of the table columns and rows, you can use the mouse to drag the lines where you need them. To widen an entire column or row, be sure to select the entire column or row before dragging the lines. To use the mouse, move the cursor over the table border until the mouse pointer changes to two parallel lines, then hold down the left mouse button and drag the line to the desired width or height. You can also select the column or row and then right-click on the table to open the shortcut menu. Choose Table Properties and fill in the appropriate information to specify the exact size of the table cells. Make sure the correct column or row is indicated in the dialog box before making changes.

Adding and Moving Rows and Columns

Adding rows and columns to your table is easy. Here are a few tips for adding cells:

- Add rows as you type by simply pressing the **Tab** key at the end of the last row.
- *Insert* rows or columns within a table using the icon on the Standard toolbar. When you select a row or column, the Insert Table icon changes to Insert Row or Insert Column respectively. Rows will be added above the insertion point; columns will be added to the left of the insertion point.
- You can also select options using the Insert Table drop-down list from the Tables and Borders toolbar (Figure 13-12).

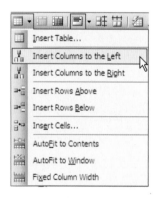

FIGURE 13-12 Insert rows or columns using the Insert Table drop-down menu on the Tables and Borders toolbar.

- To move an entire column or row, select the entire row or column and then drag the selection to a new position within the table.

You can insert more than one row or column at the same time. In an existing table, select the number of rows or columns corresponding to the number of rows or columns you want to insert, and then click the icon as above. For example, if two rows are selected, the icon will insert two rows into the table instead of one.

Aligning Tables with the Margin

Tables can be aligned with the margin as if they were paragraphs: left, right, or center. Select the entire table (Table > Select > Table) then press the corresponding paragraph alignment command. You can also select the table using the shortcut **ALT+Shift+Num5** (also written as **ALT+Clear**). If you simply set the insertion point within the table or select a few rows or columns and then apply the alignment command, the command will be applied to the *selected cells*—not the table itself.

Deleting Table Information

Follow these guidelines for deleting table information:

- To delete a table's *contents*, select the applicable cells and press **Delete**.
- To delete actual rows or columns, you need to use the delete commands associated with the table (not just the **Delete** key). To delete rows or columns, place your insertion point anywhere in the row or column to be deleted and go to Table > Delete and choose Cell, Row, or Column. You can also right-click and choose Delete.
- To delete the entire table, place the insertion point anywhere in the table and choose Table > Delete > Table. If you simply press Delete while a table is selected, Word will delete the table's *contents*.

To make it easier to remove rows and columns, assign shortcut keys to these commands: TableDeleteRow and TableDeleteColumn. See page 394 for instructions.

The easiest way to delete a table and its contents is to select the table and at least one additional paragraph mark (either above or below the table) and click **Delete**. Including a paragraph mark above or below the table will cause Word to delete the table and its contents.

Managing Table Breaks

Tables will divide wherever a page break occurs. You can make adjustments to the table to make sure that the information appears correctly when the table spans a page break. Use these guidelines for managing table breaks:

- By default, Word allows a page break to divide a row between the two pages. To prevent a table row from breaking across pages, place the insertion point in the row or select all rows so none will split across the page break. Select Table > Table Properties > **Row**. Clear the check mark at *Allow row to break across pages*.

(Continued)

- To split a table into two tables, set the insertion point *below* the intended break and press **CTRL+Shift+Enter**.
- To insert a paragraph above a table, set the insertion point in the top row and press **CTRL+Shift+Enter**. This is particularly helpful if the table begins at the top of a page and you need to insert text above the table.
- To break a table at a given point *and* force a page break, set the insertion point in the row that you want to appear on the next page and press **CTRL+Enter**.

Converting Text to Tables

A great way to alphabetize or otherwise reorganize data (eg, names and addresses) is to convert text to a table and then sort by columns. As long as each set of data is formatted consistently (ie, all addresses use four lines with one line between), you can easily convert the text to a table and then back to text again. Follow these steps:

1. Review the data to be tabulated and make sure the data is formatted consistently. Each set of data that will span a row should contain the same number of lines (insert blank lines to represent no data where necessary).
2. Select the text to be formatted as a table and choose Table > Convert > Text to Table.
3. Select the number of columns, which should correspond to the number of lines in each data set.
4. Select a character for separating the data (ie, paragraph mark) so Word will know how to separate the text into columns.
5. Conversely, you can remove text from a table format by selecting a table and choosing the opposite command: Table > Convert > Table to Text.

Using Tables as Spreadsheets and Logs

Tables are perfect for sorting and calculating. You can maintain a list of referring physicians, for example, and sort the list by name, address, or any other parameter. To do this, select the column that you want to use as the basis of your sort and choose Table > Sort. Make selections within the dialog box to determine how to sort the data.

You can alphabetize a simple list of items (eg, drug names) without converting the list to a table. Type each name on a separate line and then select the list. Choose Table > Sort and choose *Sort by: Paragraphs*.

You can also use tables to sum a column of numbers, which is a great way to tally line counts. To sum the total of a column or row, insert a blank column or row at the end of the table and place the cursor in the last cell. Click the summation icon Σ (TableAutoSum) on the <u>Tables and Borders</u> toolbar (Figure 13-10). If you use the TableAutoSum command often, copy the icon to the <u>Standard</u> toolbar or assign a shortcut key to the command (see Chapter 15).

> Make sure there is an entry in every cell of the row or column to be added or your totals will not be correct. Place a zero in blank cells to prevent summation errors.

See a list of helpful table commands and shortcut keys on page 349.

Creating Tables

To create a simple table, follow these steps:

1. Set the insertion point where you want to insert a table.
2. Go to **Insert** > <u>Table</u> > **Table**. A grid will appear.
3. Move the mouse over the grid to select the number of columns and rows you need and click the left mouse button to insert the table. You can always add or remove columns or rows once the table is placed.

> If you use a table occasionally but not in every report, create a table and store it in AutoText to quickly insert when needed.

Working with Tables

If you are familiar with using tables in Word 2003, you can still use many of the right-click menu options and shortcut keys for managing tables. Word 2007 also has an extensive set of controls on the ribbon. Use **Table Tools** that appears when the cursor is located within a table. **Table Tools** includes two tabs: **Design** and **Layout** as shown in Figure 13-13.

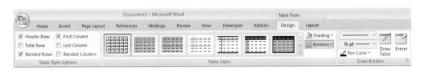

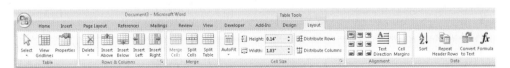

FIGURE 13-13 Table Tools includes two separate tabs on the ribbon for managing tables.

When formatting tables, you must specify exactly what part of the table you want to format. Here are tips for working with tables:

- To select rows with the mouse, double-click just to the left of the row and the entire row will backlight.
- To select an entire column, hover the mouse just over the top border/gridline until you see a down-pointing arrow and then click.
- You can also choose an option from the **Select** button (**Layout** > Table).
- To select cells with the keyboard, hold down the Shift key and press Left/Right or Up/Down.

When working with tables, the "select" commands will select the table's *contents*, not the table itself. Applying commands to the selection will affect the contents only.

If you will be working with tables often, assign shortcut keys to the commands: TableSelectRow and TableSelectColumn (see Chapter 15). TableSelect is already assigned to **ALT+Shift+Num5** (number 5 on the number pad).

Applying Paragraph and Font Formatting

You can preset the font and paragraph format within individual cells, rows, or columns. For example, if you format a column with bold and all caps, you will not have to press Caps Lock or CTRL+B when you type text in that column, even if you add more rows. Select the applicable row or column and press the shortcut key to apply the font format.

Paragraphs within cells can be formatted in the same way as paragraphs outside of a table. To change the horizontal alignment (justified, left, right, centered), use the same paragraph alignment shortcut keys (CTRL+J, CTRL+L, CTRL+R, CTRL+E).

Cells can also be formatted with automatic numbering. Select the column or row and click the numbering icon on the **Home** tab. As each new column or row is inserted, the numbers will increment.

To count the number of rows (items) in a long table, insert a column and apply numbering to that column. Each cell in the column will be numbered, so you can easily determine the number of rows.

The AutoCorrect feature includes the option to automatically cap the first word in a table cell. This option is turned on by default, but if you prefer to start table cells with a lowercase word, you can change this setting. Click **ALT, T, A** and remove the check mark at *Capitalize first letter of table cells*.

Aligning Text Vertically

Text within a table can be aligned vertically at the top, center, or bottom of the cell. By default, Word aligns text in a table to the upper left of a cell. To set the vertical alignment, right-click and choose Cell Alignment and then select the icon corresponding to your desired format (see Figure 13-14). You can also select an alignment scheme using Layout > Alignment.

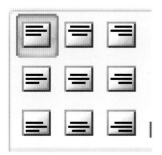

FIGURE 13-14 Choose an alignment icon to place the text vertically and horizontally within the table cell.

Formatting Borders

By default, tables have a black, ½ pt, single, solid-line border that will print. Here are tips for managing table borders:

- To manage table borders, click Design > Table Styles > Borders (and select from the drop-down menu) or select options from Design > Draw Borders (Figure 13-15). As always, you can place your insertion point anywhere in the table and right-click. Select Borders and Shading from the right-click menu to open the **Borders and Shading** dialog box (see Figure 13-11). Select the options and press Enter.

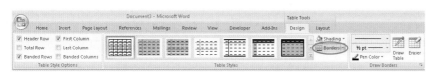

FIGURE 13-15 Change borders using the Draw Borders group on the Design tab.

- Remove all table borders by pressing **CTRL+ALT+U**.
- Apply borders to individual cells, a row, or the entire table. Use the grid in the **Borders and Shading** dialog box to apply borders to the *selected cells*.
- Even with borders removed, Word will show you light gray gridlines to define the table cells. If you do not want to see these gridlines on your screen, you can hide them by clicking View Gridlines under Layout > Table.

With gridlines displayed, tables can sometimes appear differently than when viewed without gridlines. Check your table layout using Print Preview (CTRL+F2) before finalizing the document.

Adjusting Cell Height and Width

To set the width and height of the table columns and rows, you can use the mouse to drag the lines where you need them. To use the mouse, move the cursor over the table line until the mouse pointer changes to two parallel lines, then hold down the left mouse button and drag the line to the desired width or height. To widen an entire column or row, be sure to select the entire column or row before dragging the lines. You can also set the height and width of cells, columns or rows using the tools in the Cell Size group under **Layout**.

Adding and Moving Rows and Columns

Adding rows and columns to your table is easy. Here are a few tips for adding cells:

- Add rows as you type by simply pressing the **Tab** key at the end of the last row.
- *Insert* rows or columns within a table using icons on the Rows and Columns group on the **Layout** tab (Figure 13-16). Set your insertion point in the table and click the corresponding button on the **Layout** tab.

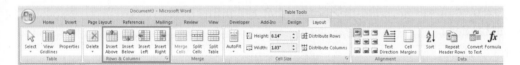

FIGURE 13-16 Use the insert buttons on the Layout tab to insert additional rows or columns.

- To move columns or rows, select the entire row or column and then drag the selection to a new position within the table.

You can insert more than one row or column at one time. In an existing table, select the number of rows or columns corresponding to the number of rows or columns you want to insert, then click the icon as above. For example, if two rows are selected, the icon will insert two rows into the table instead of one.

Aligning Tables with the Margin

Tables can be aligned with the margin as if they were paragraphs: left, right, or center. Select the entire table (**Layout** > Table > **Select** > Select Table) then press the corresponding paragraph alignment command. You can also select the table using the shortcut **ALT+Shift+Num5** (also written as **ALT+Clear**). If you simply set the insertion point within the table or select a few rows or columns and then apply the alignment command, the command will be applied to the selected cells—not the table itself.

Deleting Table Information

Follow these guidelines for deleting table information:

- To delete a table's *contents*, select the applicable cells and press Delete.
- To delete actual rows or columns, you need to use the delete commands associated with the table (not just the Delete key). To delete actual rows, columns, or the entire table, place your insertion point anywhere in the row or column to be deleted, go to Layout > Rows and Columns > Delete and select the part of the table to be deleted.
- You can also delete cells using the right-click menu. Set your insertion point, right-click and choose Delete Cells.

To make it easier to remove rows and columns, assign shortcut keys to these commands: TableDeleteRow and TableDeleteColumn. See page 403 for instructions.

The easiest way to delete an entire table and its contents is to select the table and at least one paragraph mark (either above or below the table) and click Delete.

Managing Table Breaks

Tables will divide wherever a page break occurs. You can make adjustments to the table to make sure that the information appears correctly when the table spans a page break. Use these guidelines for managing table breaks:

- By default, Word allows a page break to divide a row between the two pages. To prevent a table row from breaking across pages, place the insertion point in the row or select all rows so none will split across the page break. Select Layout > Table > Properties > Row. Clear the check mark at *Allow to break across pages*.
- To split a table into two tables, set the insertion point *below* the intended break and press **CTRL+Shift+Enter.**
- To insert a paragraph above a table, set the insertion point in the top row and press CTRL+Shift+Enter. This is particularly helpful if the table begins at the top of a page and you need to insert text above the table.
- To break a table at a given point *and* force a page break, set the insertion point in the row that you want to appear on the next page and then press **CTRL+Enter.**

WORD 2007

Converting Text to Tables

A great way to alphabetize or otherwise reorganize data (eg, names and addresses) is to convert text to a table and then sort by columns. As long as each set of data is formatted consistently (ie, all addresses use four lines with one line between), you can easily convert the text to a table and then back to text again. Follow these steps:

1. Review the data to be tabulated and make sure the data is formatted consistently. Each set of data that will span a row should contain the same number of lines (insert blank lines to represent no data where necessary).

2. Select the text to be formatted as a table and choose `Insert` > `Table` > Convert Text to Table.

3. Select the number of columns, which should correspond to the number of lines in each data set.

4. Select a character for separating the data (ie, paragraph mark) so Word will know how to separate the text into columns.

5. Conversely, you can remove text from a table format by selecting a table and taking the opposite approach: `Table Tools` > `Layout` > Data > `Convert to Text`.

Using Tables as Spreadsheets and Logs

Tables are perfect for sorting and calculating. You can maintain a list of referring physicians, for example, and sort the list by name, address, or any other parameter. To do this, select the column that you want to use as the basis of your sort and click `Table Tools` > `Layout` > Data > `Sort`.

You can alphabetize a simple list of items (eg, drug names) without converting the list to a table. Type each name on a separate line and then select the list. Choose `Home` > Paragraph > `Sort`.

You can also use tables to sum a column of numbers, which is a great way to tally line counts. To sum the total of a column or row, insert a blank column or row at the end of the table. Place the insertion point in the last cell of the column or row to be totalled and go to `Table Tools` > `Layout` > Data > `Formula`. The default formula displayed will be the summation formula. If you use this command often, add the icon to the Quick Access toolbar or assign a shortcut key to TableAutoSum.

Make sure there is an entry in every cell of the row or column to be added or your totals will not be correct. Place a zero in blank cells to prevent summation errors.

Table Commands

Table 13-1 lists helpful shortcut keys for working with tables.

Table 13-1	Helpful Shortcut Keys for Working with Tables
Shift+any arrow key	Extend a selection to adjacent cells
Shift+Up or Down	Select a column
CTRL+Shift+F8, Arrow keys	Extend a selection
Shift+F8	Reduce the selection size
ALT+Shift+Num5 (5 on the number pad)	Select an entire table
ALT+double-click within the table	Select an entire table
CTRL+J	Justify text within a cell
CTRL+E	Center (text within a cell or center the table if entire table is selected)
CTRL+L	Left align (text within a cell or left align the table if entire table is selected)
CTRL+R	Right align (text within a cell or right align the table if entire table is selected)
Enter	Create a new paragraph within a cell
Tab	Move to next cell in a row
CTRL+Tab	Insert a tab within a cell
Down	Next row
ALT+Home	First cell in a row
ALT+End	Last cell in a row
ALT+Page Up	First cell in a column
ALT+Page Down	Last cell in a column
Arrow Up	Previous row
CTRL+ALT+U	Remove borders
Delete	Delete cell contents
CTRL+Shift+Enter	Split a table without creating a page break
CTRL+Enter	Split a table and create a page break

Useful Table Commands

Refer to this list of command names for assigning shortcut keys to helpful table commands (see also Chapter 15).

TableAutoSum

TableDeleteColumn

TableDeleteRow

TableDeleteTable

TableInsertRow

TableInsertColumn

TableSelectColumn

TableSelectRow

TableSelectTable

TableSort

TableToOrFromText

Critical Thinking Questions

1. Describe the AutoFormat As You Type feature as it applies to numbering.

2. Explain why an automatic numbered list will continue to automatically number the next list item even when Automatic numbered lists is disabled in the AutoFormat As You Type dialog box.

3. Why do you think Word prevents the user from selecting the number fields of an automatic numbered list?

4. Define promote and demote.

5. Describe the difference between selecting table components vs table contents.

6. Explain how tables can help control complex layouts.

7. Create a document containing a table as in the sample layout shown on page 424.

8. Create a template using automatic numbered lists as in the sample layout shown on page 422. Be sure to include empty fields.

9. Make a list of ten physicians and their mailing addresses. Convert the list to a table and then alphabetize the list by the physicians' last name.

10. Type a simple list of 20 keywords chosen from the first few chapters of this text. Use the Sort command to sort the keywords alphabetically.

CHAPTER 14

Editing Made Easy

OBJECTIVES

▶ Use Word's spelling and grammar tools, including the Custom dictionary.

▶ Use Zoom, Formatting Marks, and Reveal Formatting to facilitate proofreading.

▶ Use shortcut keys for editing.

▶ Use Find as well as Find and Replace to aid with editing.

▶ Use Undo and Redo to reverse unwanted actions.

▶ Differentiate the Office Clipboard from Windows Clipboard.

▶ Use Comments and Track Changes for questions and feedback.

▶ Use Word's reference tools to improve accuracy.

KEYWORDS

Comments
Custom dictionary
electronic dictionary
electronic drug references
electronic references
electronic spell checker
Extend mode
Find
Find and Replace
Grammar Settings dialog box
Look up (Research)
Main dictionary
Office Clipboard
Print Preview
query
Redo
search modes
Spelling and Grammar dialog box
Spelling and Grammar shortcut menu
Undo

Shortcut Keys

ALT+F7	**CTRL+F**
F7	**CTRL+H**
F8	**Esc**
CTRL+D	**F4**
CTRL+Q	
CTRL+Spacebar	**Shift+F3**
CTRL+F2	**Shift+F5**
CTRL+Z	**CTRL+Shift+O**
CTRL+Y	

Spelling and Grammar

Creating an accurate medical record is what we all strive for, and proofreading for spelling errors is one of the most important tasks for producing top quality documents. Word has a built-in spelling and grammar checker that is tremendously useful, but *it cannot replace human judgment and discernment.* The suggestions offered in the **Spelling and Grammar** dialog or shortcut menu are based purely on possible spelling combinations; *they have no basis in context or meaning!* Never assume Word's spell check suggestions are correct for the given context. Word often makes suggestions for correcting the spelling by splitting the misspelled text into two words or hyphenating the words. These suggestions are purely guesses and have no basis in accepted usage. *Do not accept Word's suggestion to split or hyphenate terms without confirmation from a reputable resource.*

To quickly and accurately spell check medical documents, install an **electronic spell checker** such as Stedman's Electronic Medical Spellchecker that includes medical and pharmaceutical terms. This software will work seamlessly with the spell checking tool already built into Word. Spell checkers are updated on a yearly basis to include new terms.

Spell Check Methods

Word will mark misspelled words with a red sawtooth line and possible grammar errors with a green sawtooth line. Word 2007 will mark possible misused words (eg, their and there, here and hear) with a blue sawtooth line. A red X over the book icon 📖 on the Status Bar tells you there are still spelling or grammar errors in the document. A check mark appears when spelling and grammar checking is complete 📖. A pencil appears as if it were writing on the book icon 📖 to indicate Word is currently evaluating the document for spelling and grammar errors.

There are two main approaches to making spelling and grammar corrections:

Spelling and Grammar dialog box: When you are ready to spell check your entire document, press **F7** to open the **Spelling and Grammar** dialog box (Figure 14-1). You can also go to Tools > Spelling and Grammar (Word 2003) or Review > Spelling and Grammar (Word 2007). After you make each correction, Word will bring up the next sentence with a misspelled word or grammatical error. Edit the text directly in the upper pane or select a correction from the suggestion pane, and then click a command button to complete the edit (see below). You can also click into the document itself to make changes and then return to the dialog box. The dialog box will remain displayed, but you can drag it out of the way while you work within the document space. This will pause the spell check routine; click Resume to continue.

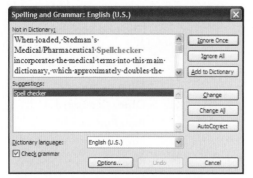
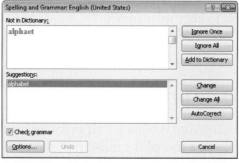

FIGURE 14-1 The Spelling and Grammar dialog box displays the error, suggestions for correcting the error, and options for managing the error. The dialogs in both Word 2003 (left) and Word 2007 (right) are almost identical.

Spelling and Grammar shortcut menu: If you prefer to make corrections using the shortcut menu rather than the dialog box, press **ALT+F7** and Word will jump to the next misspelled word and simultaneously open the shortcut menu (see Figure 14-2). Use the arrow keys to move up and down the shortcut menu and press Enter to make your selection. If no suggestions are given or you do not like any of the options, press Esc to close the menu and try to spell the word another way. Press ALT+F7 again and the insertion point will jump to the next error.

Mouse: Right-click on the misspelled word and the shortcut menu will appear. Left-click on one of the suggested spellings or choose an option from the menu.

Application key: Place the insertion point anywhere within the misspelled word and press the Application key to reveal the shortcut menu. Use the arrow keys to move up and down the shortcut menu and press **Enter** to make your selection.

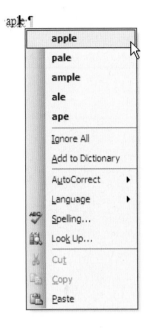

FIGURE 14-2 Spell check right-click menu.

Spell Check Options

When you identify a misspelled word, you can do more than simply correct the spelling. Your options vary slightly depending on whether you open the shortcut menu or the dialog box. On the shortcut menu (Figure 14-2), below the suggested spellings, you can choose one of the following:

Ignore All: This will instruct Word to ignore this and any other occurrence of this word in this document only. Examples include an unusual spelling of a patient's name or a doctor's name that you do not want to add permanently to your dictionary.

Add to Dictionary: Selecting this option will add the current word to your Custom dictionary so Word will no longer mark it misspelled in any document. If you accidentally add a word to your Custom dictionary and you recognize this immediately, press **CTRL+Z** to remove the word from the dictionary. If you later realize that you have incorrectly added a word, you can edit the Custom dictionary file. (Learn more about the Custom dictionary below.)

AutoCorrect: This option may have slipped by you, but it is quite handy if you come upon a word that you typically misspell. When you choose this option, the list of suggested spellings appears a second time. Click on the correct spelling, and Word will make the correction in your document and automatically add the word to your AutoCorrect list—all in one quick click!

Spelling: This command will open the **Spelling and Grammar** dialog box (Figure 14-1), which may list more spelling suggestions than the shortcut menu. In addition, there are several commands that are not available on the shortcut menu.

The **Spelling and Grammar** dialog box offers the above options as well as the following:

|Change|: Replaces the error with the selected suggestion.

|Ignore Once|: Ignores this one occurrence of the word in this document only. It will remove the sawtooth line but will not change the spelling of the word.

|Change All|: Changes all instances of this word to the selected suggestion—for this document only.

|Undo|: Reverses the last change.

|Undo Edit|: Reverses the last edit that you made in the upper pane of the **Spelling and Grammar** dialog box.

|Ignore Rule|: Tells Word to stop marking grammar errors based on the current rule—for this document only.

|Next Sentence|: Skips the current error without making any changes.

|Explain|: Displays a pop-up box with a description of the grammar error and suggestions for correcting the error.

|AutoCorrect|: Changes the current word to the selected suggestion and creates an AutoCorrect entry for the incorrect/correct word pair. Be sure to select the appropriate suggestion before clicking |AutoCorrect|.

|Options|: Opens the dialog for changing options for the spelling and grammar feature (see page 142 in Word 2003 and 162 in Word 2007).

Check Grammar: Remove this check mark to exclude grammar errors and only check spelling.

Be very careful when using the **Spelling and Grammar** dialog box. The buttons change based on your actions and the current error. It's easy to click the wrong command based on its position without realizing the command button changed.

Be sure to review suggested settings in the **Spelling and Grammar** dialog box explained on page 142 (Word 2003) or the **Proofing** dialog box (Word 2007) on page 162.

Custom Dictionary

As Word spell checks a document, it references the **Main dictionary** file. When loaded, Stedman's Electronic Medical and Pharmaceutical Spellchecker incorporates the medical terms into this dictionary. If Word encounters a word that does not appear in the lexicon, the word is marked with a red sawtooth line. The main dictionary cannot be opened or edited, so any new words added during a spell check are added to a separate file called the **Custom dictionary.** This list is automatically created the first time you click Add in the **Spelling and Grammar** dialog box or shortcut menu. Examples of words to add to the Custom dictionary include doctors' names, hospital and clinic names, new drugs, and equipment.

Be sure to check the capitalization of the word before adding a new word to the Custom dictionary. Words starting a sentence will be in title case, but may not need to be capped otherwise. If you add a capitalized word to the list, Word will mark it incorrect if you subsequently type it in lowercase.

Be extremely careful about adding new words to your Custom dictionary. Only add new drugs and new terminology after thoroughly researching and confirming the spelling. Word's reference list is extremely accurate, so do not blithely assume the reference list is wrong and add a new word to your list. Also, it's better to choose Ignore rather than Add when spell checking patient names. Adding names to your Custom dictionary may cause you to assume the wrong spelling of a medical eponym.

If you have a Custom.dic file in the Proof folder (see paths on page 71), it is the previous Custom.dic file left over from Word 2003. The current Custom.dic file should be located in the UProof folder.

Edit the Custom Dictionary

The Add command on the **Spelling and Grammar** dialog box and shortcut menu places new words in the Custom dictionary so they will be recognized by the spell checker as correctly spelled. It's fairly easy to accidentally add words to the list, so it is important to be able to edit this list. To edit the dictionary, follow these steps:

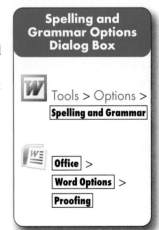

Spelling and Grammar Options Dialog Box

Tools > Options > Spelling and Grammar

Office > Word Options > Proofing

1. Open the **Spelling and Grammar** dialog box.
2. Click Custom Dictionaries to open the **Custom Dictionaries** dialog box (Figure 14-3).
3. To add or remove words from your list, select Modify (Word 2003) or Edit Word List (Word 2007). Add or delete words as necessary.

Add (on the **Custom Dictionary** dialog box) will allow you to retrieve a dictionary file from another folder and add it to your list of custom dictionaries. New will create a new custom dictionary file. Word allows you to run several custom dictionaries at one time, although you may never really have a reason to do this.

It is important to back up the Custom.dic file(s), just as you do the Normal.dot and your AutoCorrect list. See page 71 for details. You will also want to move this file to a new computer.

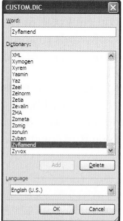

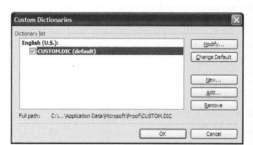

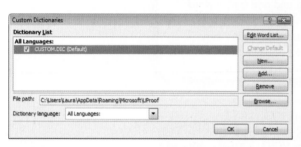

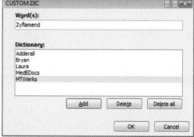

FIGURE 14-3 Add or remove words from your Custom dictionary list using the Custom Dictionaries dialog box. Word 2003's dialog boxes are shown above and Word 2007's below.

Exclusion Dictionary

Both Word 2003 and Word 2007 can use an Exclusion dictionary. This reference list will cause Word to mark a word as misspelled even if the word is spelled correctly. This will help call attention to words that are commonly mistyped yet pass the spell check because they are legitimate words. Examples include `form` and `from`, `trial` and `trail`, `rape` and `drape`.

You can also use AutoCorrect to bold words that you commonly mistype (see page 266) or you can add these words to the Exclusion dictionary; either way, you call extra attention to the word so you can double-check for accuracy. Directions for creating an Exclusion dictionary can be found in the Special Projects section on page 446.

Grammar

The grammar feature in Word is very helpful, but it is important to remember that the grammar checker presents *suggestions* for correcting the grammar; you should carefully evaluate the suggestions and never blindly accept all suggestions. Medical reports often contain sentence fragments, especially in the review of systems or the physical exam section. They are often dictated in the passive voice as well. These common dictation styles cause the grammar checker

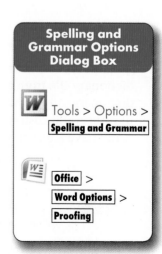

Spelling and Grammar Options Dialog Box

Tools > Options > **Spelling and Grammar**

Office > **Word Options** > **Proofing**

to needlessly flag quite a lot of text. And like the boy who cried wolf, grammar suggestions become annoying and are ignored.

The best approach is to customize the grammar checker so it marks grammar issues relevant to your work and ignores items that are standard or acceptable in medical reports. To customize the grammar settings, follow these steps:

1. Open the **Spelling and Grammar** dialog box.

2. Change the *Writing Style* to *Grammar only* and then click **Settings** to open the **Grammar Settings** dialog box (see Figure 14-4).

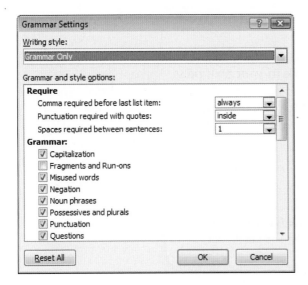

FIGURE 14-4 Change Grammar Settings so Word only marks relevant grammar and style issues.

3. Set the *Require* options to check commas, punctuation marks, and spaces between sentences according to your employer's or client's style guide. Setting these three options *does not automatically correct the document*; rather, it marks variations from your settings with a green sawtooth line. These options can serve as helpful reminders when changing habits such as the spacing between sentences.

4. Place a check mark next to the *Grammar* options you would like Word to mark. Most likely, you will want to remove the check mark at *Fragments and Run-ons*. Removing *Style* issues from the grammar checking routine will cut down on the majority of the annoying green lines.

Language

The Office applications have the ability to work in more than one language. In Word, different languages can be applied to different paragraphs in the same document. If more than one language is enabled, the current language will display on the Status Bar. Word has the option to automatically detect the current language and adjust the language tools accordingly. For example, if you type Mèniére disease, Word *may* detect a new language (French) and switch to French for spell checking. To make sure this does not happen, turn off automatic language detection.

To disable automatic language detection, go to Tools > Language > Set Language and remove the check mark at *Detect language automatically*. Learn more about language tools in Word's Help section using keywords "enabled languages."

To disable automatic language detection, go to Review > Proofing > Set Language > *Detect language automatically*. Learn more about language tools in Word's Help section using keywords "enabled languages."

Also be aware that it is possible to turn off spell checking for a single paragraph or for a particular style. If you see obviously misspelled words in your text, press **Shift+F1** to examine the formatting. Look for the attribute *Do not check spelling or grammar*. Click the link associated with the attribute (which will open the **Language** dialog box) and remove the check mark at *Do not check spelling or grammar*.

Electronic spell check is not a substitute for a complete review of the document for misused words, incorrect syntax, incorrect words or phrases, and formatting problems. Documents must be spell checked *and* proofread!

I prefer to spell check a document while proofreading. I do not use the **Spelling and Grammar** dialog box, but rather right-click on misspelled words as I encounter them while proofreading the entire document. Making spelling and grammar corrections while proofreading keeps the errors in context, makes it easier to make changes directly in the document, and combines two routines into one.

Proofreading

Proofreading a completed document is very important, and there are several ways Word can make this task easier and more efficient:

- To decrease eyestrain, increase the zoom to 125% to 150% (depending on the size of your monitor) so the characters appear larger on the screen. Change the zoom settings back to about 95% to 100% before delivering the document; otherwise, the next person to open the document may mistake the larger zoom setting for a change in formatting.
- Reveal formatting marks so you can easily see problems with character spacing and paragraph spacing.

- Troubleshoot formatting problems using the **Reveal Formatting** task pane (Shift+F1). Click any of the links in the **Reveal Formatting** task pane to open a related dialog box to make changes. Learn more about this task pane on page 223.
- View the entire document one last time using **Print Preview** (CTRL+F2). This view displays headers, footers, headings, and overall layout of the document exactly as it will print. You will be surprised by how many layout problems you can see in Print Preview that are easily overlooked in other document views.

When we read, our brain usually focuses on "chunks" of 3–4 words at a time—we do not normally focus on single words. Our brain fills in the gaps so the chunks of words make sense. Unfortunately, the brain does not always fill in the gaps correctly. This is why it is difficult to catch mistakes when proofreading—our brain is capable of making up words that do not actually exist on the page. The brain is even more prone to making assumptions when reading familiar text, such as text that was just transcribed.

To prevent your brain from clustering too many words at one time, you can change the margins—temporarily—so that the text is displayed in a narrow column. Create a macro that sets the left margin at 4 inches, leaving a 3- to 4-inch column of text. Create a second macro that returns the margins to the correct setting after proofreading.

To force your eyes to focus on each word, move the insertion point one word at a time. Either use the mouse to click on each word or use CTRL+Right to move word by word through the document. The idea is to make sure you are matching each word you *read* to each word you *see*. Forcing your brain to focus on each word (instead of chunks of words) will greatly improve your proofreading accuracy. While you want your eyes to focus on each word, you still want your brain to "listen in context." Be careful that you do not get caught up in verifying each individual word and fail to pay attention to syntax and meaning.

 The shortcut key CTRL+Right works well for moving through a document word by word, but this shortcut key takes your fingers off the home keys. If you use this shortcut key for proofreading, consider assigning the command WordRight to another key combination that keeps the fingers on or close to the home position.

Quality Assurance Review

If you are a quality assurance (QA) editor, you surely understand the need to work quickly and efficiently. The key to editing quickly is to create macros to accomplish routine editing tasks. Combining several keystrokes into one macro saves a few seconds, and over the course of the day those few seconds add up to minutes or even hours. Working efficiently will also reduce physical and mental fatigue.

Evaluate your work carefully, taking special note of command sequences you use repeatedly. Create macros for these tasks to reduce the number of keystrokes needed. Encourage your staff to standardize the way they mark blanks or questions within the document (eg, five underscore characters for blanks and double question marks ?? for questions) and then create macros for finding those marks and placing the insertion point. Find more ideas under Special Projects. For questions, training, or feedback, try using Comments (see page 375) and Track Changes (see page 376).

QA editors should make it a habit to recheck spelling based on the dictionary files on their own computer. During the original spell check routine (by the MT), a spelling error may be marked Ignore or not marked at all because of an incorrect entry in the Custom dictionary. When the document is opened on a subsequent computer, Word does not automatically mark errors again because the spell check status is "complete." Click the **Recheck Document** button on the **Spelling and Grammar** dialog to run the spell check routine again using the Main dictionary and Custom dictionary on the current computer.

Since it takes several clicks to get to the **Recheck Document** button, assign this command to a toolbar or a shortcut key (look for ToolsSpellingRecheckDocument under *All commands* in the **Customize Keyboard** dialog box).

Editing

Editing typically refers to changes made to a document after the document is typed, but the techniques described here can be used to make changes to a document at any point in the transcription or editing process. Many of these techniques are applicable to editing regardless of how the first draft was created—transcription or speech recognition technology.

Mouse Techniques

When proofreading a document that does not require extensive editing, the mouse can be quite useful. Here are a few tips for using the mouse for proofreading:

- Use the scroll wheel on the mouse to quickly move up and down the page.
- To quickly select a line of text, place the mouse pointer next to the line in the left margin and click once. Double-click in the margin to select the paragraph.
- Place the insertion point over a word and double-click to select the word; click three times to select the paragraph.
- You can also move text with the mouse. Select the text and then drag the text to a new location.
- To *copy* selected text, hold down the **CTRL** key while dragging with the mouse.

- You can also combine mouse techniques with Extend mode (explained below) to easily select a long sequence of text—especially text that spans a page break.

To get the best use of the mouse while proofreading, customize the right-click shortcut menus to include tasks that you typically use while proofreading. Think about the kinds of changes you make on a routine basis and add a command or macro to your right-click menu to accomplish that task quickly. Consider adding the following commands and macros to your right-click menu:

- the command to change case (capitalize a word)
- a macro to insert a hyphen (replace the space between words with a hyphen to punctuate compound modifiers)
- a macro to delete to the end of the sentence
- a macro to change a comma to a period (and capitalize following word)

See page 393 for instructions on customizing shortcut menus and also page 444 in Special Projects for more ideas on modifying shortcut menus.

> Another idea for proofreading and editing quickly is to create a customized toolbar with common editing commands. Word 2003 allows you to "float" a toolbar in the middle of your screen so it is always near your mouse cursor. Learn more about creating a custom toolbar on page 388.

> Word 2007 no longer provides tools for modifying right-click menus or creating customized toolbars, but it will accept modified shortcut menus and toolbars created in previous versions of Word and brought over in the Normal.dot file or other template files. If you have access to a copy of Word 2003, create customized menus and toolbars and then copy the template to the computer running Word 2007. If you use a template other than the Normal.dot, add the template as a global template (see page 469) so you can access the customizations at all times.

Shortcut Keys for Editing

There are a few shortcut keys that are essential for editing documents with the keyboard. First, review the list of keystrokes for moving the cursor and selecting text listed on pages 189-190. At first the list may appear daunting, but you will notice there is a pattern. Here are a few tips:

- The basic set of keys to navigate the document include: Up, Down, Right, and Left; Page Up and Page Down; Home and End.
- Each of the navigation keys can be modified by pressing the CTRL key at the same time. The CTRL key will cause each command to increment. In other words, Right and Left normally move one *character*. Adding the CTRL key will move the insertion point over one *word*.
- Adding the Shift key to any navigation key will select text.

Below is a list of essential keyboard commands for editing. The actual command name for each shortcut is given in parentheses. Use these command names to locate the command in the **Customize Keyboard** dialog box if you want to reassign the shortcut key (see Chapter 15).

F4 (EditRedoOrRepeat): This command repeats the last action, including formatting commands and typing text. If you have typed a line of text and would like to repeat that line of text, simply press F4. To apply bold formatting to several words, press the bold command the first time, then click on each word and press F4. The shortcut keys ALT+Enter and CTRL+Y have the same function as F4.

Shift+F3 (ChangeCase): This command changes the case of a word or selected words. You can also use this command to capitalize the current word while you are still in the middle of typing the word. Change case toggles between initial cap (title case), all uppercase, and all lowercase. Set the insertion point anywhere within a word (you do not have to select the entire word) and press the shortcut. Repeat until the word is formatted appropriately.

You can also select several words at one time and change the case. If you include a period in the selection, this command will toggle to sentence case (ie, only the first word will be capitalized). This command works well for creating editing macros to correct missed capitalization or to change commas to periods (and cap the following word).

Shift+F5 (GoBack): This command moves the insertion point to the previous revision or to the last insertion point before the document was closed. Press the command repeatedly to cycle through the last three edit points. This shortcut is helpful if the dictator edits a previous section of the dictation and then returns to the current heading (eg, adds a comment to the medication list and then returns to plan). You can also use this if you back up several words to make an edit and want to move the insertion point back to where you left off. This command can also be helpful when creating macros.

CTRL+Q (ResetPara): This command removes direct paragraph formatting (strips any manual formatting and returns the paragraph to the underlying style). This particular command is helpful if you have applied the incorrect formatting and you want to strip the formatting and start again. Review information on the Normal style and direct formatting on page 222.

CTRL+Spacebar (ResetChar): This command removes character formatting. It can be helpful to remove bold or underline formatting or to remove several character formatting attributes at one time. If you use this command and the font changes unexpectedly, review information on default fonts and direct formatting on page 222.

F8 (ExtendSelection): This command turns on Extend mode, which is a clever tool for selecting text. Learn more ways to use Extend mode below.

CTRL+Z (EditUndo): Reverses anything *you* have done or any *automatic actions taken by Word*. By far, Undo is the most useful command and will save you more time and frustration than any other command/shortcut key. Learn more ways to use Undo on page 372.

CTRL+D (FormatFont): This shortcut key opens the **Font** dialog box so you can make several character changes at one time.

Esc: Use this key to cancel an action or close a dialog box.

 Two other helpful commands that you may want to assign to shortcut keys include SentLeft and SentRight. These commands move the cursor to the beginning and end of sentences respectively.

Extend Mode

Next to Undo, **Extend mode** (**F8**) is probably the most clever feature in Word. Extend mode gives you precise control over the selection of text and will revolutionize the way you edit documents. Extend mode essentially "locks" the keyboard in select mode, so you can use the keyboard to quickly and precisely select any amount of text.

Press **F8** to activate Extend mode. EXT (Word 2003) or Extend Selection (Word 2007) displays on the Status Bar while the mode is active. Press **F8** again, and the word containing the insertion point will be selected. Press a third time and Word will select the sentence (regardless of length). Press **F8** a fourth time and Word will extend the selection to the entire paragraph. Now, apply any command using a shortcut key or the mouse. The command will be applied and Extend mode will be turned off. There is no faster way to delete words, phrases, or sentences. If that is all you could do with Extend, it would still be a great tool, but you can do much more! Note these methods for using Extend mode:

- Press **F8** once to turn on Extend and then press any *character* key. Word will extend the selection from the insertion point to the next occurrence of that character. Press another key to continue to select text.
- Press **F8** once to turn on Extend and then press any *navigation* key. Word will extend the selection in the direction or the distance of the navigation key used. Press another key to continue to select text.
- **F8 Period** will select to the end of a sentence.
- **F8 Enter** will select to the end of the paragraph.
- **F8 Spacebar** will select to the next space, which makes this a very easy way to select one word at a time.
- Press **F8** and then click the mouse anywhere in the document to extend the selection. Click the mouse in the middle of the selection to deselect text below the mouse click.
- As long as Extend mode is on, you can continue to extend the selection using any character or navigation key on the keyboard. Apply any command and Word will simultaneously turn off Extend mode.

(Continued)

- Press **Esc** to turn off Extend but keep the text selected. To de-select text without applying a command, press the **Left** or **Right** arrow key. If you start typing with text selected, the selected text will be replaced. If you accidentally delete characters, press **CTRL+Z**.

- **F8** followed by **F11** will select to the next field (empty field or data field).

- To shrink a selection, use **Shift+F8**.

- Use **CTRL+Shift+F8** to select columns or rows in a table.

- Combine Extend mode with the Find feature (see below) to create macros for deleting specific blocks of text. Set the insertion point, press **F8** then **CTRL+F**, type a word and press **Enter**. Word will select from the insertion point to the first occurrence of the *Find what* text. This technique works perfectly for recording a macro to delete specific text from the standard text of a template or boilerplate because it defines a very specific point for ending the selection.

Create macros using the Extend mode to delete sentences or parts of sentences. **F8** three times followed by **Delete** will remove a sentence. **F8 Period Delete** will remove the last part of a sentence. These macros will turn three- and four-keystroke operations into a single keystroke, or better yet, eliminate a cumbersome mouse technique.

Editing Speech Recognition Drafts

Editing a draft created by speech recognition technology takes a somewhat different approach than editing traditionally-transcribed documents. Properly reviewing a speech recognized (SR) draft requires the editor to listen to the entire audio file and compare each word in the audio to each word in the document. Inserting or changing punctuation is also quite common. In addition, there will be varying degrees of formatting required. Editing an SR draft is best accomplished by maintaining the hands in the home position on the keyboard and moving the insertion point through the document at the same pace as the audio playback.

Many of the editing commands already discussed above will be of great benefit to the SR editor, but there are other editing commands that can be created using macros that will greatly enhance the editor's speed (techniques for creating the editing macros referenced below are described in the Special Projects section). Use the following ideas for increasing your efficiency when editing SR drafts:

- Create macros for moving through a document one word at a time. You might create a macro that moves the insertion point one word at a time (setting the insertion point at the beginning of each word) or you may prefer to *select* one word at a time.

- Create macros for performing the most common editing tasks. Typical tasks include inserting a period and capitalizing the next word, inserting a period and ending a paragraph, converting plain text to heading format and inserting a colon (eg, change history of present illness to **HISTORY OF**

PRESENT ILLNESS:), inserting a comma, or changing a comma to a period and capitalizing the next word.

- Assign the most common editing commands, such as deleting words and adjusting punctuation, to shortcut keys that combine the **CTRL** key with the home keys (A, S, D, F, J, K, L). This maintains your hand position over the home keys, making it easy to alternate between typing text and executing common commands.

- Assign shortcut keys so that the simplest key combinations are used while the sound file is playing (or while the foot is on the pedal). **CTRL**-key combinations are probably the easiest key combinations to strike repeatedly and accurately. **ALT**-key combinations are also fairly easy to use. Use multiple-key combinations (eg, **ALT+Shift+**x) for commands that are executed when you are not tracking the audio.

- Reassign Word's built-in editing commands so they are easier to strike. For example, the command to change the case, as described above, is an incredibly useful command, but **Shift+F3** (the native key assignment) is awkward and moves the fingers away from the home position. See Chapter 15 for instructions on customizing key assignments.

Many of the commands used for editing speech-recognized drafts are also useful for educators and quality assurance editors. Any situation requiring extensive editing or tracking the audio with the text (often referred to as a full audit) will benefit from the same editing techniques used in speech recognition.

Word Count

Word includes a word count tool that tallies characters, characters with spaces, words, paragraphs, and lines. Lines, in this context, refers to a line of text, regardless of the amount of text on the line, and also includes blank lines. To display the dialog box, go to Tools > Word Count (Word 2003) or Review > Proofing > Word Count (Word 2007).

To track your character or word counts, display the Word Count toolbar. In Word 2003, go to View > Toolbars > Word Count. Choose which count to display. Word 2007 will display the word count (but not the character count) on the Status Bar (right-click and choose Word Count). Click the word count on the Status Bar to see character, word, line, and paragraph counts.

Find and Replace

You can quickly search for words, phrases, symbols, formatting marks, or styles using **Find** (CTRL+F). Or you can easily replace text and/or formatting using

Find and Replace (CTRL+H). For example, you can correct gender by replacing she with he (and vice versa), replace dysphagia with dysphasia, or change formatting (eg, replace *Present Illness* with **PRESENT ILLNESS**).

Find Text

To search for specific text or characters within a document, follow these steps:

1. Press **CTRL+F** to open the **Find** dialog box.
2. Click **More** to expand the box, as shown in Figure 14-5.

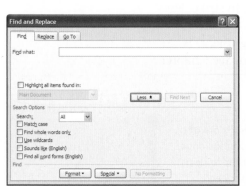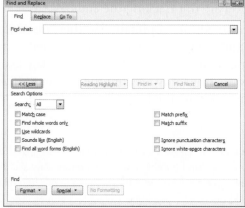

FIGURE 14-5 Use the Find dialog box to locate text within the document.

3. In the *Find what* box, enter the search text.
4. Select applicable *Search Options* to customize your search (this is optional). The option to *Ignore white-space characters* (Word 2007) will locate the search text when written as one word or two (eg, follow up or followup).
5. Fine tune a search using wildcard characters (this is optional). For example, use the asterisk (*) wildcard to substitute for a string of unknown characters, or use a question mark to substitute for a single character (eg, s*d finds "sad" and "started"; s?d would find "sad" and "sod"). Be sure to place a check mark at *Use wildcards* if you use asterisks or question marks to represent unknown characters; otherwise, Word will literally search for asterisks and question marks in the document.
6. Click **Find Next**. Word will jump to the next occurrence of the search text and select that text. Press **Esc** to close the dialog box or click within the document space to keep the dialog box open while you edit the document.
7. To select all items that match the search criteria, click *Highlight all items found in: Main Document* (Word 2003) or *Find in: Main Document* (Word 2007). Once the words are selected, close the **Find** dialog. You can copy (**CTRL+C**) or apply formatting to all the selected words at one time (even

if the words are scattered throughout the document). If you copy the words, you can then paste them into a document to create a list of words that have been "gathered" throughout the document.

8. Word often retains the formatting characteristics in the *Find what* box. Before starting a new search, be sure to click No Formatting to clear the formatting criteria.

 Be sure to use the option *Find whole words only* when searching for words such as he or she. Otherwise, Word will also locate words *containing* he and she (eg, the, father, mother, sheath, brushes, etc).

 Once you have filled out the **Find** dialog box and clicked Find next, you can close the dialog box and continue to "find next" using Shift+F4 (RepeatFind). You can also click the Find next or Find Previous buttons (the Browse by buttons) at the bottom of the Vertical scroll bar (see page 125).

Find Formatting

Word can find text based on formatting criteria such as character and paragraph formatting, styles, and highlighting. Word allows you to search for specific formatting with or without specific search text (ie, you can search for *any* word with specific formatting characteristics). To search using formatting criteria, follow these steps:

1. To search for text based on formatting only, leave the *Find what* box blank.

2. With the cursor in the *Find what* box, click Format and select the appropriate dialog box (see Figure 14-6).

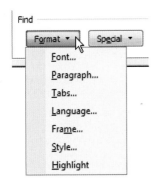

FIGURE 14-6 Use the dialog boxes listed under Format to create a search based on a specific format or style.

3. Make the appropriate format selections from one or several of the formatting dialog boxes (eg, Font, Paragraph, Styles). After making your

(Continued)

selection, press **Enter** to return to the **Find and Replace** dialog box. You can also press the shortcut key for a formatting command (eg, **CTRL+B**) instead of opening the formatting dialog. Formatting characteristics will be listed just below the *Find what* box.

4. Click **Find Next** to jump to the next occurrence, or choose *Highlight all items found in: Main Document* (Word 2003) or *Find in: Main Document* (Word 2007) to select all occurrences at once.

> You can take advantage of the **Find** feature to select all occurrences of a particular format or style to create a log sheet or to gather specific information within a single document. Learn more on page 466.

Find and Replace Text

Find and Replace (**CTRL+H**) allows you to search for specific words and/or formatting and replace those instances with something else—either the same words with different formatting or different words. To replace text, or even delete text, follow these steps:

1. Press **CTRL+H** to open the **Replace** dialog box (Figure 14-7). In the *Find what* box, enter the search text and/or format.

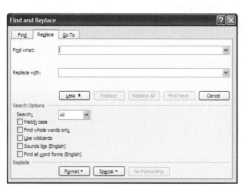
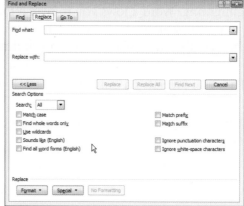

FIGURE 14-7 Use the Replace dialog to replace text, reformat text, or delete text.

2. In the *Replace with* box, enter the replacement text and/or format.

3. Select other search options by clicking **More** to expand the dialog.

4. To review each occurrence before replacing, click **Find Next** and then click **Replace** to perform the find/replace function on that selected text. Click **Replace All** to find and replace all occurrences without reviewing each replacement first.

5. To search for text and delete that text, leave the *Replace with* box empty or type a single space (**Spacebar**).

If you type multiple patient reports in the same file and they all have the same date, you can use Find and Replace to enter the correct date in all reports at one time. When you set up a template, include a date marker such as three asterisks (***) or a pound sign (#) in place of the date. When you finish transcribing all of your reports, use Find and Replace to substitute the date marker with the current date.

Find Special Characters

You can easily search for and replace special characters, formatting marks, and document elements such as page breaks and white space. Click Special to select from a list of possible characters (Figure 14-8). When you make a character selection, a code will be entered into the *Find what/Replace box* (eg, ^t represents a tab character, ^p represents a paragraph mark). If you already know the code, you can type it directly into the *Find what/Replace* box. Finding paragraph marks and replacing with a space (**Spacebar**) is an easy way to take the paragraph breaks out of email text that you have copy/pasted from an email message to a Word document or from a PDF file into Word. Learn other ways to take advantage of special characters in Special Projects starting on page 454.

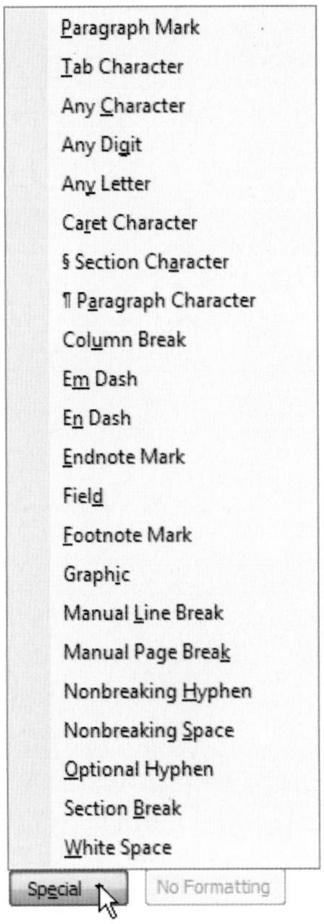

Paragraph Mark
Tab Character
Any Character
Any Digit
Any Letter
Caret Character
§ Section Character
¶ Paragraph Character
Column Break
Em Dash
En Dash
Endnote Mark
Field
Footnote Mark
Graphic
Manual Line Break
Manual Page Break
Nonbreaking Hyphen
Nonbreaking Space
Optional Hyphen
Section Break
White Space

Special   No Formatting

FIGURE 14-8 The Find and Replace dialog box includes a list of special characters that can be used to find and replace specific text, symbols, formatting marks, etc.

Use **Find and Replace** to quickly repair formatting. For example, use this technique to clean up a paragraph that was originally formatted with tab characters and then subsequently edited, thereby scattering tab characters throughout the paragraph. See page 216 for an example. To fix these paragraphs, select the entire paragraph and press **CTRL+H**. Type ^t (the symbol for a tab character) in the *Find what* box and leave the *Replace with* box blank. Click [Replace All]. The tab characters contained in the selected paragraph will be deleted. Word will ask if you want to continue searching the rest of the document; answer [No].

Undo and Redo

An absolutely indispensable command in Word is **Undo (CTRL+Z)**. This command will reverse almost any action. It will even undo automatic actions performed by Word! Here are tips for using Undo and its opposite command Redo:

- On the <u>Standard</u> toolbar/<u>Quick Access</u> toolbar, click the Undo icon (arrow curved to the left) to undo the last action.

- Click the down arrow next to Undo to display a list of the most recent actions. Drag the mouse down the list to select a range of actions to undo all at once (Figure 14-9). You have to undo actions in reverse order and you cannot skip an action to undo.

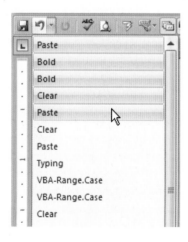

FIGURE 14-9 Select a range of actions to undo at one time.

- You can also click **CTRL+Z** repeatedly until you step back through as many actions as necessary.

- If you step back too far, use **Redo (CTRL+Y)** to reverse the Undo command. The Redo icon (the arrow curved to the right) will be available after you have used Undo. The Redo command will also have a drop-down list of actions that you can redo.

Use the Undo command:

- to undo an AutoCorrect entry on a one-time basis (eg, revert b.i.d. to bid)
- to reverse automatic capitalization (eg, to change Cc: to cc:)
- to reverse automatic numbering
- to change a border back to a signature line
- to delete the last few words typed
- to replace text that was accidentally deleted
- to reverse an accidental addition to the Custom dictionary
- when you press the wrong command or an "unknown" command
- when the cat walks across your keyboard!

You cannot use Undo to revert to the previous zoom setting or return to the previous document view.

Office Clipboard

When you use the Copy command, the selected item is "stored" on the Windows Clipboard where it is available to be pasted into any other application. This allows the transfer of items (text or objects) within the same file or between separate files or folders. The Windows Clipboard is limited to one item at a time. Each time the Copy or Cut command is used, the previous item is replaced with the newly copied item. Sometimes it is helpful to be able to "collect" text or graphics from various places and paste them either individually or together.

In addition to the Windows Clipboard, Office includes its own clipboard capable of storing up to 24 separate items. Once copied, items stored in the **Office Clipboard** can be inserted individually or all at once. Although there are two separate clipboards for storing copied items (the Windows Clipboard and the Office Clipboard), the last item copied always goes to both clipboards, so it is available no matter where you want to paste. Clearing the Office Clipboard will also clear the Windows Clipboard.

Follow these steps to use the Office Clipboard:

1. Press **CTRL+C** twice to open the **Office Clipboard** task pane (Figure 14-10).
2. Select an item to be copied and press **CTRL+C**. Items copied from any of the Office programs (Word, Outlook, Excel, etc) will be placed on the Office Clipboard as long as the task pane is open in at least one of the Office programs.
3. To paste a single item, select the item from the task pane and click Paste from the item's drop-down menu. To paste all items, click Paste All.

Click Options at the bottom of the **Clipboard** task pane to control the way the Office Clipboard behaves. The Office Clipboard will collect items only while the task pane is displayed unless you choose Collect Without Showing Office Clipboard under Options. The Windows Clipboard is always functional, regardless of the options you choose for the Office Clipboard.

Word also allows you to select text from various places in the document at the same time and copy all of these selections with a single copy command. Hold

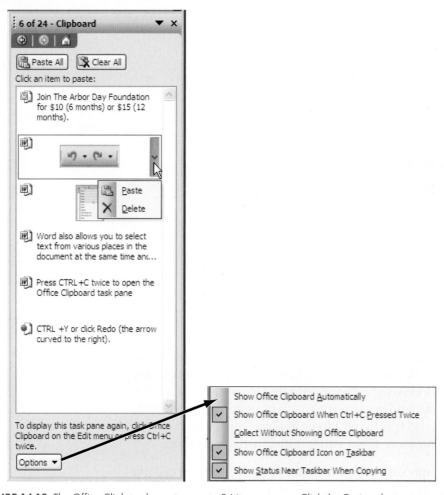

FIGURE 14-10 The Office Clipboard can store up to 24 items at once. Click the Options button to control the Office Clipboard's behavior.

down the **CTRL** key while selecting words or phrases scattered throughout the document, then press **CTRL+C** to copy. As mentioned above, you can also use Find to select words scattered throughout a document and select them all at once.

When you use the paste command, a Paste Options icon will appear immediately below the pasted object/text. Click the icon to display a menu of paste options, as shown in Figure 14-11. To display the menu using the keyboard, press **ALT+Shift+F10** while the button is visible.

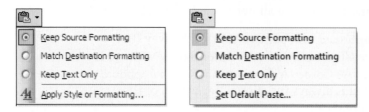

FIGURE 14-11 The Paste Options icon opens a drop-down menu. Choose how you would like to format text that has been pasted. The menu from Word 2003 is shown on the left and Word 2007's menu is shown on the right.

Comments

The **Comments** feature in Word is a useful tool for providing feedback to MTs or for "flagging" reports with questions for the quality assurance staff, dictator, or facility. Learn more about using Comments on the accompanying CD.

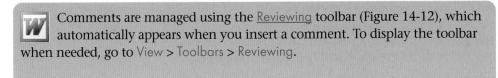
Comments are managed using the Reviewing toolbar (Figure 14-12), which automatically appears when you insert a comment. To display the toolbar when needed, go to View > Toolbars > Reviewing.

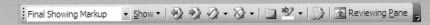

FIGURE 14-12 The Reviewing toolbar is used to manage comments as well as tracked changes.

To insert a comment, set the insertion point on the line related to the comment or select several words. Go to Insert > Comment (**ALT, I, M**). Depending on your settings, a pane will open across the bottom of the display or a balloon will appear in the margin. Type a comment in the designated space. A comment marker will also insert, which consists of brackets with the user's initials and a comment number. Use the following tips to help manage comments:

- Use the Comments pane instead of balloons, since balloons in the margin "shrink" the text to accommodate both the balloons and the text. To use the Comments pane instead of balloons, open the Show menu on the Reviewing toolbar and choose Balloons > Never.

- Click the Reviewing Pane button on the toolbar to toggle the reviewing pane open and closed, or right-click on the comment marker and choose Edit Comment.

- To view the comment as a ToolTip, go to Tools > Options > View and place a check mark at Screen Tips. With this option selected, the comment will appear in a pop-up box when you hover the mouse over the comment marker.

- To delete comments, delete the comment marker from the document, right-click the comment marker and choose Delete Comment, or right-click the comment in the Reviewing pane and choose Delete Comment.

- To print the document with comments, open the **Print** dialog box. In the Print what box, choose Document showing markup. To print comments on a separate document, choose List of markup.

Comments are managed using the **Review** tab, <u>Comments</u> and <u>Tracking</u> groups (Figure 14-13).

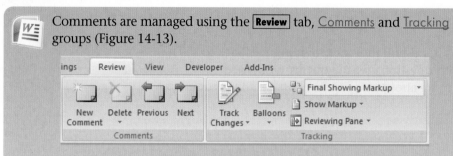

FIGURE 14-13 The Review tab is used to manage comments.

To insert a comment, set the insertion point on the line related to the comment or select several words. Click **ALT, I, M** or go to **Review** > <u>Comments</u> > **New Comment**. Depending on your settings, a pane will open on the left side of the display or a balloon will appear in the margin. Type a comment in the designated space. Press **Esc** to move from the balloon back to the document space. Press **F6** to move from the comments pane to the document space. A comment marker will also insert, which consists of brackets with the user's initials and a comment number. Use the following tips to help manage comments:

- Use the Comments pane instead of balloons, since balloons in the margin "shrink" the text to accommodate both the balloons and the text. To use the Comments pane instead of balloons, click **Balloons** (in the <u>Tracking</u> group) and choose Show All Revisions Inline.

- Click the **Reviewing Pane** button on the <u>Tracking</u> group to toggle the reviewing pane open and closed. Open the Reviewing Pane drop-down menu and choose whether to display the pane vertically or horizontally.

- To delete comments, delete the comment marker from the document. You can also right-click the comment marker and choose Delete Comment, or select the comment marker and click Delete on the ribbon.

- To print the document with comments, open the **Print** dialog box. In the *Print what* box, choose *Document showing markup*. To print comments on a separate document, choose *List of markup*.

Track Changes

Track Changes is a tool for marking changes to a document. You may find Track Changes to be useful for training and feedback. When Track Changes is enabled, deletions are marked with strikethroughs and insertions display in a different color, as shown in Figure 14-14. A vertical line displays in the left margin to indicate lines that contain edits; this is especially useful for lines that contain easily missed edits such as a change in punctuation.

¶
Since·we·are·unable·to· ~~visual~~ ·visualize·the·fundus·of·her·uterus·secondary·to·her·having·a·
retroverted·uterus,·we· ~~will~~ ·would·recommend·a·hysteroscopy·to·evaluate·her·endometrial·
cavity.··I·would·also·like·to·perform·an·endometrial·biopsy·to·insure·that·infection·is·not·the·
etiology·for·her·loss.··She·had·a· ~~torch·tighter~~ TORCH·titer[LLB2]·performed·that·was·within·
normal·limits.··Because·she·has·————two·alleles·that·are·positive·for·the·MTHFR·mutation,·I·
would·advise·placing·her·on·Folgard·treatment.··¶
¶

FIGURE 14-14 An excerpt of a report showing edits marked with the Track Changes feature. A comment marker is also shown with the initials LLB.

Commands for controlling Track Changes are found on the Reviewing toolbar in Word 2003 (View > Toolbars > Reviewing) and the **Review** tab in Word 2007. Track Changes has a tremendous functionality. If your circumstances would benefit from this tool, learn more about Track Changes on the accompanying CD.

It's surprisingly easy to accidentally invoke Track Changes (the shortcut key is **CTRL+Shift+E**). If text is suddenly marked with strikethroughs or displayed in a different color, you have inadvertently turned on revision marks. Press **CTRL+Shift+E** to toggle off or click TRK on the Status Bar. Use **CTRL+Z** to reverse the changes made while track changes was enabled or click Accept Changes (blue check mark) on the Reviewing toolbar/**Review** tab.

Be sure to turn off Track Changes before delivering a document to the client. This setting "follows" the document, so changes will continue to be tracked when the document is opened on another computer.

Reference Tools

Honing your research skills is absolutely essential to increasing your speed and productivity in transcription. Of all the techniques taught in this book, none will improve the quantity and quality of your work as much as a foundational knowledge of terminology and disease processes. When you combine this knowledge with electronic search skills, you will be able to produce more accurate documents in much less time.

Transcription is a production-driven profession, but accuracy is paramount. If confirming information is laborious or time-consuming, you will be tempted to put it off or not do it at all. Make searching for information fast and easy and you won't be tempted to sacrifice quality for quantity. This section will introduce search techniques that will greatly decrease the time you spend researching and ensuring the accuracy of your documents.

Dictionary and Thesaurus

Word includes a dictionary and a thesaurus as part of the **Look Up (Research)** feature (**CTRL+Shift+O**), so confirming the meaning of an English word is quick and easy. Here are several tips for using Look Up:

- Simply place the insertion point anywhere in the word and press CTRL+Shift+O (the letter o). You can also right-click on the word and choose Look up. The definition will appear in the **Research** task pane (Figure 14-15).

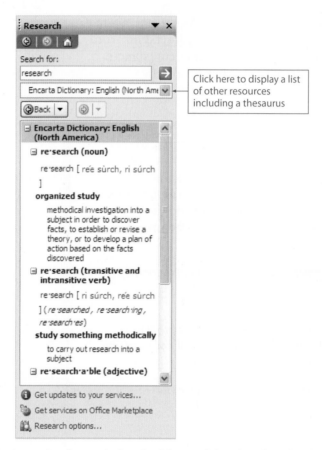

FIGURE 14-15 The Research task pane displays the definition of the selected word. A thesaurus is also available from the drop-down list of resources.

- Look up synonyms for the word by clicking Shift+F7.
- Press CTRL+F1 to close the task pane in Word 2003. Press CTRL+Spacebar, C to close the task pane in Word 2007.

Electronic References

Electronic references, such as Stedman's Electronic Medical Dictionary, Stedman's Electronic Word Books, and Quick Look Electronic Drug Reference are amazingly fast, simple, and powerful tools for finding terms, confirming definitions, and researching drug names, dosages, and indications. Electronic references offer ways of searching that are not possible with printed materials. Electronic references allow searches using the end of a word or part of a word, as well as searches based on the definition, concept, or words contained within the definition. Quick Look Drug Reference can be searched using keywords, indications, dosage, or partial spellings.

Electronic resources contain the same content as their corresponding printed version and often contain bonus features. Electronic references are stored in database format, so the information can be sorted, filtered, and searched in numerous ways. They also offer easier readability compared to the small print of traditional bound materials. Electronic resources allow you to:

- search for terms in numerous ways (partial word, meaning, sounds-like)
- retrieve information faster
- copy words from the reference directly into the document for efficiency and accuracy
- take your references with you, especially if you work while traveling or work in more than one location
- reduce the amount of desktop space needed for open books
- reduce the amount of bookshelf space needed within arm's reach of your desk

The ability to use electronic resources will serve you well throughout your career in medical documentation, whether you work as a traditional transcriptionist, a quality assurance editor, a speech recognition editor, transcription manager, service owner, or any emerging role that may develop as a result of the EHR. The increased speed and efficiency of electronic searches will help you produce more documents in less time with better accuracy, and that will always translate into higher income. Practical skills acquired using electronic reference materials will also translate directly into any work you may do in the electronic health record. These fundamental database skills will be vital to your ongoing success in the field of healthcare documentation.

Most electronic resources are sold on CD and are intended to be installed on your computer's hard disk. The easier it is to look up information, the more likely you are to confirm the information and the less likely you are to assume or guess. After installing your electronic resources, spend a few minutes creating shortcuts and placing those shortcuts where they are easily accessible.

I create shortcuts to my electronic references and place those shortcuts on my Start menu. This approach gives me two-keystroke access to most of my references at all times—without minimizing windows. Since I have quite a few electronic references, I group them together in a single folder (and place a shortcut to the folder on the Start menu). Review instructions in Chapter 3 for adding shortcuts to your Start menu.

Electronic Medical Dictionaries and Word Lists

An **electronic dictionary** is not the same as an electronic spell checker. A dictionary provides spelling, pronunciation, etymology, and definitions. Electronic spell checkers, on the other hand, work with your transcription software to check spelling only. Electronic word lists give the correct spelling but do not include pronunciations or definitions. Documentation specialists should invest in each of these tools, as each one plays an important role in the documentation process.

Electronic references offer several **search modes** for locating information. The modes are similar across various software products, but depending on the type of reference, the modes have slightly different names. Refer to the help files within your specific reference software to learn how to change to a different search mode. The following provides a basic overview of search modes:

Index mode provides an alphabetized list for scanning, much like you would scan the index of a book. Simply type the word you are looking for and the indexed list will scroll to the entry.

Search Index, also called Search on Headword or Search on Entry, allows you to search against the indexed list of terms using wildcard characters to replace unknown characters.

To search for information contained within the definition or subentry, use Search, Search on Definition, or Search on Entry.

Table 14-1 summarizes the types of search modes you may encounter and gives examples of queries that can be used with the different search modes.

Electronic Drug References

Properly transcribing drugs is one of the most challenging aspects of medical transcription, and an up-to-date drug reference is absolutely essential. **Electronic drug references** contain information on medications, indications, dosages, trade and generic names, and other pertinent information. The information is stored as a database, so these references are extremely useful for searching. Electronic drug references allow you to search against the end of the word, part of the word, keywords, indications, and even the drug dose. For example, a search using 5 & headache would list drugs dispensed in 5 (mcg or mg) that include the word headache as an indication. This approach narrows the list of possible drugs to a smaller list that is easier to scan, especially if you have an idea of the beginning sound of the drug. Table 14-2 lists sample searches using Quick Look Electronic Drug Reference.

Internet Search

Search engines have become an indispensable tool for researching new terms, medical phrases, drugs, and equipment names. Google has traditionally been the most-used search engine, outpacing the other market forerunners Yahoo! and

Table 14-1   Examples of Search Queries Using Electronic References.

Wildcard/Search command (operators)	Search Modes	Sample Query	Sample Results
Asterisk (*) to represent any number of characters	Search Index Search on Headword Search on Entry	H*p	hip, hump, hemoclip, hiccup
	Search Index Search on Headword Search on Entry	H*p*p	hemopump
	Search Index Search on Headword Search on Entry	*ase	lipase, amylase
Question mark (?) to represent any single character	Search Index Search on Headword Search on Entry	H?p	hip, hop
		H?cc?p	hiccup
Combine wildcards	Search Index Search on Headword Search on Entry	m?r*s	marasmus, mirabilis, mortis
Find entries whose content contains both words using the ampersand (&)	Search Search on Definition Search on Subentry	Cholesterol & athero*	atherosclerosis, cholesterol embolism
Find entries whose contents contain the first word and exclude entries containing the second word (NOT)	Search Search on Definition Search on Subentry	Cholesterol NOT atherosclerosis	lipoprotein, low-fat diet
Fuzzy search using tilde (~) based on a concept	Search Search on Definition Search on Subentry	helper~	Entries including helper, holder, retractor

Microsoft Live Search. Google can be used to locate most any information, including local business names, schools, hospitals, referring physician addresses, as well as new terms and phrases.

Place a shortcut to Google on your Start menu (see instructions on page 106). When you use the shortcut, the cursor will default to Google's search box so you can immediately type your search query. You may also choose to make Google your Home page. Go to http://www.Google.com and click on Help to learn how to make Google your home page in your particular browser.

The **query** is made up of words or phrases that best describe the information you need. The key to any successful search, regardless of the search engine you use, is

Table 14-2   Sample drug searches using Quick Look Electronic Drug Reference.

Wildcard/Search command (operators)	Sample Query	Sample Results
Wildcard to replace beginning of word	*tor	Lipitor, Eltor, Crestor, Florastor
	*amine	Desipramine, Bonamine, chlorpheniramine, thiamine
Fuzzy search (sounds like) using tilde (~)	Anaprox~	Anadrol, Anaplex, Anaspaz, Monodox, etc.
	acedil~	Acetasol, acetaminophen (and all entries containing acetaminophen), Aci-jel
Find entries whose content contains both words using the ampersand (&)	diuretic & HCT	Diuretics which contain HCT (hydrochlorothiazide)
Find entries whose contents contain the first word and exclude entries containing the second word (NOT)	diuretic NOT HCT	All diuretics that do not contain HCT (hydrochlorothiazide)
Exclude drugs dispensed in milligrams	40 NOT mg	All drugs dispensed in 40 mcg or ml
Find entries which include two parameters but do not include the third	120 & diuretic NOT HCT	All diuretics dispensed in 120 (mg, mcg, ml) that do not contain hydrochlorothiazide
Fuzzy search with ampersand (&)	40 & anaprox~	Drugs sounding like Anaprox including 40 in the content (40 mg, mcg)
Keyword	Hypertension	Drugs used to treat hypertension

the query. The query should be as specific as possible, yet not so specific that you exclude your search target. As you gain experience searching, you will improve your ability to create highly relevant queries that will hone in on the needed information quickly and accurately.

To improve your search results, use several keywords in the query. An asterisk can be used in place of missing words, and quotation marks can be used to keep words together in the exact order (ie, a phrase). Combine keywords, quotation marks, and asterisks to decipher partial phrases (see examples below).

Here are some examples of queries you can use with Google:

- `"left * hypertrophy"` (left <u>ventricular</u> hypertrophy)
- `EKG "* flutter"` (<u>atrial</u> flutter)
- `"recurrent pregnancy loss" "* anticoagulant"` (<u>lupus</u> anticoagulant)
- `How many inches in a centimeter` (converts inches to centimeters)
- `Beta-blockers are used to treat *` (sites listing indications for beta-blockers)

- `Vitamin * supports *` (which vitamin supports which metabolic function?)
- `Safesearch:erectile dysfunction` (excludes sites with adult content)
- `124*584` (multiplies 124 by 584)
- `"cardiac arrest" "elevated enzymes" diagnostic` (sites listing diagnostic tests for evaluating cardiac arrest)
- `"reference range" hematocrit +female` (normal range for hematocrit in females)

Evaluate the search results by examining several key points. First, look at the Search Results bar to see how many hits (references) were found. A really good search should have thousands of hits. A small search result usually indicates the word or phrase is wrong or not commonly accepted. An obscure term may only have 100 or so hits, but certainly a result with fewer than 100 hits should be confirmed with reliable sources.

When referencing medical terms and phrases, give the most credence to sites maintained by major medical centers (eg, Mayo Clinic, Cleveland Clinic), government agencies, and medical journals. The National Institutes of Health (NIH) and the National Library of Medicine (NLM) maintain archives of peer-reviewed articles on PubMed, which are very reliable sources of medical information. NIH and NLM also maintain a patient-friendly site at http://MedlinePlus.gov.

To confirm the accuracy of the information, always cross-reference terms found on the Web to your trusted resources, such as Stedman's Medical Dictionary, Stedman's word books, Quick Look Drug Reference, or a collegiate dictionary. Even reliable sites can contain typos, as many sites are maintained by web masters who are adept at managing websites but are not trained in medical terminology. The following types of websites should *never* be used as a definitive source of information:

- online pharmacies
- consumer organizations
- patient advocacy sites
- private physician's websites
- public bulletin boards and discussion forums
- distributors of medical equipment or supplies (unless it is the manufacturer of the actual product you are researching)
- PowerPoint presentations published online

Critical Thinking Questions

1. Why is it important to confirm the spelling and meaning of words suggested by the spell checker?

   _____

   _____

2. Step through the following:

   a. Open Word.

   b. Type a paragraph of text, purposely misspelling several words and leaving out commas or periods.

   c. Right click on the misspelled words using the Application key and correct the spelling using the Arrow keys and the Enter key to select the correct word.

   d. Right click on the grammar errors (marked with a wavy green line) and correct the grammar. Do this without using the mouse.

3. What is the Custom dictionary and how does Word use it?

   _____

   _____

4. Explain Extend mode.

   _____

   _____

5. Describe how you can combine Extend and Find to select specific blocks of text.

   _____

   _____

6. Describe how Find and Replace can be used to delete the same character or symbol throughout a document.

   _____

   _____

7. What is the difference between an electronic spell checker and an electronic dictionary?

   _____

   _____

8. Use CTRL+Shift+O and Shift+F7 to look up the definitions of affect, effect, elute, elude, elicit and illicit.

_____

_____

9. Proofread Exercise B. Navigate the document using the keyboard and correct the errors using only the keyboard. Place the mouse several feet away from the keyboard to keep you from reaching for the mouse.

10. Describe five different ways you can take advantage of Undo and give specific examples of how you have used this command to complete your exercises.

_____

_____

11. Compare and contrast the Office Clipboard and the Windows Clipboard.

_____

_____

12. Use a phrase search to determine the accuracy of the following excerpts

a. I have discussed with them as well whether to perform a hemizona essay.

_____

_____

b. She had a clomiphene citrate challenge test that had a day-10 FSH of 14.8. At the time, we observed 5 antral follicles.

_____

_____

c. Regarding her recurrent pregnancy loss, would also recommend evaluating male carry type, antiphospholipid antibodies, and lupus anticoagulant.

_____

_____

d. Infertility workup shows normal prothrombin, anticardiolipin antibodies, and protein CNS activities.

_____

_____

CHAPTER 15

Customizing Word

OBJECTIVES

▸ Customize the Word interface to increase efficiency.

▸ Assign shortcut keys to commonly used commands.

KEYWORDS

Customize dialog box

Customize Keyboard dialog box

**customize mode
(Word 2003 only)**

Shortcut Keys

ALT+CTRL+Num+

ALT+CTRL+–

WORD 2003

Customizing Word 2003

Modifying Word to operate to your specifications is a great way to increase your productivity. Any time spent customizing Word will be rewarded many times over. Although many commands are already available on menus, toolbars, and dialog boxes, there are many more commands that can be assigned to a shortcut key and/or placed on a new or different menu or toolbar. You can change existing toolbars or menus, including many of the right-click menus, or you can create your own. The sky is the limit! Before you begin customizing, you may find it helpful to print a list of commands already available in Word (see page 183 for instructions). Customizing toolbars, menus, and shortcut keys is simple once you understand a few basic concepts. (See also page 16 which shows the Add/Remove buttons for toolbars.)

Customize Dialog Box

Most customizations are accomplished through the **Customize** dialog box (Figure 15-1). The dialog box is used two ways. First, simply having the **Customize** dialog box open puts Word in **customize mode** and changes the function of the right mouse button. This allows you to make changes to existing toolbar buttons and menu commands (see details below). For other changes, you will actually use the dialog box, which has four major components:

> Toolbars: Use to create new toolbars and to display toolbars that you want to customize.

Customize Dialog Box

Right-click on any toolbar and choose Customize.

Press ALT, T, C.

Double-click in an empty area to the right of the toolbars.

WORD 2003

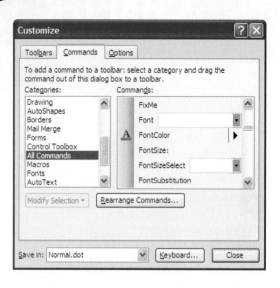

FIGURE 15-1 The Customize dialog box is used to customize menus, toolbars, and shortcut keys.

Options: Use to change the overall behavior of menus and toolbars (see page 152).

Commands: Use to place commands on menus and toolbars. This dialog lists all of Word's 400+ commands sorted into categories.

The **Commands** tab of the **Customize** dialog box is divided into two panes. The left pane lists *Categories* and the right pane lists specific *Commands*. The categories include each of the main menus on the *Menu* bar as well as other categories such as *Macros, Fonts, Styles, AutoText, Built-in menus*, and *New menus*. The category list also includes *All Commands*.

Commands may be found under more than one category, and of course, all of them are listed under *All Commands*. To locate a command, select the *Category* in the left-hand pane, then find the specific *Command* in the right-hand pane. Once you have located the specific command you need, simply drag and drop the command onto a toolbar, shortcut menu, or drop-down menu. This doesn't seem very intuitive, but it really does work! More detailed information on customizing menus and toolbars is given below.

Often the hardest part of customizing Word is locating the command you need. Carefully examine the command names listed in the *Commands* pane and note the icon. Oftentimes the icon will help you identify the command you are looking for. Some commands listed in the *Commands* pane will have the same name, but they are not actually duplicates. Commands listed with an ellipsis will open a dialog box. Those listed with a right-pointing arrow will open a submenu. Some commands listed represent text boxes or drop-down selection lists (see Figure 15-1 for examples).

Customizing Toolbars

To simply rearrange existing toolbar buttons, press the **ALT** key while dragging the button either to a new location on the same toolbar or another toolbar. To *copy* a button to another toolbar, display both toolbars and hold down **CTRL** and **ALT** while dragging the button to the other toolbar. To remove a button from a toolbar, press and hold **ALT** while dragging the button "off the screen."

To change the icon associated with a button or change the name of a button, display the **Customize dialog box** to put Word in customize mode. Ignore the dialog box and right-click *directly on the button you want to change*. This will open the Customize menu (Figure 15-2).

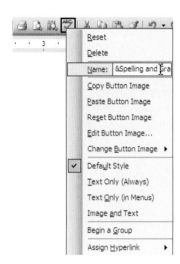

FIGURE 15-2 Use the Customize menu to change the icon, text, hot key, or other aspects of a toolbar button.

You can perform any of the following:

- Rename a button: type a new name for the button in the Name box. Place an ampersand in front of the letter that you want to designate as the hot key for that button (although you may never actually use hot keys for toolbar buttons).

- Change the button image: select Change Button Image to display a pick-list of icons. Select an icon to change the icon associated with the button. Edit button image allows you to tweak the image associated with the button.

- Change the way the button appears: choose whether to display the button image, the button name, or both. Choose Text Only or Image and Text. This Read button, for example, has both image and text `Read` .

- Sort buttons: Begin a Group inserts a faint horizontal gray line in the toolbar to visually separate icons into related groups.

- Link to another item: Assign Hyperlink allows you to associate a button with a link that will open another document, go to a web page, or start an email message.

- Reset the button: click Reset to discard your changes and restore the button to its original settings.

Remember, the key to customizing a toolbar button is to have the **Customize** dialog box open, even though you do not actually interact with the dialog. Drag the dialog box off to the side if you need to move it out of the way. Press **Esc** to close the menu or dialog box without making changes.

Add a Macro to a Toolbar

You can add macros to toolbars just like any other command. To do this, follow these steps:

1. Open the **Customize** dialog box and select the `Commands` tab.

2. Select *Macros* from the *Category* pane and choose the specific macro from the *Command* pane. The name you assigned to the macro will be listed at the end of the full macro name, so it is sometimes hard to read the entire name (see Figure 15-3).

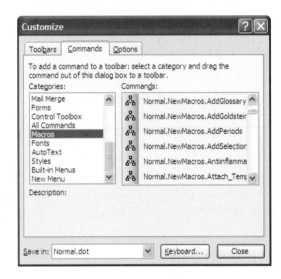

FIGURE 15-3 Macros are listed with the full macro name in the Commands pane of the Customize dialog box.

3. Drag the macro name out of the right-hand pane and drop it onto a toolbar.

4. The name will be very long, so the toolbar button will be very wide. Right-click the new button and rename the macro button or choose an icon (image).

5. Press **Enter** to accept the changes and close the *Customize* menu.

If you have accessed the **Customize** dialog box by way of the **Record Macro** dialog (ie, just before actually recording your macro), click `Close` on the **Customize** dialog box. The **Record Macro** dialog box will still be open. Click `OK` to close the **Record Macro** dialog and proceed to record your macro.

Create a Custom Toolbar

Word allows you to build your own toolbars containing icons of your choosing. To create a new toolbar, follow these steps:

1. Open the **Customize** dialog box as above and select the `Toolbars` tab.

2. Click `New`.

3. In the **New Toolbar** dialog box (Figure 15-4), type a name for your new toolbar and designate a template (*Make toolbar available to*). If you would like it available at all times, choose Normal.dot. Click `OK`.

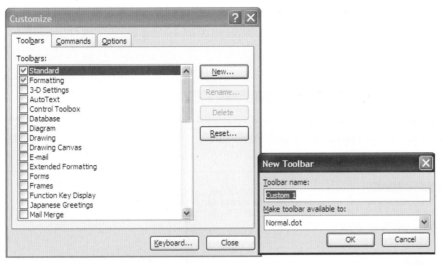

FIGURE 15-4 Use the Toolbars tab on the Customize dialog box to create your own toolbars. Click New to display a dialog for naming your new toolbar.

4. A small square will appear on your screen. This is your new, empty toolbar. Drag copies of existing buttons from any other toolbar or menu to this new toolbar (hold down **CTRL** while dragging to *copy*) or choose commands from the Commands tab of the **Customize** dialog box. Locate the command on the Commands tab and drag the command out of the *Command* pane and place it on your new toolbar. You can also drag and drop macros, styles, fonts, and AutoText entries onto this new toolbar. Select the appropriate category and then choose the specific macro, style, font, or AutoText entry.

5. Repeat these steps until you have all the buttons you want on the toolbar.

6. Some button names may be quite long, so right-click the button to display the Customize menu and type a shorter name for the button. To add space between the button names, type spaces at the beginning and end of each button name. Follow directions as above for customizing the buttons on your new toolbar. Figure 15-5 shows two customized toolbars.

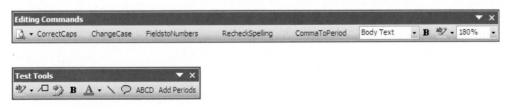

FIGURE 15-5 Two customized toolbars with styles, macros, and other tools for accomplishing specific tasks.

Arrange Toolbars

Toolbars themselves can also be rearranged. Grab any toolbar by its handle (see page 16) and drag the toolbar to a new position. Toolbars can be moved to the left and right side of a document or placed just above the Status Bar. Toolbars can also "float" in the document space and be resized as a horizontal box or a long bar. Figure 15-6 shows various ways to display toolbars.

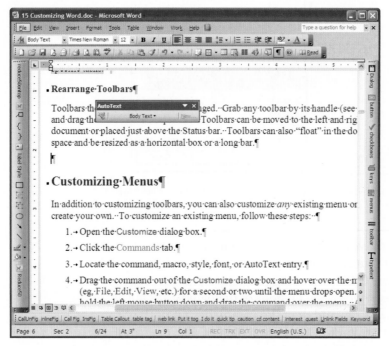

FIGURE 15-6 Toolbars can be placed on any edge of the document or float in the document space.

Customizing Menus

In addition to customizing toolbars, you can also customize *any* existing menu or you can create your own. To customize an existing menu, follow these steps:

1. Open the **Customize** dialog box.
2. Click the **Commands** tab.
3. Locate the command, macro, style, font, or AutoText entry.
4. Drag the command out of the **Customize** dialog box and hover over the menu heading (eg, File, Edit, View, etc.) for a second or two until the menu drops open. Continue to hold the left mouse button down and drag the command over the menu. A black bar will appear, indicating the location of the command once the mouse button is released.
5. To move the command, simply grab it with the mouse again and drag it to a new position on the menu.
6. Right-click the new command and edit the name if you wish. Type an ampersand in front of one of the characters in the command name to designate the hot key.

You can also customize the Menu bar itself by dropping commands directly onto the Menu bar.

Add a New Menu to the Menu Bar

To create an entirely new menu to add to your <u>Menu</u> bar, open the **Customize** dialog box and follow these steps:

1. Click the Commands tab.
2. Specify a template to store the new menu by selecting the template name from the *Save in* drop-down box. You must be working in a document based on a template to store a new menu in that particular template.
3. Under *Categories*, choose *New Menu*.
4. Drag *New Menu* from the right-hand pane and drop it on the <u>Menu</u> bar.
5. Right-click and rename the new menu. Type an ampersand in front of one of the letters to designate a hot key.
6. Drag commands, macros, AutoText, or any other item and drop them on the new menu as described above under customizing menus.

Customize a Shortcut Menu

Shortcut menus appear when you right-click text or graphics or click the Application key. They are "context sensitive," so a different menu will appear depending on the item that you click. In Word, there are three categories of shortcut menus: Text, Table, and Draw. There are over 40 different shortcut menus in all, but you will typically use only a few of these, mostly those in the Text category and possibly some under the Table category. You cannot create new shortcut menus or delete shortcut menus, and you cannot reassign them to a different category, but you can delete individual commands or add new commands to the shortcut menus provided by Word.

To make changes to these shortcut menus, locate the shortcut menu you want to change. For example, to modify the shortcut menu that appears when you click on text, choose the *Text* menu under the *Text* category (see below). To modify the shortcut menu associated with spelling and grammar functions, modify the spelling and grammar menus (also in the Text category). If you are not sure which menu to choose, look carefully at the commands available and use that information to identify the exact menu you want to modify.

To add commands to a shortcut menu, follow these steps:

1. Open the **Customize** dialog box.
2. Select Toolbars.
3. Place a check mark at *Shortcut Menus*. The small <u>Shortcut Menu</u> toolbar will appear as in Figure 15-7, displaying the three categories of shortcut menus.
4. Choose a category: *Text*, *Table*, or *Draw* as displayed in Figure 15-7. (This same figure shows part of the list of shortcut menus available under the Text category.)

(Continued)

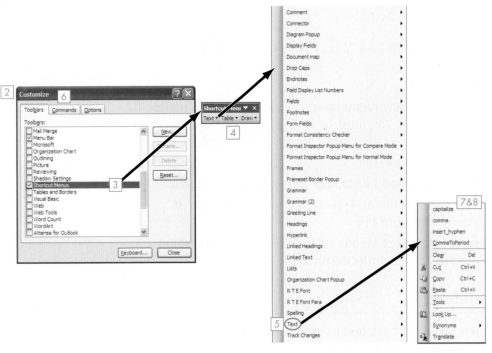

FIGURE 15-7 Place a check mark at Shortcut Menus to open the Shortcut Menu toolbar. Click Text to open the list of shortcut menus available for working with text.

5. From the list of shortcut menus, select the specific shortcut menu you want to change. (Figure 15-7 shows the Text shortcut menu found under the Text category with changes made.)

6. With the shortcut menu displayed, click the **Commands** tab in the **Customize** dialog box. You may need to use the mouse to move boxes around so you can access the commands on the **Customize** dialog box. (Sometimes the screen can get crowded!)

7. Select the specific command or macro and drag to the displayed shortcut menu. Drag the command up or down to position it on the menu.

8. Right-click the command to change the name and/or assign an icon.

9. To delete a command from the shortcut menu, right-click on the command and choose Delete.

Adding macros to shortcut menus is a great way to shortcut editing tasks. Consider modifying the following menus under the Text category: Spelling, Grammar, Grammar (2), Lists, and Text. If you use Tables, modify the following under the Tables category: Table Cell, Table Text, and Whole Tables. See also Special Project on page 444.

Customizing Shortcut Keys

The best way to customize Word and increase your efficiency is to create shortcut keys that work for *you*. You can reassign shortcut keys or you can assign shortcut keys to commands that do not already have a key assignment. You can

WORD 2003

assign a shortcut key to a command, macro, font, AutoText entry, style, or a commonly used symbol. Shortcut keys must start with either **ALT** or **CTRL** and can also include the **Shift** key or any combination of the three. The function keys (F keys) can be used alone or combined with **CTRL**, **Shift**, and **ALT**.

Follow these steps to assign a shortcut key:

1. Open the **Customize** dialog box and click Keyboard to open the **Customize Keyboard dialog box** as in Figure 15-8.

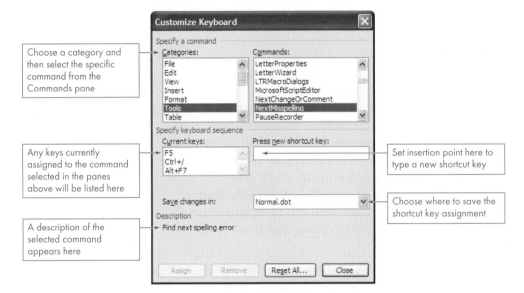

FIGURE 15-8   Use the Customize Keyboard dialog box to assign or reassign shortcut keys.

2. In the *Save changes in* box, choose the template to store the shortcut key. Selecting Normal.dot will make the change available in all templates. You can assign the same key combination to different commands if you store them in different templates.

3. Select a *Category* from the left-hand pane. If you do not know the category of the particular command, select *All commands*.

4. In the *Commands* box, click the name of the command. Read the *Description* in the lower part of the dialog to make sure you have selected the command you need.

5. In the *Press new shortcut key* box, type the new shortcut key combination exactly as you intend to use it (eg, press the modifier key—don't spell out ALT). If that key combination is already assigned to another command, Word will display a message under the *Current keys* box. You can choose to overwrite an existing shortcut key if you like your new key assignment better. If you choose not to overwrite the key, click **Backspace** to remove the first key combination and type another.

6. Once you have selected a shortcut key, click Assign. The dialog box will remain open. You can make another key assignment or click Close.

 Be sure you click Assign before closing the **Customize Keyboard** dialog box. The shortcut key assignment will not "stick" if you do not click Assign before clicking Close (and it's really easy to forget to click Assign!).

Word has already assigned many shortcut key combinations (see page 183 for instructions on printing a master list). Consider these ideas for assigning shortcut keys:

- Start with simple key combinations first such as **ALT**+any number or letter. Most of the **CTRL** key combinations are already assigned to commonly used commands, so you may not want to overwrite the **CTRL** key combinations.

- Most punctuation keys can be used, such as **ALT+,** (comma), **ALT+.** (period), and **CTRL+/** (forward slash).

- Use the number pad keys, which are not considered the same as the numbered keys across the top of the keyboard.

- If necessary, you can use multiple modifier keys to expand the number of shortcut keys. For example, you can use the combination **ALT+CTRL+Shift+M** or even append another letter to the end (**ALT+CTRL+Shift+M, A**). To use the multi-key combinations, press and hold the modifier keys while you press the first character key. Release those keys and press the second character. In the above example, hold down **ALT+CTRL+Shift** and press **M**. Release these keys and press **A**. Note: if you append an additional key to your shortcut, such as the A in **ALT+CTRL+Shift+M, A**, you cannot use the shortcut key **ALT+CTRL+Shift+M** (without another letter to follow), as this combination is now considered a prefix and must be followed by another key to distinguish from **ALT+CTRL+Shift+M, A**.

- Always test your key combinations right away to make sure they really do work and do not conflict with any other keystrokes already in use.

- Assign keys according to the way you will use them. Assign simple and easy-to-hit shortcuts to commands that you will use while "the foot is on the pedal." Assign more awkward key combinations for commands that you use when "the foot is off the pedal."

Assign a Shortcut Key to a Macro

Assigning shortcut keys to macros is similar to assigning keys to other commands. Follow these steps:

1. Open the **Customize Keyboard** dialog box (as above).

2. In the *Save changes in* box, choose the template to store the shortcut key. Selecting Normal.dot will make the change available in all templates. Be sure to store the key assignment in the same template that contains the macro itself. You can assign the same key combination to different commands if you store them in different templates.

3. In the *Categories* pane, choose *Macros*.

4. In the *Macros* pane, select the name of the macro (Figure 15-9). Assign the shortcut key as described above (starting at step 5).

If you have accessed the **Customize Keyboard** dialog box by way of the **Record Macro** dialog (ie, just before actually recording your macro), click Assign and then click Close . The **Record Macro** dialog box will still be open. Click OK to close the **Record Macro** dialog and proceed to record your macro.

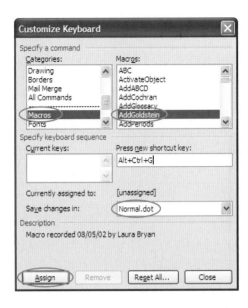

FIGURE 15-9 Select the Macros category and then the specific macro name to assign a shortcut key for running your macro.

Remove Shortcut Keys

To remove an assigned shortcut key, locate the command in the **Customize Keyboard** dialog box. The currently assigned shortcut(s) will appear in the *Current keys* box (Figure 15-10). There may be more than one key assignment. Select a key assignment from the *Current Keys* box and click **Remove**.

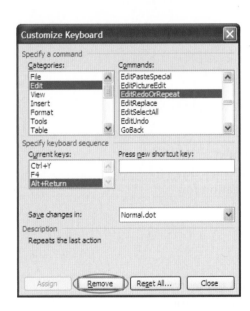

FIGURE 15-10 Use the Customize Keyboard dialog box to remove a key assignment.

Remember, pressing the **ALT** key by itself will activate the <u>Menu</u> bar. Holding down the **ALT** key while pressing another key will issue a command. If you try to use a shortcut key using the **ALT** key and nothing happens, look at your <u>Menu</u> bar to see if it has been activated. Press **Esc** and try your shortcut key again.

Assign a Shortcut Key to a Symbol

To assign a shortcut key that will insert a symbol, follow these steps:

1. Choose Insert > Symbol (**ALT, I, S**) to open the **Symbol** dialog box
    (Figure 15-11).

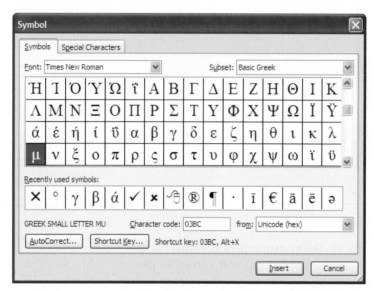

FIGURE 15-11   Open the Symbols dialog box to select a symbol to be assigned to a shortcut key.

2. Select a symbol from the grid and click **Shortcut Key**.
3. The **Customize Keyboard** dialog box will open.
4. Select a template in the *Save changes in* box (optional).
5. In the *Press new shortcut key* box, type the key combination you want to
    use and click **Assign**.

Some symbols will already have shortcut keys assigned (as indicated next to the
Shortcut Key button in the **Symbols** dialog box), but the key assignments may be
too tedious to use. There's no harm in assigning a simpler key combination for
symbols you use often.

Shortcuts for Customizing

As you may have discovered, it can be difficult to locate the command name in
order to assign the command to a shortcut key, but Word offers a clever trick for
assigning shortcut keys to commands already located on toolbars and menus.
Follow these steps to assign a shortcut key to a command already located on a
menu or toolbar:

1. Press **ALT+CTRL+Num+** (the plus sign on the number pad). This will
    convert the cursor to a double figure-of-eight ⌘.
2. Use this new cursor to select any icon or command name displayed
    on a toolbar or one of the menus on the <u>Menu</u> bar. When you make a

selection, the **Customize Keyboard** dialog box will open with the specific command already selected in the *Commands* box.

3. Type a new shortcut key and click [Assign].

4. Press **Esc** to cancel this action and return to the regular pointer/insertion point.

To quickly remove commands from a menu, press **CTRL+ALT+-** (hyphen). The cursor will change to a large minus sign (–). Use this modified cursor to click on the command you would like to remove from a menu. *Be careful! The undo option is not available here.* Press **Esc** to cancel this action and return to the regular pointer/insertion point.

Printing a List of Custom Key Assignments

To print a list of *your own key assignments*, open a document based on a specific template (if you have stored key assignments in a specific template) or simply open a document based on the Normal.dot. Press **CTRL+P** to open the Print dialog box. In the *Print What* box, choose *Key assignments*. A list of key assignments will be sent straight to the printer to be printed. (To print a list of all key assignments, see instructions on page 183.)

Commands to Assign to Shortcut Keys

See page 409 at the end of this chapter for a list of helpful commands that you might want to assign to shortcut keys.

Customizing Word 2007

Modifying Word to operate to your specifications is a great way to increase your productivity. Any time spent customizing Word will be rewarded many times over. Although many commands are already available on menus, ribbons, and dialog boxes, there are many more commands that can be assigned to a shortcut key and/or placed on the Quick Access toolbar.

If you have worked in previous versions of Word, you may be a bit disappointed with the customization limitations in 2007. The ribbon and the menus are far less amenable to customizing than the toolbars and menus in Word 2003. Word 2007 does allow you to fully customize your shortcut keys, just as in previous versions. So, your best strategy as a transcriptionist is still to work with shortcut keys.

The only truly customizable part of the Word 2007 interface is the Quick Access toolbar. There are tools available for customizing the ribbon, but it requires knowledge of XML. If you have customized a previous version of Word, you can use your previous Normal.dot file or other template files that contain customized toolbars and right-click menus, but you cannot modify shortcut menus or create new toolbars using the Word 2007 interface.

Customizing the Quick Access Toolbar

Right-click the down arrow at the right-hand end of the <u>Quick Access</u> toolbar (Figure 15-12) to make the following changes:

- Add a commonly used command. Choose from a list of common commands to add to the <u>Quick Access</u> toolbar.
- Place the <u>Quick Access</u> toolbar above or below the ribbon. Choose the appropriate option from the menu (Show Above or Below the Ribbon).
- Hide the ribbon. Choose Minimize the Ribbon to hide or display the ribbon. You can also toggle CTRL+F1.

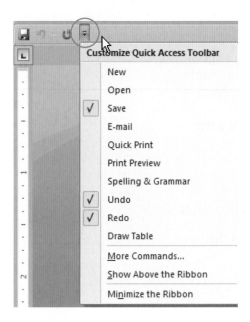

FIGURE 15-12 Click the down arrow at the end of the Quick Access toolbar to modify the toolbar.

Modify the Quick Access Toolbar

To add a new command to the <u>Quick Access</u> toolbar, locate the actual command on the ribbon or a drop-down menu and right-click the command. Choose Add to Quick Access Toolbar (Figure 15-13). To remove a command, right-click on the command to be removed and choose Remove from Quick Access toolbar.

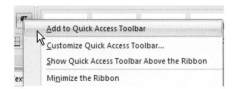
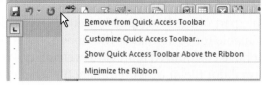

FIGURE 15-13 Right-click any command on the ribbon or drop-down menu to add to the Quick Access toolbar or right-click a command already on the Quick Access toolbar to remove it.

WORD 2007

Using the Customize Dialog Box

You can also use the **Customize dialog box** to add, remove, or rearrange commands on the <u>Quick Access</u> toolbar. Right-click on the <u>Quick Access</u> toolbar and choose Customize Quick Access Toolbar. This will open the **Customize** dialog box shown in Figure 15-14.

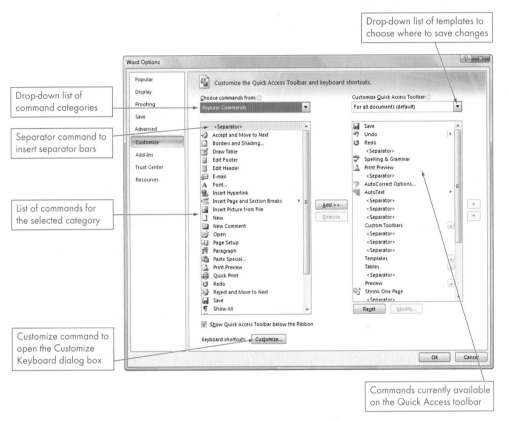

FIGURE 15-14   Use the Customize dialog box to add, remove, and rearrange commands on the Quick Access toolbar.

Here are several tips on customizing the <u>Quick Access</u> toolbar:

- The easiest way to add a command is to locate the command on the ribbon and right-click (as above), but you can also select the command from the dialog (see next bullet point).

- To locate the command, open the drop-down list at *Choose commands from* and choose a ribbon or category that contains the specific command you need. Select the specific command name from the command list. Click **Add** to place the command on the <u>Quick Access</u> toolbar.

- Use the **Up** and **Down** arrows on the right side of the dialog to move commands to a new position on the toolbar.

- Some commands will add a drop-down list, a gallery, a check box, a text box, or other types of controls. Look at the command name listed in the left pane. Commands with an ellipsis will open a dialog box, commands with a right-pointing arrow will open a menu, a down-pointing arrow will open a menu or gallery, etc.

(Continued)

- Select *Separator* (in the left-hand pane) and click **Add** to insert a faint vertical line. Use the Separator to visually separate buttons into groups on the toolbar. The groups are simply there to make the commands easier to locate.

- Add multiple separators to add space between the commands on the toolbar. The buttons themselves are small and are set close together, making it difficult at times to distinguish the buttons (see Figure 15-15). You cannot add names to the buttons or otherwise change the size or look of the buttons. To distinguish buttons, hover the mouse over a button to see a description.

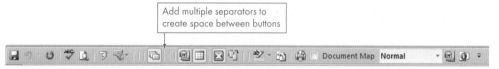

FIGURE 15-15 A customized Quick Access toolbar.

Add a Macro to the Quick Access Toolbar

You can add macros to the <u>Quick Access</u> toolbar just like any other command. Follow these steps:

1. Right-click on the <u>Quick Access</u> toolbar and choose *Customize Quick Access Toolbar*. This will open the **Customize** dialog box.

2. Select *Macros* from the *Choose commands from* list and then choose the specific macro. The name you assigned to the macro will be listed at the end of the full macro name, so read from the end of the macro name (see Figure 15-16).

3. Select the macro and click **Add**. The macro will appear in the right-hand pane.

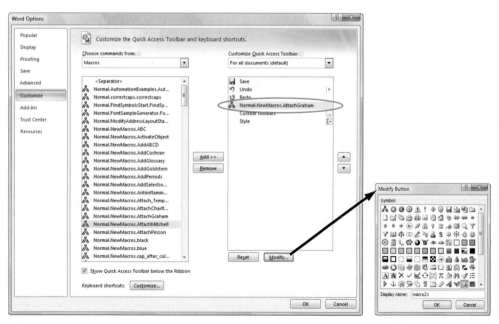

FIGURE 15-16 Use the Customize dialog box to add buttons for running macros. Click the Modify button to assign a custom icon to the macro.

4. Select $\boxed{\text{Modify}}$ and choose an icon to associate with your macro. If you do not select an icon, your macro will appear with the generic macro icon and it will be difficult to identify, especially if you have more than one macro on your <u>Quick Access</u> toolbar.

5. At the bottom of the **Modify** dialog, type a shorter name for your macro. This name will appear as a ToolTip when you hover over the macro's button on the <u>Quick Access</u> toolbar.

If you have accessed the **Customize** dialog box by way of the **Record Macro** dialog (ie, just before actually recording your macro), click $\boxed{\text{OK}}$ on the **Customize** dialog box. The **Record Macro** dialog box will still be open. Click $\boxed{\text{OK}}$ to close the **Record Macro** dialog and proceed to record your macro.

Customizing Shortcut Keys

The best way to customize Word and increase your efficiency is to create shortcut keys that work for *you*. You can reassign shortcut keys or you can assign shortcut keys to items that do not already have a key assignment. You can assign a shortcut key to a command, macro, font, AutoText entry, style, or a commonly used symbol. Shortcut keys must start with either **ALT** or **CTRL** and can also include the **Shift** key or any combination of the three. The function keys (F keys) can be used alone or combined with **CTRL**, **Shift**, and **ALT**. Follow these steps to assign a shortcut key:

1. Open the **Customize** dialog box (right-click the <u>Quick Access</u> toolbar and choose Customize Quick Access Toolbar) and click $\boxed{\text{Keyboard}}$ to open the **Customize Keyboard dialog box** as in Figure 15-17.

(Continued)

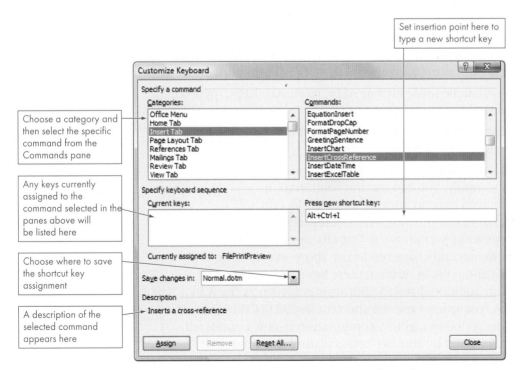

FIGURE 15-17 Use the Customize Keyboard dialog box to assign or reassign shortcut keys.

2. In the *Save changes in* box, choose the template to store the shortcut key. Selecting Normal.dot will make the change available in all templates. You can assign the same key combination to different commands if you store them in different templates.

3. Select a *Category* from the left-hand pane. If you do not know the category of the particular command, select *All commands*.

4. In the *Commands* box, click the name of the command. Read the *Description* in the lower part of the dialog to make sure you have selected the command you need.

5. In the *Press new shortcut key* box, type the new shortcut key combination exactly as you intend to use it (eg, press the modifier key—don't spell out ALT). If that key combination is already assigned to another command, Word will display a message under the *Current keys* box. You can choose to overwrite an existing shortcut key if you like your new key assignment better. If you choose not to overwrite the key, use Backspace to remove the first key combination and type another.

6. Once you have selected a shortcut key, click Assign . The dialog box will remain open. You can make another key assignment or click Close .

Be sure you click Assign before closing the **Customize Keyboard** dialog box. The shortcut key assignment will not "stick" if you do not click Assign before clicking Close (and it's really easy to forget to click Assign !).

Word has already assigned many shortcut key combinations (see page 183 for instructions on printing a master list). Consider these ideas for assigning shortcut keys:

- Start with simple key combinations first such as ALT+any number or letter. Most of the CTRL key combinations are already assigned to commonly used commands, so you may not want to overwrite the CTRL key combinations.

- Most punctuation keys can be used, such as ALT+, (comma), ALT+. (period), and CTRL+/ (forward slash).

- Use the number pad keys, which are not considered the same as the numbered keys across the top of the keyboard.

- If necessary, you can use multiple modifier keys to expand the number of shortcut keys. For example, you can use the combination ALT+CTRL+Shift+M or even append another letter to the end (ALT+CTRL+Shift+M, A). To use the multi-key combinations, press and hold the modifier keys while you press the first character key. Release those keys and press the second character. In the above example, hold down ALT+CTRL+Shift and press M. Release these keys and press A. Note: if you append an additional key to your shortcut, such as the A in ALT+CTRL+Shift+M, A, you cannot use the shortcut key ALT+CTRL+Shift+M (without another letter to follow), as this combination is now considered a prefix and must be followed by another key to distinguish from ALT+CTRL+Shift+M, A.

- Assign keys according to the way you will use them. Assign simple and easy-to-hit shortcuts to commands that you will use while "the foot is on the pedal." Assign more awkward key combinations for commands that you use when "the foot is off the pedal."

Assign a Shortcut Key to a Macro

Assigning shortcut keys to macros is similar to assigning keys to other commands. Follow these steps:

1. Open the **Customize Keyboard** dialog box (as above).

2. In the *Save changes in* box, choose the template to store the shortcut key. Selecting Normal.dotm will make the change available in all templates. Be sure to store the key assignment in the same template that contains the macro itself. You can assign the same key combination to different commands if you store them in different templates.

3. In the *Categories* pane, choose *Macros*.

4. In the *Macros* pane, locate the name of the macro (Figure 15-18). Assign the shortcut key as described above (starting at step 5 on page 404.

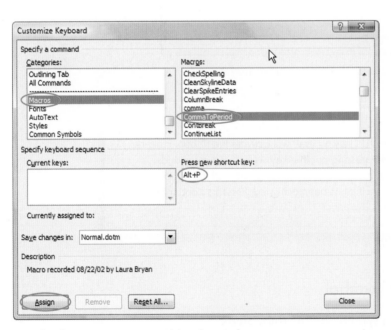

FIGURE 15-18 Select the Macros category and then the specific macro name to assign a shortcut key for running your macro.

If you have accessed the **Customize Keyboard** dialog box by way of the **Record Macro** dialog (ie, just before actually recording your macro), click **Assign** and then click **Close**. The **Record Macro** dialog box will still be open. Click **OK** to close the Record **Macro** dialog and proceed to record your macro.

Remove Shortcut Keys

To remove an assigned shortcut key, locate the command in the **Customize Keyboard** dialog box. The currently assigned shortcut(s) will appear in the *Current keys* box (Figure 15-19). There may be more than one key assignment. Select a key assignment from the *Current Keys* box and click Remove.

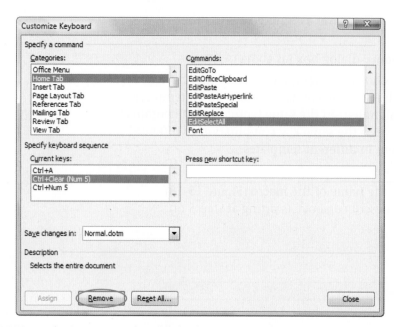

FIGURE 15-19 Use the Customize Keyboard dialog box to remove a key assignment.

Remember, pressing the **ALT** key by itself will activate the ribbon. Holding down the **ALT** key while pressing another key will issue a command. If you try to use a shortcut key using the **ALT** key and nothing happens, look at your ribbon to see if it has been activated. Press **Esc** and try your shortcut key again.

Assign a Shortcut Key to a Symbol

To assign a shortcut key to insert a symbol, follow these steps:

1. Choose Insert > Symbol > More Symbols or **ALT, I, S** to open the **Symbol** dialog box (Figure 15-20).
2. Select a symbol from the grid and click Shortcut Key.
3. The **Customize Keyboard** dialog box will open.
4. Select a template in the *Save changes in* box (optional).
5. In the *Press new shortcut key* box, type the key combination you want to use and click Assign.

WORD 2007

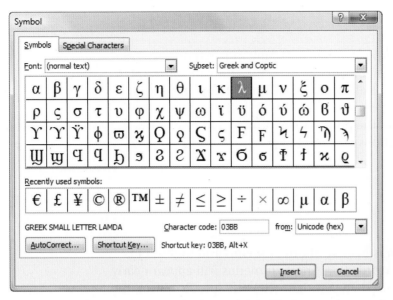

FIGURE 15-20 Select a symbol in the Symbols dialog box and click Shortcut Key to assign a shortcut to the symbol.

Some symbols will already have shortcut keys assigned (as indicated next to the [**Shortcut Key**] button), but the key assignments may be too tedious to use. There is no harm in assigning a simpler key combination for symbols you use often.

Shortcuts for Customizing

As you may have discovered, it can be difficult to locate the command name in order to assign the command to a shortcut key, but Word offers a clever trick for assigning shortcut keys to commands already located on ribbons and menus.

1. Press **ALT+CTRL+Num+** (the plus sign on the number pad). This will convert the cursor to a double figure-of-eight ⌘.

2. Use this new cursor to select any icon or command name displayed on the ribbon. When you make a selection, the **Customize Keyboard** dialog box will open with the specific command already selected in the *Commands* box.

3. Type a new shortcut key and click [**Assign**].

4. Press **Esc** to cancel this action and return to the regular pointer/insertion point.

Printing a List of Custom Key Assignments

To print a list of *your own key assignments*, open a document based on a specific template (if you have stored key assignments in a specific template) or simply open a document based on the Normal.dotm. Press **CTRL+P** to open the **Print** dialog box. In the *Print What* box, choose *Key assignments*. A list of custom key assignments will be sent straight to the printer to be printed. (To print a list of all key assignments, see instructions on page 183.)

Importing Changes from 2003

Fortunately, if you have created personalized shortcut menus and toolbars in Word 2003, you can use them in Word 2007. Shortcut menus will appear nearly the same as they do in Word 2003. When you right-click the specific object, the same shortcut menu will appear, although Word 2007 may add a few more commands.

Any customized toolbars brought over from Word 2003 will also be available but not in the same way you used them in Word 2003. You cannot make them float in the middle of the display and you cannot rearrange the icons or move the toolbar to any other position. Custom toolbars can be found under the **Add-Ins** tab (see Figure 15-21). Click the arrows at the right and/or left end of the ribbon to see more toolbars. You can also add a button to the Quick Access toolbar to display the custom toolbars. In the **Customize** dialog box, under *All Commands*, choose *Custom Toolbars*.

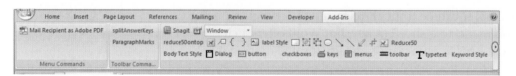

FIGURE 15-21 Customized toolbars created in Word 2003 will be displayed under the Add-Ins tab in Word 2007 as a collection of buttons, not as toolbars.

Word 2003 stores custom toolbars in template files, so to use the toolbars in Word 2007, move the template files to the new computer. If you have migrated to Word 2007 (Word 2003 was previously installed on this PC), the template files will already be on your computer. Open documents based on these templates to use the custom toolbars. You can also make the toolbars and menus available by adding the templates as global templates (see page 468).

Helpful Commands to Assign to Shortcut Keys and Toolbars

There are many commands already available in Word, but some are difficult to find. Although they are listed alphabetically under *All commands* in the **Customize Keyboard** dialog box, many are not listed the way you might expect. Below is a list of useful commands the way they appear in the *Commands* list of the **Customize** dialog box:

EditAutoText	Opens the **AutoText** dialog box (works in both versions, but displays **AutoText** dialog as it appears in Word 2003)
EditClear	Same as Delete
SentLeft	Moves the cursor to the beginning of the sentence
SentRight	Moves the cursor to the end of the sentence
TableDeleteRow	Deletes row containing insertion point
TableDeleteColumn	Deletes column containing insertion point
ToolsWordCount	Displays word, character, and line counts for current document
ToolsAutoCorrect	Displays the **AutoCorrect** dialog box
ToolsOptions	(Word 2003) Opens the **Options** dialog box
ToolsCustomize	(Word 2003) Opens the **Customize** dialog box
ToolsCustomizeKeyboard	Opens the **Customize Keyboard** dialog box
GoToHeaderFooter	
CloseViewHeaderFooter	
ToggleHeaderFooterLink	Removes "Same as previous" command from a Header
ShowPrevHeaderFooter	
ShowNextHeaderFooter	
ViewHeader	
ViewFooter	
FileCloseAll	Closes current file or all files currently open
FilePageSetup	Opens the **Page Setup** dialog box
GoToNextPage	
GoToPreviousPage	

RestartNumbering

InsertNewComment

InsertSectionBreak   Opens the **Break** dialog box for inserting
                                    page and section breaks

FormatNumberDefault   Apply automatic numbering using the default
                                    format

ToolsSpellingRecheckDocument

ParaKeepWithNext   Keeps paragraphs together when they
                                    approach a page break

Sometimes you can work backwards to discover a command name. If you
know the shortcut key but do not know the official command name, type
the shortcut key into the *Press new shortcut key* box (in the **Customize
Keyboard** dialog box) and look below to see the command name
associated with that shortcut key (under *Currently assigned to*).

Critical Thinking Questions

1. Explain how customizing Word can increase productivity.

   _____

   _____

2. Why do you think there are commands in Word that are not already assigned to a toolbar, menu, or ribbon?

   _____

   _____

3. Record three separate macros to delete a sentence, part of a sentence, and part of a paragraph and assign these to shortcut keys.

   _____

   _____

4. List the different features in Word that can be customized.

   _____

   _____

5. List three ways to open the Customize dialog box.

   _____

   _____

6. Where can you find a list of over 400 commands that can be added to menus and toolbars?

   _____

   _____

7. How would you decide whether to create a toolbar button or assign a shortcut key to a command?

   _____

   _____

8. Describe how to use the shortcut key ALT+CTRL+Shift+A, M

   _____

   _____

9. How do you access the Customize Keyboard dialog box?

   _____

   _____

10. Assign a shortcut key to the following commands:

   a.   SentLeft

   b.   SentRight

   c.   TableDeleteRow

   d.   TableDeleteColumn

   e.   ToolsAutoCorrect (to open the AutoCorrect dialog box)

The questions below pertain to Word 2003 (only):

11. Explain how Word changes behavior when the Customize dialog box
    is open.

    _____

    _____

12. Describe a simple method of moving an icon to a new location on a
    toolbar.

    _____

    _____

13. Describe a simple method of copying an existing icon from one toolbar
    to another toolbar.

    _____

    _____

14. Add a new command or macro to the Text/Text shortcut menu.

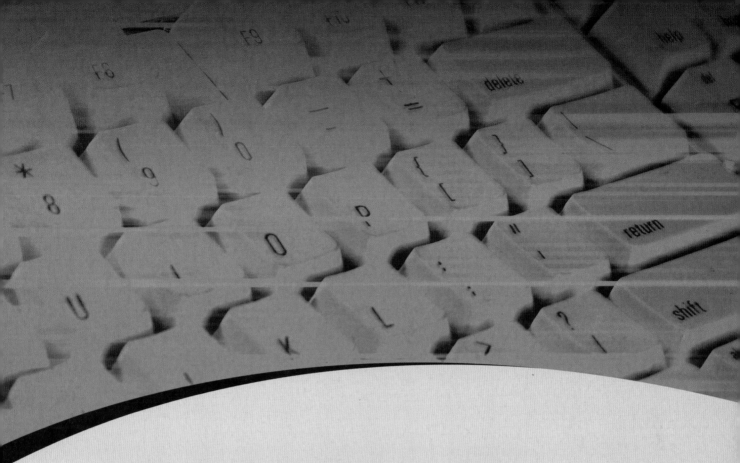

SECTION III

Applying What You
Have Learned

SECTION II

CHAPTER 16

Putting It Together

OBJECTIVES

▸ Formulate a personal action plan for implementing the techniques described in this text.

▸ Troubleshoot common problems encountered while using MS Word.

▸ Apply the features described throughout this text to your daily work.

▸ Format report layouts, including headers and footers, using formatting commands and tables.

A Plan of Action

This chapter outlines an approach to implementing the techniques described throughout this text and provides a variety of sample layouts that you can use as models for creating your own templates.

Create a Plan

The list below gives you a stepwise plan for implementing the techniques described throughout this text. Not all the steps described below will apply to every user. Some transcriptionists will be working within a documentation/transcription platform that incorporates other software along with MS Word, so some of the file management suggestions may not apply. Transcriptionists working independently or as business owners would most likely follow the majority of the steps.

1. Study the images and labels in Chapter 1 and Chapter 4 so you are familiar with the terminology used to describe Windows' elements and the objects in the Word interface. This will make it infinitely easier to interact with technical support, troubleshoot computer problems, and to understand both written and verbal instructions.

2. Organize the files and folders you already have on your computer. Create a folder system for storing projects, research notes, references, and bookmarks. If you do not work on a transcription platform with file management built in, create folders for sorting your transcription work, research notes, and reference files.

(Continued)

3. If you maintain a transcription folder for storing your work on a daily basis, consider changing the default working folder from **My Documents** (Windows XP)/**Documents** (Windows Vista) to your designated transcription folder (page 33 in Windows XP and page 49 in Windows Vista.).

4. Locate the program data files on your computer (see page 71) and implement a method for routinely backing up these files.

5. Create shortcuts to your most-used programs, files, and folders. Place shortcuts in strategic areas, such as the Start menu, Quick Launch bar, or **(My) Documents** so you always have one- or two-click access to items you use daily. Create shortcuts that use unique hot keys so you can reduce mouse clicks.

6. Change the way toolbars and menus behave (Word 2003, page 152) and move the Quick Access toolbar (Word 2007) below the ribbon if you prefer (page 165).

7. Review the **Options** dialog boxes (Chapter 5) and make the necessary changes. Take special note of the options marked with shading. Pay special attention to the options in the **Spelling and Grammar** dialog box and the **AutoFormat As You Type** dialog box.

8. Make a list of shortcut keys that you would like to implement starting with commands that you use the most. Select two or three shortcuts and write them on a sticky note to place on your monitor. Every few days, replace these hints with several more. Make a point of implementing a few shortcut keys at a time—if you attempt to do them all at once you will be frustrated.

9. Set up report layouts for the major report types that you transcribe. Be sure to include headings, subheadings, date lines, address lines, signature lines, and standard text. Apply as much formatting to the layout as possible to reduce formatting tasks while you are transcribing. Add empty fields for quickly navigating standard text.

10. Create template files (dot files) using the report layouts created in Step 9. Be sure to set default fonts and default page margins.

11. Create AutoText entries for phrases, paragraphs, and other elements that are needed regularly but not in every report (ie, text that is not part of the template's standard text). Save entries in their corresponding template (dot) file.

12. Create AutoCorrect entries for shortcuts that you use in all reports such as abbreviations and acronyms as well as entries with formatting (eg, superscript, subscript, bold, mixed case).

13. Create macros to streamline routine tasks and to quickly edit standard text as you transcribe. Create macros to change options that you routinely adjust based on specific work. Create macros to enhance proofreading and to create log sheets if necessary.

14. Customize the Word interface (especially Word 2003) to reduce clutter and make the items you routinely use easily accessible. Remap shortcut keys so they are easier to reach or easier to remember.

Top Ten Suggestions for Working with Word

Follow these tips to improve your proficiency and to help avoid some of the most common pitfalls in MS Word.

1. Make a commitment to spend five minutes each day learning something new about Word or Windows.

2. Turn off automatic features as explained in Chapter 5, especially in the **AutoFormat As You Type** dialog box. Enable features one at a time as you become accustomed to managing them.

3. Work with formatting marks displayed, even if they are initially distracting.

4. If you switch between different fonts on separate reports, be sure to set the default font.

5. Learn about the Normal.dot and its importance to operating Word.

6. Use actual formatting commands (indent, hanging indent, etc) to format your documents, and especially avoid using **Tab** to create indents and hanging indents.

7. Use AutoText, AutoCorrect, or a third-party text expander to memorize text shortcuts (not the Macro recorder). Use macros to record a series of *commands* for formatting, editing, and other tasks.

8. Use shortcut keys as much as possible—it is much faster than picking up the mouse. The first shortcut key to learn is **CTRL+Z** (the Undo command).

9. Use Print Layout so you can see the entire document, including headers, footers, white space, and "edges" of the page.

10. Keep a positive attitude. Word is a world-class word processor and absolutely can do *anything* you want it to do. Believe it or not, Word is very flexible—so be patient and know that if you don't like the way it behaves, there is a way to change it.

Top Three Ways to Avoid Problems

These three guidelines will help you avoid overall problems with your computer.

1. Use your computer for transcription *only* and *never* allow other members of your household to use your computer. Load only the programs you need to transcribe documents, communicate with coworkers and clients, and maintain your business. Maintain a separate computer for hobbies, music, and personal business.

2. Use the Internet and email carefully. Remember, "free" Internet downloads are never really free. Even the most innocent freebies (coupon offers, smiley faces, toolbars) are really just Trojan horses (gift on the outside, trouble on the inside) and will wreak havoc on your computer's performance. Never click on links from inside email messages to make account or password changes; log onto the website directly instead.

3. Keep data files backed up! Problems *will* strike—it's not a matter of *if*, but *when*.

Sample Formats

The following pages give examples of formatting approaches for a variety of documents and layouts. Use these as examples for formatting your documents. Pay close attention to the formatting marks in these images.

Incorrect Formatting for Hanging Indents

This report shows incorrect formatting techniques using the tab key. This report would be incredibly tedious to transcribe and even more frustrating to edit. A single edit would force every line to be adjusted. This approach requires 60 or more additional keystrokes compared to using formatting commands.

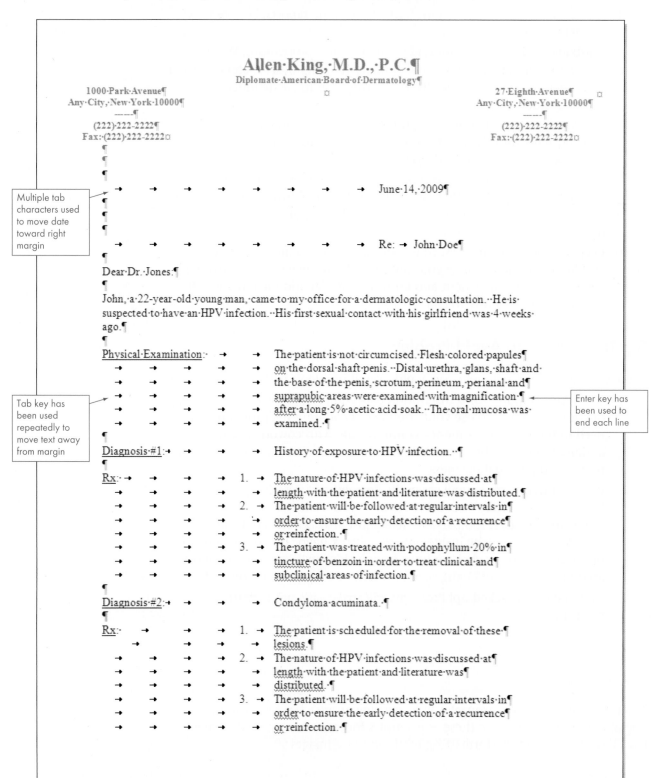

Multiple tab characters used to move date toward right margin

Tab key has been used repeatedly to move text away from margin

Enter key has been used to end each line

Correct Formatting for Hanging Indents

This is the same as the report on the facing page, but this version has actual formatting commands applied. This report is easily edited, since the formatting commands ensure correct formatting as text is added or removed.

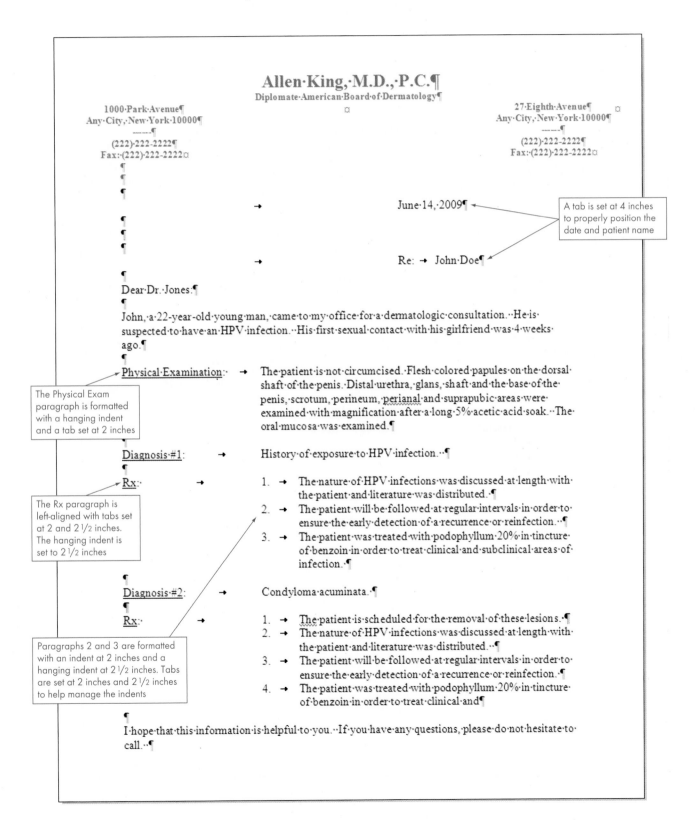

Allen·King,·M.D.,·P.C.¶
Diplomate·American·Board·of·Dermatology¶

1000·Park·Avenue¶
Any·City,·New·York·10000¶
-----¶
(222)-222-2222¶
Fax:·(222)-222-2222▯

27·Eighth·Avenue¶
Any·City,·New·York·10000¶
-----¶
(222)-222-2222¶
Fax:·(222)-222-2222▯

→ June·14,·2009¶

A tab is set at 4 inches to properly position the date and patient name

→ Re:·→ John·Doe¶

Dear·Dr.·Jones:¶

John,·a·22-year-old·young·man,·came·to·my·office·for·a·dermatologic·consultation.··He·is·suspected·to·have·an·HPV·infection.··His·first·sexual·contact·with·his·girlfriend·was·4·weeks·ago.¶

Physical·Examination:· → The·patient·is·not·circumcised.·Flesh·colored·papules·on·the·dorsal·shaft·of·the·penis.·Distal·urethra,·glans,·shaft·and·the·base·of·the·penis,·scrotum,·perineum,·perianal·and·suprapubic·areas·were·examined·with·magnification·after·a·long·5%·acetic·acid·soak.··The·oral·mucosa·was·examined.¶

The Physical Exam paragraph is formatted with a hanging indent and a tab set at 2 inches

Diagnosis·#1:· → History·of·exposure·to·HPV·infection.··¶

Rx:· → 1.· → The·nature·of·HPV·infections·was·discussed·at·length·with·the·patient·and·literature·was·distributed.·¶
2.· → The·patient·will·be·followed·at·regular·intervals·in·order·to·ensure·the·early·detection·of·a·recurrence·or·reinfection.··¶
3.· → The·patient·was·treated·with·podophyllum·20%·in·tincture·of·benzoin·in·order·to·treat·clinical·and·subclinical·areas·of·infection.·¶

The Rx paragraph is left-aligned with tabs set at 2 and 2 1/2 inches. The hanging indent is set to 2 1/2 inches

Diagnosis·#2:· → Condyloma·acuminata.·¶

Rx:· → 1.· → The·patient·is·scheduled·for·the·removal·of·these·lesions.·¶
2.· → The·nature·of·HPV·infections·was·discussed·at·length·with·the·patient·and·literature·was·distributed.··¶
3.· → The·patient·will·be·followed·at·regular·intervals·in·order·to·ensure·the·early·detection·of·a·recurrence·or·reinfection.·¶
4.· → The·patient·was·treated·with·podophyllum·20%·in·tincture·of·benzoin·in·order·to·treat·clinical·and·¶

Paragraphs 2 and 3 are formatted with an indent at 2 inches and a hanging indent at 2 1/2 inches. Tabs are set at 2 inches and 2 1/2 inches to help manage the indents

I·hope·that·this·information·is·helpful·to·you.··If·you·have·any·questions,·please·do·not·hesitate·to·call.··¶

SOAP Note Template

This is an example of a SOAP note template with multiple boilerplates set one after another. Instructions for formatting this report type are found on page 219.

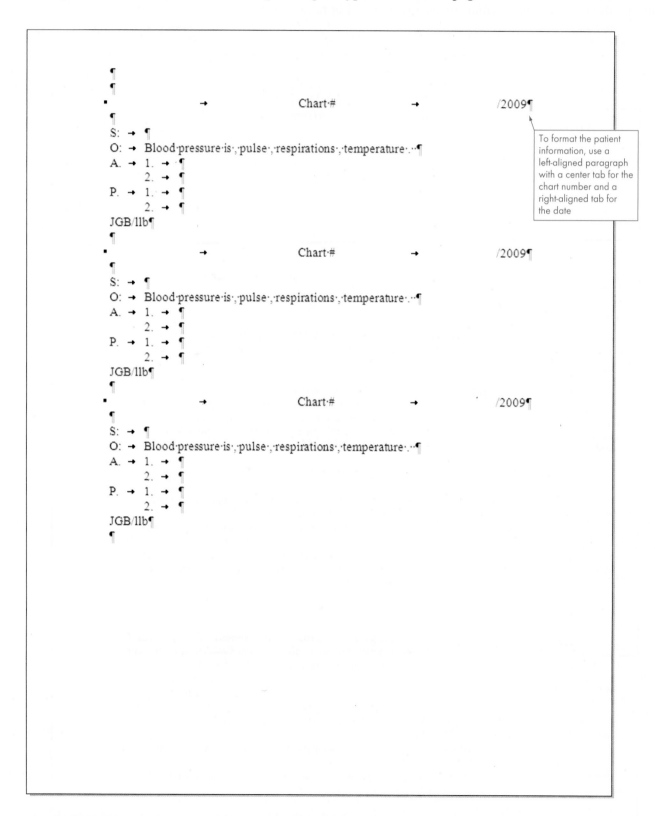

SOAP Note

This example shows two reports transcribed using the template on the facing page.

John Doe → Chart #12345 → 6/7/2009

S: → The patient is seen in followup. She underwent cardiac catheterization which was totally normal. Echocardiography was also totally normal. Lab from Dr. Smith was reviewed that demonstrated an HDL cholesterol of 56, LDL 172. Triglycerides were 70. The patient has had no further chest pain. She remains fatigued. Medications and lab were reviewed.

O: → Blood pressure is 100/64, pulse 64, respirations 16, temperature 98.2 °F. The patient is alert, oriented, and in no apparent distress. Skin is warm and dry. PERRLA. There is no xanthelasma noted. No thyromegaly or jugular venous distention seen. Carotids are equal bilaterally. Heart rate and rhythm are regular without murmur, S3, or S4. Lungs are clear to auscultation with normal respiratory effort. Abdomen is soft without organomegaly or bruit. No guarding or rebound. Extremities are warm without edema.

A. → 1. → No evidence of myocardial disease.
    2. → Hypothyroidism.
    3. → Hyperlipidemia.
    4. → Exogenous stressors.

P. → 1. → The patient was counseled to lose weight.
    2. → Dietary counseling was given.

JGB/llb

Jane Doe → Chart #8765 → 6/10/2009

S: → The patient is seen in followup. Her cardiac monitor demonstrated only isolated singlet PVCs. She was not symptomatic with most of them. Echocardiography showed mild mitral valve prolapse, otherwise it was normal. The patient did not have her lab drawn.

O: → Blood pressure is 100/66, pulse 88, respirations 16, weight 178 lb. The patient is alert, oriented, and in no apparent distress. Skin is warm and dry. PERRLA. There is no xanthelasma noted. No thyromegaly or jugular venous distention seen. Carotids are equal bilaterally. Heart rate and rhythm are regular without murmur, S3, or S4. Lungs are clear to auscultation with normal respiratory effort. Abdomen is soft without organomegaly or bruit. No guarding or rebound.

A. → 1. → Palpitations, singlet PVCs, benign.
    2. → Pregnancy.
    3. → Mild mitral valve prolapse.

P. → 1. → The patient was reassured as to the benign nature of her palpitations.
    2. → The patient is to follow up with Dr. Chambers.

JGB/llb

Alternative Template for SOAP Note using a Table

The next two figures show an alternative method of formatting a SOAP note using tables. The first figure is the template and the second figure shows the final report as it will print. The table borders are hidden, so it does not appear as a table when the document is printed.

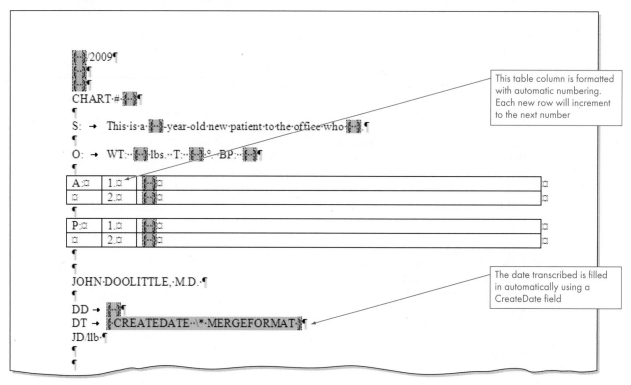

Office Consultation Template (Version 1)

This office consultation template uses empty fields throughout the standard text to quickly navigate the template.

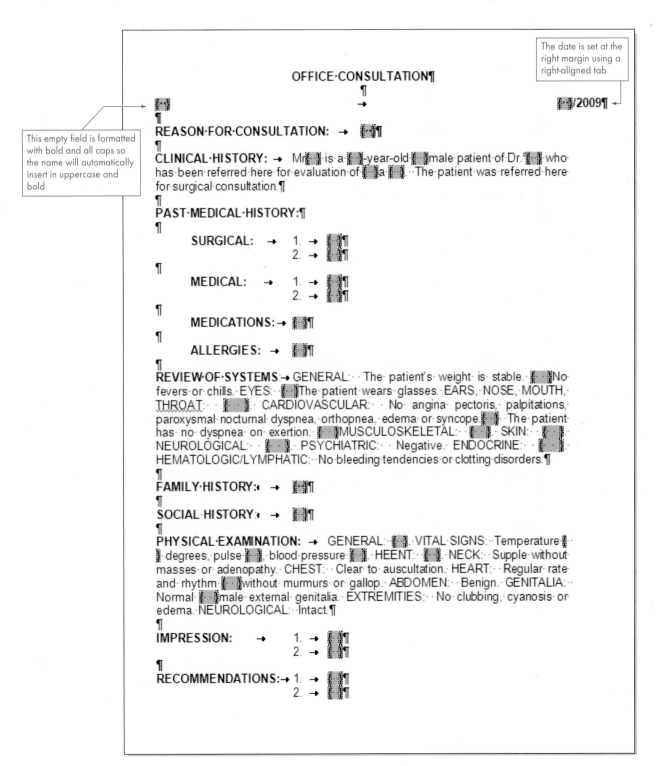

The date is set at the right margin using a right-aligned tab

This empty field is formatted with bold and all caps so the name will automatically insert in uppercase and bold

Office Consultation Template (Version 2)

This office consultation note is similar to the Office Consultation version 1, but the Past Medical History is formatted using tables instead of deep indents.

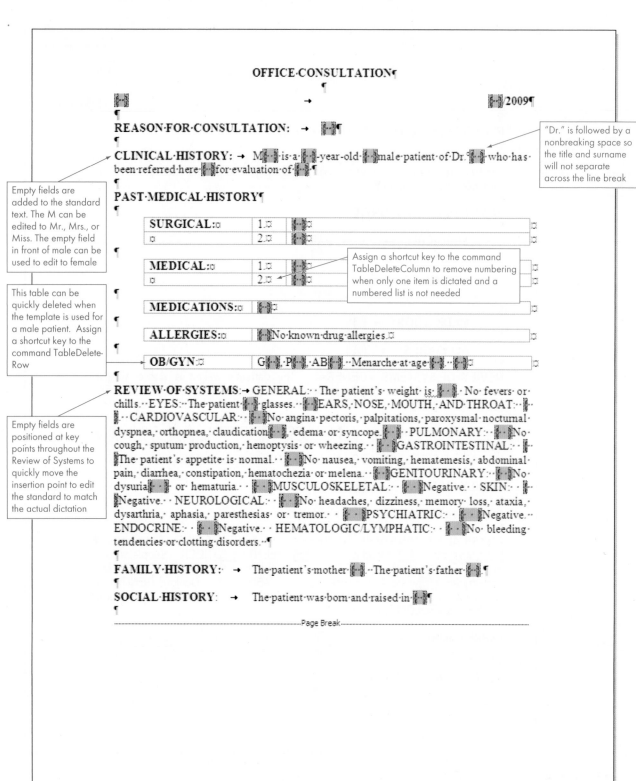

Office Consultation Report using Tables

This figure shows an office consultation as it will print. The template on the facing page was used to create this report.

OFFICE CONSULTATION

JOHN DOE   1/10/2009

REASON FOR CONSULTATION: Left inguinal hernia.

CLINICAL HISTORY: Mr. John Doe is a quite active 75-year-old white male patient of Dr. Herbert who has been referred here for evaluation of a left inguinal hernia. Mr. Doe believes that the hernia has been present for at least 2-3 months. It is increasing in size and is becoming more tender. The hernia reduces when the patient assumes a recumbent position. The patient has no history of prior hernias. His bowel movements have been normal. He has had no obstructive symptoms. The patient has problems with his prostate. He has recently had a PSA test which was elevated at 6.5. Digital prostate exam by Dr. Fine revealed no abnormalities. The patient will be undergoing followup of his PSA. The patient is a long-term smoker and has a chronic cough.

PAST MEDICAL HISTORY:

SURGICAL:	1.	Vasectomy in 1956.
	2.	The patient had cystoscopic extraction of kidney stones in 1985.
MEDICAL:	1.	Asthma/COPD.
	2.	No history of myocardial infarction, congestive heart failure, hypertension, cerebrovascular accident, diabetes mellitus, asthma, deep vein thrombosis, pulmonary embolism or cancer.
MEDICATIONS:	None.	
ALLERGIES:	No known drug allergies.	

REVIEW OF SYSTEMS: GENERAL: The patient's weight is stable. No fevers or chills. EYES: The patient wears glasses. EARS, NOSE, MOUTH, THROAT: The patient has problems with sinusitis. He wears dentures. He has had his tonsils removed. CARDIOVASCULAR: No angina pectoris, palpitations, paroxysmal nocturnal dyspnea, orthopnea, claudication, edema or syncope. PULMONARY: The patient denies coughing on the patient questionnaire, but on questioning states he does have a chronic cough. No hemoptysis. The patient has wheezing.

FAMILY HISTORY: The patient's mother died of heart failure at age 85. The patient's father died of cancer at age 65.

SOCIAL HISTORY: The patient was born and raised in Arkansas.

Operative Report Template

This operative report uses a table to manage the deep indents.

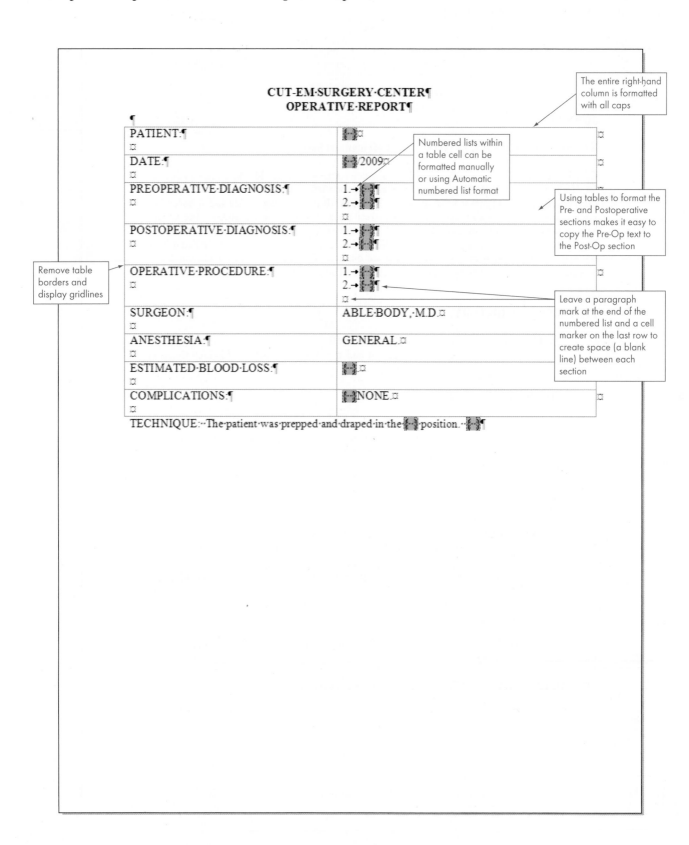

Operative Report

This sample shows a completed operative report using the template on the facing page.

CUT-EM SURGERY CENTER
OPERATIVE REPORT

PATIENT: DOE, JANE

DATE: 5/20/2009

PREOPERATIVE DIAGNOSIS:
1. MULTIPLE INTRAEPITHELIAL VULVAR LESIONS INVOLVING THE VULVAR FOURCHETTE, CONFLUENCE OF RIGHT LABIA MAJORA AND MINORA, CONFLUENCE OF THE LEFT LABIA MAJORA AND MINORA.
2. HYMEN RING SKIN TAG AT APPROXIMATELY 12 O'CLOCK.

POSTOPERATIVE DIAGNOSIS:
1. MULTIPLE INTRAEPITHELIAL VULVAR LESIONS INVOLVING THE VULVAR FOURCHETTE, CONFLUENCE OF RIGHT LABIA MAJORA AND MINORA, CONFLUENCE OF THE LEFT LABIA MAJORA AND MINORA.
2. HYMEN RING SKIN TAG AT APPROXIMATELY 12 O'CLOCK.

OPERATIVE PROCEDURE:
1. BIOPSY AND CAVITRON ULTRASONIC ASPIRATION (CUSA) REMOVAL OF VULVAR INTRA-EPITHELIAL LESIONS.
2. RESECTION OF HYMEN SKIN TAG LESION WITH PRIMARY CLOSURE.

SURGEON: ABLE BODY MD

ANESTHESIA: GENERAL.

ESTIMATED BLOOD LOSS: LESS THAN 50 ML.

COMPLICATIONS: NONE.

TECHNIQUE: The patient was prepped and draped in the lithotomy position. Acetic acid was placed on the vulva after it was prepped and a thorough colposcopic examination was done. The abnormal lesions were noted in the vulvar fourchette and extending in a horseshoe-like configuration along the confluence of the left labia majora and minora to the confluence of the right labia majora and minora. Representative biopsy was taken and submitted for permanent histologic evaluation. The remainder of that abnormal area was vacuumed off with the Cavitron ultrasound aspirator machine set at 70% aspirate, 70%

Physical Therapy Template

A well-planned template can make a physical therapy report much easier to transcribe.

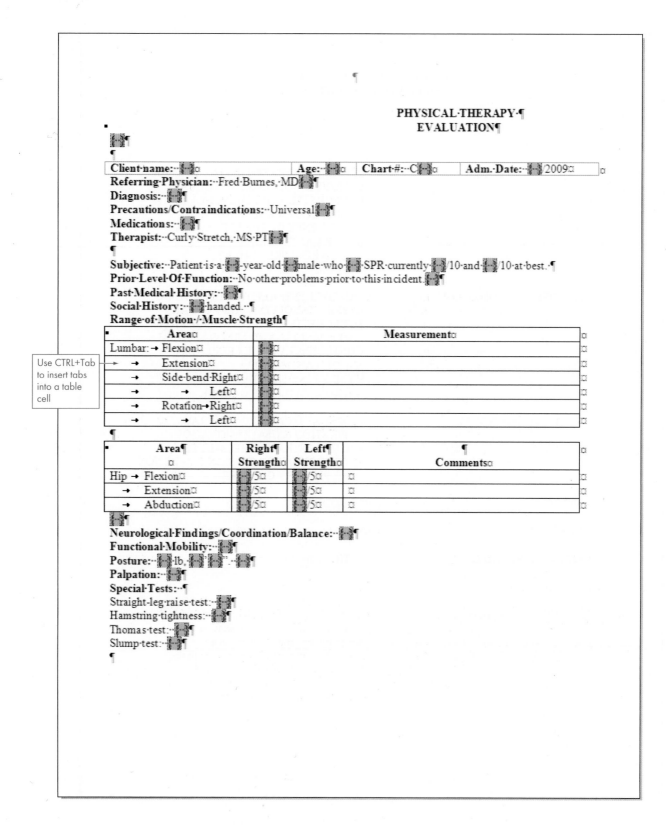

PHYSICAL·THERAPY·¶
EVALUATION¶

Client·name:··{·}¤	Age:··{·}¤	Chart·#:··C{·}¤	Adm.·Date:··{·}·2009¤	¤

Referring·Physician:··Fred·Burnes,·MD{·}¶
Diagnosis:··{·}¶
Precautions/Contraindications:··Universal{·}¶
Medications:··{·}¶
Therapist:··Curly·Stretch,·MS·PT{·}¶

Subjective:··Patient·is·a·{·}-year-old·{·}male·who·{·}·SPR·currently·{·}/10·and·{·}/10·at·best.··¶
Prior·Level·Of·Function:··No·other·problems·prior·to·this·incident.{·}¶
Past·Medical·History:··{·}¶
Social·History:··{·}-handed.··¶
Range·of·Motion·/·Muscle·Strength¶

Area¤	Measurement¤	¤
Lumbar:·→·Flexion¤	{·}¤	¤
→ Extension¤	{·}¤	¤
→ Side·bend·Right¤	{·}¤	¤
→ → Left¤	{·}¤	¤
→ Rotation→Right¤	{·}¤	¤
→ → Left¤	{·}¤	¤

> Use CTRL+Tab to insert tabs into a table cell

Area¶ ¤	Right¶ Strength¤	Left¶ Strength¤	¶ Comments¤	¤
Hip·→·Flexion¤	{·}/5¤	{·}/5¤	¤	¤
→ Extension¤	{·}/5¤	{·}/5¤	¤	¤
→ Abduction¤	{·}/5¤	{·}/5¤	¤	¤

Neurological·Findings/Coordination/Balance:··{·}¶
Functional·Mobility:··{·}¶
Posture:··{·}·lb,·{·}{·}··{·}¶
Palpation:··{·}¶
Special·Tests:··¶
Straight-leg·raise·test:··{·}¶
Hamstring·tightness:··{·}¶
Thomas·test:··{·}¶
Slump·test:··{·}¶
¶

Physical Therapy Report

This figure shows a transcribed physical therapy report using the template shown on the facing page.

PHYSICAL THERAPY
EVALUATION

Client name: Pete Rose   **Age:** 39   **Chart #:** C12815   **Adm. Date:** 03/09/2009
Referring Physician: Fred Burnes, MD
Diagnosis: Lumbar sprain
Precautions/Contraindications: Universal
Medications: Celebrex
Therapist: Curly Stretch, MS PT

Subjective: Patient is a 39-year-old male who was the restrained driver in a motor vehicle accident on March 2, 2007. Patient was rear ended. Patient noted low back pain at that time. Patient continues with low back pain which is inconsistent. Pain is increased with prolonged sitting and with sit-to-stand transfers. Patient is scheduled for an MRI on April 3, 2009. SPR currently 5/10 and 0/10 at best.
Prior Level Of Function: No other problems prior to this incident.
Past Medical History: Significant only for right rotator cuff surgery in 1988.
Social History: Left handed. Coffee salesman. Married with 2 children ages 12 and 7.
Range of Motion / Muscle Strength:

Area		Measurement
Lumbar:	Flexion	Forward flexion about 2 inches from ankle joint with low back pain
	Extension	About 20° with low back pain, worse than with flexion.
	Side bend Right	Knee joint line with low back pain.
	Left	To inferior patella.
	Rotation Right	WNL
	Left	WNL

Area		Right Strength	Left Strength	Comments
Hip	Flexion	4/5	4/5	
	Extension	4-/5	4-/5	Left and right with pain
	Abduction	5/5	4+/5	Left with left-sided low back pain

Knee: Flexion, extension and dorsiflexion are all 5/5 bilaterally.

Neurological Findings/Coordination/Balance: Patient reports bilateral lower extremity pins and needles upon waking in the morning on occasion which is resolved after a couple of minutes. Patellar deep tendon reflexes are 0 bilaterally.
Functional Mobility: Difficulty with sitting, sit-to-stand transfers and driving.
Posture: 240 lbs, 5'11", rounded shoulders, muscular build, equal-height iliac crests.
Palpation: Tenderness and tightness noted in lumbar paraspinals.
Special Tests:
Straight-leg raise test: Negative.
Hamstring tightness: Positive.
Thomas test: Positive.
Slump test: Negative.

Stress Echocardiogram Template

This figure shows decorative page elements formatted with drawing objects (rectangles) and text boxes. See the video on the accompanying CD to learn more about using text boxes in MS Word.

MORDECAI N. SMITH, MD, FACC

1600 Smith Road | Suite 304 | Smith, Texas 75075
PHONE: 972.222.2222 | FAX: 972.222.2222

STRESS ECHOCARDIOGRAPHIC REPORT

Name:				DOB:		Patient ID:				
Exam Date:		Last Exam		Age	Yrs	St Type		ECHO	Exam Quality	
Gender		Location	Klein	Wt	lb	Ht	in		BSA	m²
Referring Physician				MO Disk #		Sonographer				
Cardiologist		Mordecai N Smith, MD		Indications/Reason for Echo						

BASELINE ECHOCARDIOGRAM
2D MEASUREMENTS

Chamber Dimensions		Wall Thickness	
LV end-diastolic	cm (3.5 – 5.7)	Septum	cm (0.6 – 1.1)
LV end-systole	cm (2.3 – 3.5)	Posterior wall	cm (0.6 – 1.1)
Aortic root	cm (2.0 – 3.7)	Wall Motion/Systolic Function	
LVOT	cm (1.5 – 2.5)	LV EF	%
Left Atrium	cm (1.9 – 4.0)	Wall motion	

ETT SUMMARY

Exercise duration:		Peak SBP	
Max Stage:		RPPP	
Peak Heart Rate		Symptoms	
Terminated D/T:		Baseline EKG:	
% Max Predicted HR:	%	EKG Summary:	

FINAL FINDINGS

REST IMAGES

STRESS IMAGES

INTERPRETATION

/IIb

> These section separators were created using a rectangle (drawing object) with a text box placed inside the rectangle. The text box is filled with black and the text is formatted in white

Echocardiogram with Doppler

This sample template shows how tables can be used two different ways to lay out the data and also to control the direction of the insertion point using either the **F11** key or arrow keys.

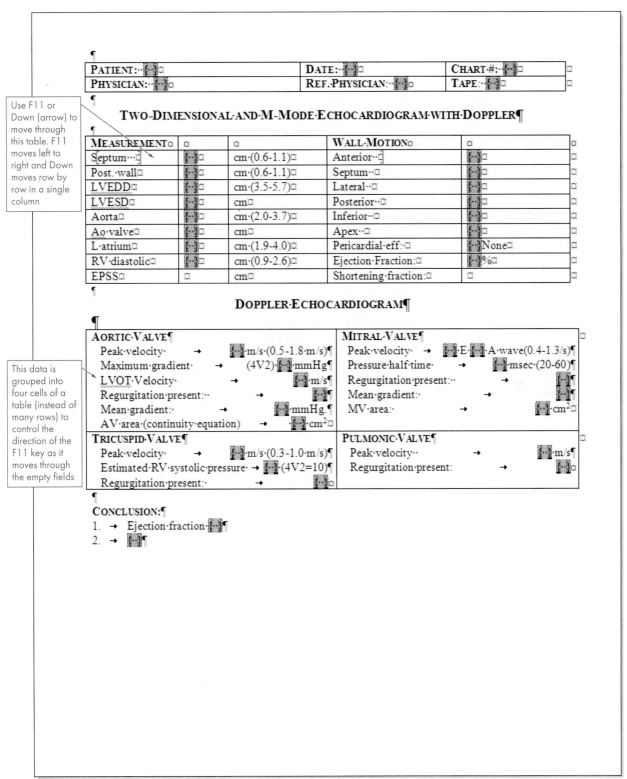

Use F11 or Down (arrow) to move through this table. F11 moves left to right and Down moves row by row in a single column

This data is grouped into four cells of a table (instead of many rows) to control the direction of the F11 key as it moves through the empty fields

Letterhead with Names in Left Margin

A column of names can be added in the left margin. Elements added *anywhere on the page while the header space is open* are considered part of the header and footer. Text boxes, tables, watermarks, and drawing objects inserted in the header will not interfere with text added to the body of the document. In Word 2003, go to Insert > Text box. Drag the cross-shaped cursor across the screen to draw a box and type text within the box. Right-click the text-box border and choose Format Text Box. In Word 2007, go to Insert > Text > Text box. Choose a format from the gallery and modify the box using commands on the ribbon. See the video on the accompanying CD to learn more about using text boxes in MS Word.

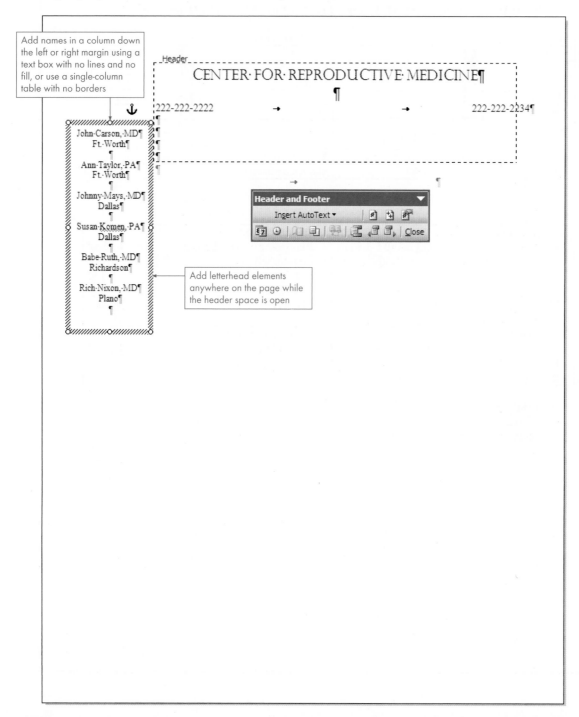

Sample Report using Letterhead in Left Margin

The letterhead template shown on the facing page was used to transcribe this report. The line around the text box is set to "no line" so it does not print.

CENTER FOR REPRODUCTIVE MEDICINE

222-222-2222   222-222-2234

John Carson, MD
Ft. Worth

Ann Taylor, PA
Ft. Worth

Johnny Mays, MD
Dallas

Susan Komen, PA
Dallas

Babe Ruth, MD
Richardson

Rich Nixon, MD
Plano

June 15, 2009

John Smith, MD
1234 Any Street Dr
Any City, ST 12345

RE: Jane Doe

Dear Dr. Smith,

It is a great pleasure that we send Jane back to you for obstetrical care. As you recall, Jane is a 36-year-old gravida 1, para 0 with an EDC of 01/12/2010. She currently has a twin gestation status post in vitro fertilization. She is on metformin treatment in the form of 1500 mg daily through the first trimester. In addition, she is also on Prometrium 200 mg t.i.d. vaginally until the end of 10 weeks of gestation. We have followed her through her first trimester, at which time she has not had any difficulties, and her fetuses have shown interval growth and development.

Please let us know if you need any additional information. Thank you for your support.

With every kind wish, I am sincerely yours,

John Carson, MD
JC/lb

Letterhead Formatted using Tables

These figures demonstrate how a single-row table can be used to lay out the addresses in a letterhead. The first figure shows the template with gridlines displayed and the second figure shows the letterhead as it will print.

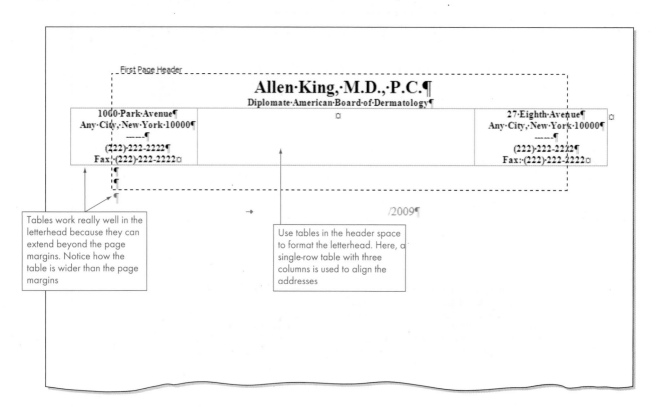

Tables work really well in the letterhead because they can extend beyond the page margins. Notice how the table is wider than the page margins

Use tables in the header space to format the letterhead. Here, a single-row table with three columns is used to align the addresses

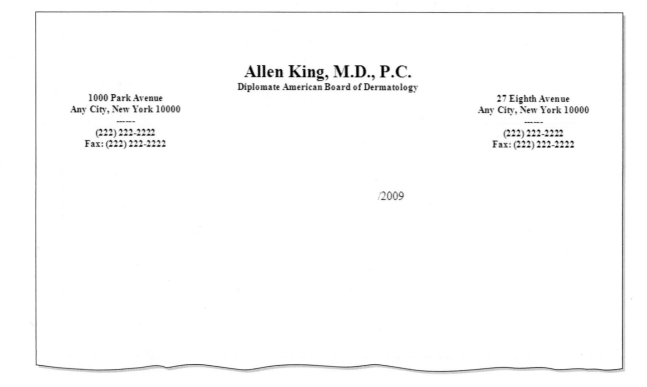

Letterhead Formatted using Text Boxes

These figures demonstrate the use of text boxes in a letterhead to lay out the addresses. Text boxes work well when the text is not the same font or font size. The second figure below shows the letterhead when printed. Information on using text boxes can be found on the accompanying CD.

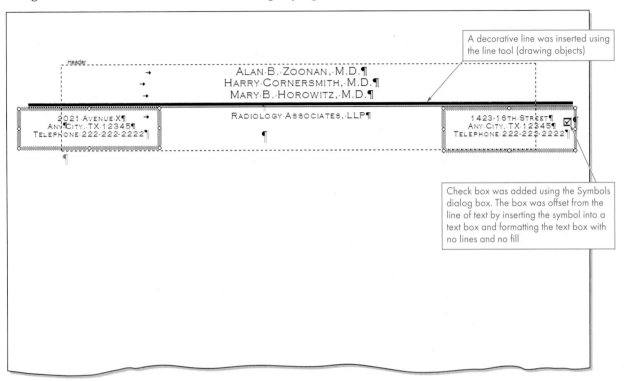

A decorative line was inserted using the line tool (drawing objects)

Check box was added using the Symbols dialog box. The box was offset from the line of text by inserting the symbol into a text box and formatting the text box with no lines and no fill

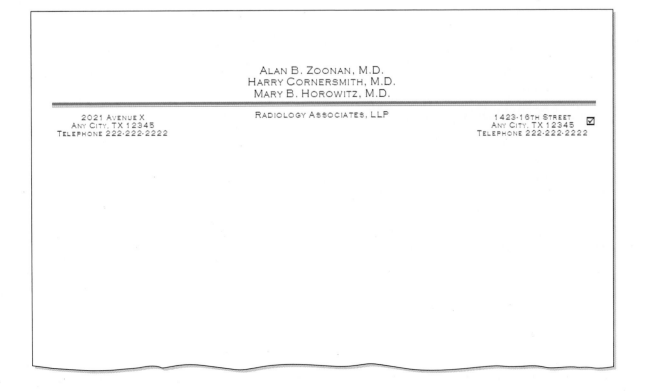

Template using Document Property Fields, Bookmarks, and Cross-references

This template uses fields from Document Properties (see page 308 for Word 2003 and page 311 for Word 2007) as well as a bookmark and cross-reference. See page 460 for instructions on using bookmarks and cross-references.

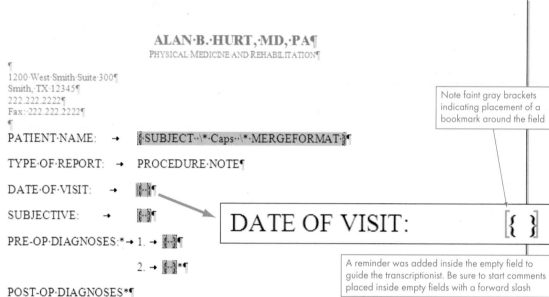

ALAN·B.·HURT,·MD,·PA¶
PHYSICAL·MEDICINE·AND·REHABILITATION¶

¶
1200·West·Smith·Suite·300¶
Smith,·TX·12345¶
222.222.2222¶
Fax:·222.222.2222¶
¶

PATIENT·NAME: → {SUBJECT··*·Caps··*·MERGEFORMAT}¶

TYPE·OF·REPORT: → PROCEDURE·NOTE¶

DATE·OF·VISIT: → {·}¶

SUBJECTIVE: → {·}¶

PRE-OP·DIAGNOSES:*→·1.·→·{·}¶

2.·→·{·}·*¶

POST-OP·DIAGNOSES·*¶

OPERATIONS: → **BOTOX·NEURECTOMIES·OF·THE·{·/RIGHT·OR·LEFT·} SUPERFICIAL·CERVICAL·PLEXUS·NERVE·#{·}·VIA·EMG· GUIDANCE·AND·FLUOROSCOPIC·GUIDANCE.¶**

PROCEDURE·NOTE: → The·patient·was·placed·in·the·prone·position·on·the·fluoroscopy· table.··The·cervical·region·was·cleansed·with·hydrogen·peroxide·solution.··The·head·was·turned· away·from·the·side·to·be·blocked.··A·Neuroline·{·}27-gauge,·{·}1¼-inch·monopolar·needle·was· inserted·along·the·posterior·border·of·the·right·and·left·sternocleidomastoid·and·midway·between· its·origin·on·the·clavicle.··The·needle·was·carefully·advanced·1·inch·superiorly·and·inferiorly· along·the·edge·of·the·muscle.··Next,·{·}0.5·cc·of·Omnipaque·{·}150·contrast·was·injected·at· each·site.··Then,·{·}250·units·of·Myobloc,·Lot·#·{·},·expiration·date·{·},·were·injected.··Sterile· technique·was·used.·¶
¶

POST·PROCEDURE·ASSESSMENT: → {·}The·patient·tolerated·the·procedure·well·and·was· released·to·the·observation·and·recovery·area·for·monitoring·of·any·possible·adverse·affects·of· the·injection·procedure.··Followup·visit·is·{·}·¶

{TITLE··*·MERGEFORMAT}¶
▪ Diplomate,·American·Academy·of·Pain·Management¶
▪ ¶
▪ ABH·¶
▪ DD:··{REF·DateofVisit··h·}¶
▪ DT:··{CREATEDATE··*·MERGEFORMAT}¶

Note faint gray brackets indicating placement of a bookmark around the field

DATE OF VISIT: { }

A reminder was added inside the empty field to guide the transcriptionist. Be sure to start comments placed inside empty fields with a forward slash

Continued·on·page·2¶

Properties Dialog Boxes

The **Document Properties** dialog (Word 2003 on top, Word 2007 on bottom) with Title and Subject filled in. Information in this dialog will automatically insert into the document using the Title and Subject fields as shown in the template on the facing page.

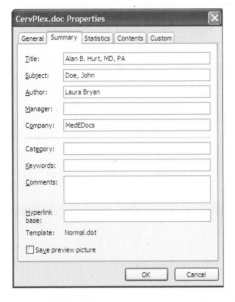

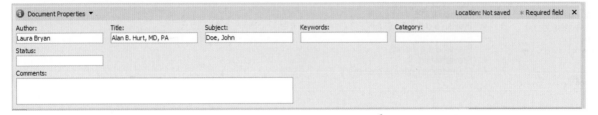

Letterhead Size and Spacing

Apply *Space above* (**Paragraph** dialog box) to the first line of a document that requires a large white space at the top of the first page in order to accommodate letterhead stationery. This technique allows the text to start far enough down the first page to accommodate preprinted stationery but does not require a section break to format a second-page header of a different size. Be sure to only apply "space above" to the first line of the template.

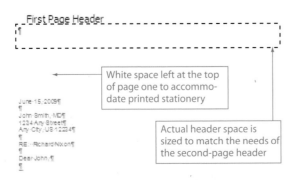

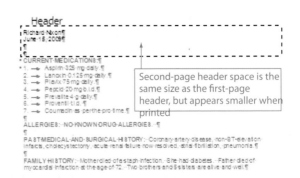

Use Keep with Next to Manage Page Breaks

Apply *Keep with next* (**Paragraph** dialog box, **Line and Page Breaks**) to prevent headings from being separated from the text they introduce. When a heading approaches a soft page break, the heading automatically moves to the next page to "keep with" the next paragraph. This command can be applied to all headings in the template.

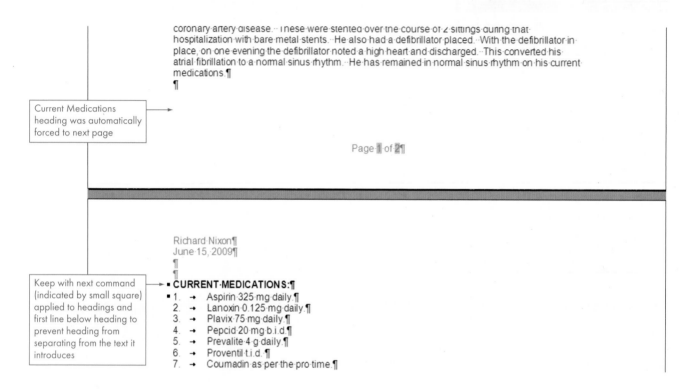

Critical Thinking Questions

1. You notice that you typed "PENECILLIN" (in all caps) but Word did not mark it as misspelled. What should you do?

   _____

   _____

2. Suddenly you have red and blue lines in your document (underscores and strikeouts). What should you do?

   _____

   _____

3. After inserting the AutoText entry "The patient returns for followup," the insertion point moves to the next line but you want the insertion point to remain on the same line to continue with the sentence. What should you do?

   _____

   _____

4. After creating an AutoText entry for "The patient comes in today," the entry does not insert into the document after typing the shortcut and pressing F3. What should you do?

   _____

   _____

5. You notice there are random words that are not capitalized even though they start a sentence. What should you do?

   _____

   _____

6. You created several macros that would be helpful to other MTs that work on the same account. How could you share these macros with them?

   _____

   _____

7. You created a template that has the office letterhead on the first page but you want to put patient information on the second page. What should you do?

   _____

   _____

8. You are using a computer workstation that belonged to another MT and you have found several spelling errors that were not marked by the spelling and grammar checker. What should you do?

   _____

   _____

9. When typing a numbered list, it always indents. What do you do if you need the list to line up at the left margin?

_____

_____

10. You created a shortcut in AutoCorrect for b.i.d., but this one time you need to type the actual word bid. What is the easiest way to solve this problem?

_____

_____

11. During a tech support call, the technician asks you what version of Windows you are running and what type of processor is installed. How do you find the answer?

_____

_____

12. The office calls and asks you to email a copy of a file that you typed about two weeks ago. The only information they can give you is the patient's last name. What do you do?

_____

_____

13. You need to devise a way to quickly access a group of folders and their files. You can use the mouse to set up the system, but you must use the keyboard to access the files on a routine basis. Explain how you could do this.

_____

_____

14. You have a list of 20 Internet sites that you use on a regular basis. How could you set up shortcuts for these so you can access them using the keyboard?

_____

_____

15. You need to locate and delete about 20 files that have the name Jones included in the file name. This folder contains over 200 files. What is the easiest way to do this?

_____

_____

16. You have been working on a file, but the program has stopped responding to the mouse and the keyboard. You can still use the mouse and keyboard in other programs. What should you do?

_____

_____

17. You have created a template that includes several standard paragraphs. About twenty percent of the time, the dictator asks you to delete part of the standard and replace it with a different standard. How can you do this with a single keystroke?

_____

_____

18. You are working in a document and suddenly every time you strike another key, more text is selected. What has happened? What should you do?

_____

_____

19. You created a new document yesterday, but you do not remember the file name or the folder. How can you find this file?

_____

_____

20. You were given a sample document for a new account. You use this document as the starting point for all new documents of that type and use Save As to rename the sample document each time you use it. You find that at least once a day you forget to rename the file before saving changes, thereby contaminating the standard text. What would be the best solution to prevent you from having to "decontaminate" your base document?

_____

_____

21. You have been working on a particularly difficult dictation during a thunderstorm. If you *must* continue working in spite of the storm, what should you do?

_____

_____

22. You accidentally pasted a large amount of text in the middle of a document. What is the easiest way to fix this?

_____

_____

23. You have been asked to proofread some documents typed by a new transcriptionist. You notice there is a misspelled word that is not marked. What should you do to check for other possible spelling errors?

_____

_____

24. Word 2003 always abbreviates the drop-down menus, making you click at the bottom of the menu to see the entire list of menu choices. What can you do to change this behavior?

   _____

   _____

25. Word 2007's default paragraph style includes spacing after the paragraph. How can you change this default style?

   _____

   _____

26. How would you set formatting in all caps and bold as part of the template so that you do not have to apply formatting while typing?

   _____

   _____

27. You have set up a series of template files (dot files) that you use regularly. You need to be able to modify these templates fairly often. Describe how you can easily access these templates.

   _____

   _____

Special Projects

The following pages contain specific projects with step-by-step instructions. Many of them combine techniques described throughout this text. Duplicate these projects or use them to inspire projects to fit your own particular needs. Many of the macros described here are also included on the CD and can be copied to your computer. Projects are marked with icons to identify a specific version's instructions. If not otherwise marked, the project is applicable to both Word 2003 and Word 2007.

Customizing

The following projects will help you customize your copy of Word to increase your efficiency.

Create a Toolbar to Streamline Customizing

When you have an extra few minutes to create some custom commands and toolbars, you can do this quickly and easily using this Customizing toolbar. Follow these steps to create the toolbar:

1. Open the **Customize** dialog box (Tools > Customize).
2. Select Toolbars.
3. Select New.
4. Type a name in the *Toolbar name* box.
5. Choose a template in *Make toolbar available to*.
6. Click OK.
7. Switch to Commands.
8. Under *Categories*, choose *All Commands*.
9. Drag any or all of the following commands to the new toolbar:
   NewToolbar (opens the **New Toolbar** dialog box)
   ToolsCustomizeKeyboard (opens the **Customize keyboard** dialog box)
   ToolsCustomizeToolbars (opens the *Commands* tab of the **Customize** dialog box)

WORD 2003

ToolsCustomizeKeyboardShortcut (changes the cursor to the Customize icon described on page 398).

ToolsCustomizeRemoveMenuShortcut (changes the cursor to the Remove icon described on page 399).

10. Right-click on each button to shorten the toolbar button name.

11. Close the dialog box.

12. When you are ready to customize Word, simply display the toolbar and click the icons to display the appropriate dialog box.

Create a Work Menu for Frequently Used Documents

Some transcriptionists find it useful to keep reference lists and notes. To make these documents more accessible, create a Work menu and place it on the Menu bar. You can also place document templates on this Work menu to quickly access your template files to make changes to the standard text.

1. Open the **Customize** dialog box.

2. Select the Commands tab.

3. From the Categories list, choose Built-in Menus.

4. From the Commands list, choose Work.

5. Drag the word Work to the Menu bar and drop it on the Menu bar next to Help.

6. Close the **Customize** dialog box.

To add documents to the Work menu:

1. Open the document you wish to place on the menu.

2. Select Work (**ALT, K**).

3. Select Add to Work Menu.

To use the Work menu:

1. Select the Work menu (**ALT, K**).

2. Arrow down to the document name or press the number corresponding to the document.

To remove documents from the Work menu:

1. Press **ALT+CTRL+-** (hyphen).

2. With the modified cursor, open the Work menu and click on the document you want to remove from the menu. This will not delete the document; it will only remove the document name from the Work menu.

Modify Shortcut Menus with Editing Commands

To increase your efficiency with editing, modify the shortcut menus with common editing commands. You can use the **Application** key to open the edit menu or you can use a right-click. If the document does not require extensive editing, you can use the mouse to track the words as you listen to the audio playback and then right-click on errors to make the correction. Place your most common editing tasks on your right-click menus to make this approach more efficient. Follow the directions on page 393 for modifying right-click menus.

You can place commands or macros on your right-click menus. Listed below are a few ideas to get you started (the actual command names are listed in parentheses along with the shortcut key).

Add these commands to the shortcut menus listed under the Text category— Grammar, Spelling, Lists, and Text:

Change Case (**Shift+F3**, ChangeCase)

Delete (**Delete**, EditClear)

Bold (**CTRL+B**, Bold)

Go to next misspelled word (**ALT+F7**, NextMisspelling)

Remove direct formatting (**CTRL+Q**, ResetPara or **CTRL+Spacebar**, ResetChar)

Add to Table shortcut menu:

Delete row (TableDeleteRow)

Delete column (TableDeleteColumn)

Hint: For commands not listed above, you can often identify the command name as it appears in the Commands list using the **Customize Keyboard** dialog box. If you know the shortcut for the command that you want to place on the shortcut menu, open the **Customize Keyboard** dialog box and type the shortcut key in the Press new shortcut key box. The command name will appear in the area below. Press **Esc** to close the dialog box.

Also, when you are in customize mode, you can drag icons from any available toolbar or commands from menus directly onto the shortcut menu.

Create the editing macros described on the following pages and drag some of these to your shortcut menus also.

Note: Choose your favorite commands carefully so your shortcut menu does not become too long and too unwieldy. You can also remove some of the native commands from the shortcut menus to make more room for your favorites. To remove a command, drag it from the menu while in customize mode.

Editing and Proofing

The following macros and projects are designed to increase your efficiency while editing.

Create Macros for "Jumping Jacks"

Some dictators are not as organized and consistent as we would like. These dictators keep the MT jumping all around the document. To quickly move to any point in a document, create macros to locate specific headings and move the insertion point. Refer to page 466 for the Seven Steps to Start a Macro and then continue with the following steps:

1. Press **CTRL+Home** to move the cursor to the beginning of the document. This will ensure that the macro runs correctly in all situations by always beginning from the same position in the document.

2. Open the **Find** dialog box (**CTRL+F**).

3. Type the heading name (eg, history of present illness) and click Find.

4. Press **Esc** to close the **Find** dialog box.

5. Press **Right** to deselect the heading and then move the insertion point to the position within that section where you typically begin transcribing. Remember to use the keyboard to move the insertion point—mouse movements will not be recorded.

6. Stop the recorder.

Create separate macros to move to all the main headings in a report. Assign shortcut keys to the macros, or use the method described on page 471 to run macros using the macro name. If you choose to run the macros by name, keep the macro name short and easy to remember (eg, HPI, ROS, PE, Plan).

Create a Spelling Exception List

Some typos will pass the spell check routine because they are still legitimate words. For example, it is easy to transpose "form" and "from" or, even worse, drop a character and type "rape" instead of "drape." There are two approaches to calling attention to these words. You can create AutoCorrect entries to append an X to these words so they are deliberately misspelled (so the red underline will draw your attention) or to apply bold formatting, causing you to double check the word. Another approach is to create an exception list for the spell checker. This has the effect of "removing" a word from the Main dictionary, so words on this list will be marked as incorrect during a spell check.

 Follow these steps for Word 2003:

1. Close Word.

2. Open Explorer (**Logo+E**) and in the Address bar, type %AppData% and press **Enter**.

3. Go to **Microsoft** > **Proof**.

4. Press **ALT, F** to open the File menu of the Explorer window. Choose New > Text Document (make sure you have not selected the Custom.dic file within the Explorer window).

5. A new file will appear in the file-list area. Name the file mssp3en.exc.

6. Open the file you just created. It should open in Notepad.

7. Type the list of words to include in your exception list. Carefully type one word per line using lowercase, and avoid inserting leading or trailing spaces.

8. Save and close the file.

9. To edit the list, open the file and add or remove words as needed. If it does not automatically open, right-click the file name, choose Open With > Notepad.

Words on your exception list will now be marked with a red sawtooth line when you type them into a document. The words will remain marked, even if you run the spell check routine and mark Ignore. These words will not appear with a sawtooth line when the document is opened on another computer.

Note: The exception list works with Stedman's Plus Medical/Pharmaceutical Spellchecker but will not work with Spellex brand spell-checking software.

 Follow these steps to add words to the exceptions list in Word 2007:

1. Locate the **UProof** folder. To do this, type `%AppData%` in the Explorer Address bar then go to **Microsoft** > **UProof**.

2. Right-click on the file named ExcludeDictionaryEN0409.lex. Choose Open With > *Select a program from a list of installed programs* > *Notepad*.

3. Type the list of words to include in your exception list. Carefully type one word per line using lowercase, and avoid inserting leading or trailing spaces.

4. Save and close the file.

5. To edit the list, open the file and add or remove words as needed. If it does not automatically open, right-click the file name, choose Open With > Notepad.

Words on your exception list will now be marked with a red sawtooth line when you type them into a document. The words will remain marked, even if you run the spell check routine and mark Ignore. These words will not appear with a sawtooth line when the document is opened on another computer.

Macros for Selecting Text

The navigation keys work very well for moving through text one word at a time or for selecting text, but if you would like, you can create additional navigation keys that work slightly differently than Shift + the navigation keys. These navigation techniques work especially well for editing speech recognized documents.

Track One Word to the Right

This particular macro will select one word at a time moving left to right. It differs from CTRL+Shift+Right in that it doesn't continue the selection—it selects one word at a time. Follow the steps on page 466 to start a macro and then continue with these steps:

1. Press Right.
2. Press F8 twice.
3. Press Esc.
4. Stop the recorder.

Assign this macro to an easy key combination that is close to the home keys. Press the shortcut key to track/select one word at a time. As you encounter a word to be edited, it will already be selected—so simply begin typing to delete/replace the word.

Track One Word to the Left

This particular macro will select one word at a time moving right to left. It differs from CTRL+Shift+Left in that it doesn't continue the selection—it selects one word at a time. Follow the steps on page 466 to start a macro and then continue with these steps:

1. Press Left twice.
2. Press F8 twice.
3. Press Esc.
4. Stop the recorder.

Macros for Deleting Text

Here are examples of macros that you can create to make editing easier. Assign these macros to easy-to-use shortcut keys or drag them to shortcut menus (as described on page 394). These macros are especially helpful for editing speech-recognized documents, but are also useful for proofreading and for quality assurance reviews. Choose the macros most useful to your particular work. For each macro described below, begin with the Seven Steps to Record a Macro (on page 466).

Delete a Word

1. Press F8 twice then press Delete.
2. Stop the recorder.

To use, place the insertion point anywhere in the word or next to the word and press your assigned shortcut key.

Delete Sentence

1. Press F8 three times then press Delete.
2. Stop the recorder.

To use, place the insertion point anywhere in a sentence and press your assigned shortcut key to remove the entire sentence.

Delete to Period (Delete Part of a Sentence)

1. Press F8 once followed by the Period and then Delete.
2. Stop the recorder.

To use, set the insertion point where you want to begin deleting and press the shortcut key. This will remove text from the insertion point to the next occurrence of a period.

Delete to Comma

1. Press **F8** once followed by the **Comma** and then **Delete**.
2. Stop the recorder.

To use, set the insertion point where you want to begin deleting and press the shortcut key. This will remove text from the insertion point to the next occurrence of a comma.

Macros for Punctuating

The following macros are designed to speed up editing tasks that involve changing punctuation. They are most useful for reviewing a document word for word for a quality assurance review or for speech-recognition editing. At first you may wonder why a simple task of inserting a comma needs to be streamlined, but you will find that this approach works really well because you do not have to "take aim" at a specific point to insert or change punctuation—you can set the insertion point anywhere in the word or directly in front of the word. If you use the navigation keys (eg, **CTRL+Right**) to move word-by-word through a document as you review the audio, you will find that you can adjust punctuation effortlessly without adjusting the position of the insertion point.

Remove an Apostrophe

Use this macro to convert eponyms from the possessive form (eg, change Crohn's to Crohn).

1. Set the insertion point in a word that contains an apostrophe.
2. Press **F8** twice (to select the word).
3. Press **Esc** (to turn off Extend mode).
4. Open **Find** (**CTRL+F**).
5. Type an apostrophe in the *Find what* box.
6. Press **Enter** (or click **Find Next**).
7. Press **Esc** (to close the **Find** dialog box).
8. Press **Delete**.
9. Stop the recorder.

To use this macro, place the insertion point anywhere in the word containing the apostrophe and press the shortcut key.

Insert Hyphen

Use this macro to quickly hyphenate a compound modifier.

1. Place the insertion point in the first word of the hyphenated pair.
2. Press **F8** twice (to select the word).
3. Press **Esc** (to turn off Extend mode).
4. Press **Right** (to move to the end of the word).
5. Press **Backspace** (to remove the space).

(Continued)

6. Press - (hyphen).

7. Stop the recorder.

To use this macro, place the insertion point anywhere in the first word of the hyphenated pair and press the shortcut key. For a compound modifier that has several hyphens, press the shortcut key repeatedly (you don't need to reset the insertion point before pressing the shortcut key).

Insert a Comma

1. Set the insertion point anywhere within a word.

2. Press **F8** twice (to select the word).

3. Press **Esc** (to turn off Extend mode).

4. Press **Right** (to remove the selection from the word).

5. Press **Left** (to move the insertion point over one space).

6. Press the **Comma**.

7. Stop the recorder.

To use this macro, place the insertion point anywhere in the word that precedes the intended comma and press the shortcut key. You don't have to set the insertion point at the end of the word. Assign the shortcut key **CTRL+,** (comma) to make it easy to use and easy to remember.

Insert a Period and Cap the Next Word

1. Set the insertion point anywhere within a word.

2. Press **F8** twice (to select the word).

3. Press **Esc** (to turn off Extend mode).

4. Press **Right** (to remove the selection from the word).

5. Press **Left** (to move the insertion point over one space).

6. Press the **Period**.

7. Press **Spacebar** (only if you transcribe with two spaces between sentences).

8. Press **Right** two times.

9. To cap the first word:

   a. Press **ALT, O, E** and choose Sentence Case (either version).

   b. In Word 2003, go to Format > Change Case > Sentence case.

   c. In Word 2007, go to Home > Font > Change Case > Sentence Case.

10. Stop the recorder.

To use this macro, place the insertion point anywhere in the word that precedes the intended period and press the shortcut key. You don't have to set the insertion point at the end of the word.

Change a Comma to a Period and Cap the Next Word

1. Set the insertion point anywhere within the word that precedes a comma.

2. Press **F8** twice (to select the word).

3. Press **Esc** (to turn off Extend mode).

4. Press **Right** (to remove the selection from the word).

5. Press **Delete** to remove the comma.

6. Press the **Period**.

7. Press **Spacebar** (only if you transcribe with two spaces between sentences).

8. Press **Right** two times.

9. To cap the first word following the period, do this:

   a. Press **ALT, O, E** and choose Sentence Case (either version).

   b. In Word 2003, go to Format > Change Case > Sentence case.

   c. In Word 2007, go to |Home| > Font > |Change Case| > Sentence Case.

10. Stop the recorder.

To use this macro, place the insertion point anywhere in the word preceding the comma and press the shortcut key. You don't have to set the insertion point at the end of the word.

Format Headings in a Speech-Recognized Document

This macro is especially useful for editing a document that was created using a speech recognition platform that does not format the report and apply formatting to the headings. This macro will begin a new paragraph, format the selected words as a heading (bold, all caps), insert a colon and two spaces following the heading, and cap the first word following the heading. This particular macro places the heading on the same line as the text that follows it. The next macro (described below) will place the heading on its own line and start the text on the line immediately following the heading. You can easily modify these macros to format the heading according to your particular specifications, such as not bold, underlined, etc.

1. Type this sample text into a document: `Patient complains of headaches history of present illness two weeks ago.` (Note: the actual content of the sample text is not really important—you just need some text to create the macro.)

2. Select the words `history of present illness` without picking up leading or trailing spaces.

3. Go through the Seven Steps to Start a Macro explained on page 466 (be sure the heading text remains selected). With the recorder on, step through the following keystrokes.

4. Press **CTRL+X** (cut the heading text from the document).

5. **Delete** (to remove the extra space).

6. **Enter** (to end the paragraph).

7. **Enter** (to insert a blank line).

8. Type a **Colon** followed by two **Spaces**.

9. Press **Shift+F3** (to cap the first word following the colon).

(Continued)

10. Press **Home** (to move the insertion point to the beginning of the line).

11. Press **CTRL+V** (to paste the heading text back into the document).

12. Press **Shift+Home** (to select the heading text).

13. To capitalize the heading, do this:

    a. Press **ALT, O, E** and choose UPPERCASE (either version).

    b. In Word 2003, go to Format > Change Case > UPPERCASE.

    c. In Word 2007, go to Home > Font > Change Case > UPPERCASE.

14. Press **CTRL+B** (to apply bold) or press the shortcut keys for any other formatting needed.

15. Press **Right** (to remove selection).

16. Stop the recorder.

To use this macro, select the text to be formatted as a heading and then press the shortcut key. The heading can be a single word or several words.

To create a macro similar to the above macro that will format the heading on its own line, follow these steps:

1. Type this sample text into a document: Patient complains of headaches history of present illness two weeks ago. (Note: the actual content of the sample text is not really important—you just need some text to create the macro.)

2. Select the words history of present illness without picking up leading or trailing spaces.

3. Go through the Seven Steps to Start a Macro explained on page 466 (be sure the heading text remains selected). With the recorder on, step through the following keystrokes.

4. To capitalize the heading, do this:

    a. Press **ALT, O, E** and choose UPPERCASE (either version).

    b. In Word 2003, go to Format > Change Case > UPPERCASE.

    c. In Word 2007, go to Home > Font > Change Case > UPPERCASE.

5. Press **CTRL+B** (to apply bold) or press the shortcut keys for any other formatting needed.

6. Press **CTRL+X** (cut the heading text from the document).

7. Press **Enter** three times (to end the paragraph and insert two blank lines).

8. Press **Delete** (to remove the extra space).

9. To capitalize the first word following the heading, do this:

    a. In Word 2003, go to Format > Change Case > Sentence case.

    b. In Word 2007, go to Home > Font > Change Case > Sentence Case.

10. Press **Up**.

11. Press **CTRL+V** (to paste the heading text back into the document).

12. Type a **Colon**.

13. Press **Right** (to move to the next line).

14. Stop the recorder.

To use this macro, select the text that will become the heading and press your assigned shortcut key.

Insert Headings in a Speech-Recognized Document

AutoText is a good tool for inserting formatted headings into a speech-recognized document. To insert a new heading in the middle of a paragraph, as shown below, include the paragraph breaks at the beginning of your AutoText entry.

To·change:¶

CHIEF·COMPLAINT:···Headaches.··The·patient·returns·today·for·a·followup·appointment·for·chronic·headaches.¶

To·this:¶

CHIEF·COMPLAINT:···Headaches.··¶

¶

HISTORY·OF·PRESENT·ILLNESS:···The·patient·returns·today·for·a·followup·appointment·for·chronic·headaches.¶

Select the two paragraph marks, the heading text, colon, and spaces as shown in this figure to create the AutoText entry.

CHIEF·COMPLAINT:···Headaches.¶

¶

HISTORY·OF·PRESENT·ILLNESS:··The·patient·returns·today·for·a·followup·appointment·for·chronic·headaches.¶

Create a Macro to Find Blanks

Editors will want to get to blanks and problem areas within a document quickly. Use this technique for locating a blank, deleting the blank, and setting the insertion point in order to fill in the missing information. Have the transcription staff use the **Underscore** key to create a blank with one space on either side of the line. Start with the Seven Steps to Start a Macro on page 466 and then continue:

1. Press **CTRL+F** to open the **Find** dialog box.
2. In the *Find what* box, type two underscore characters.
3. Click **Find Next**.
4. Press **Esc** (to close the dialog box).
5. Press **F8** (to turn on Extend mode).
6. Press the **Spacebar** (to select to the end of the blank line).
7. Press **Delete**.
8. Stop the recorder.

Create a Macro to Correct Missed Caps after a Colon

Colons are very common in medical transcription. Typically, the first word after the colon is capitalized, but this can be awkward to key. It's also easy to forget, since you may be in the habit of Word capitalizing sentences for you. The macro described below will capitalize words that follow a colon. This macro assumes that you place two spaces after a colon (but you can adjust accordingly if you use a single space following a colon). Run this macro *after you have transcribed the document* to correct any missed caps.

Start with the Seven Steps to Start a Macro on page 466 and then continue:

1. Press **CTRL+H** (to open the **Find and Replace** dialog box).
2. In the *Find what* box, type : ^$ (**Colon** followed by two spaces, **Caret, Dollar sign**). The caret+dollar sign represents "any letter," so you are searching for the occurrence of a colon followed by two spaces followed by any letter.
3. In the *Replace with* box, type ^& (**Caret, Ampersand**). This symbol represents the "find what text."
4. Select **Format** > Font.
5. Press **ALT+A** to select *All caps*.
6. Press **Enter** to close the **Font** dialog box.
7. Select **Replace All**.
8. Press **Esc** to close the dialog box.
9. Stop the macro recorder.

In the instructions above, the caret+dollar sign represents "any letter" and the caret+ampersand represents the "find what text" (ie, the text that you are searching for). These codes correspond to *Any Letter* and *Find What Text* listed under **Special**. You can type the code directly into the *Find what* and *Replace with* boxes or you can select the special characters from the menu that appears when you click **Special**.

Note: This macro adds the format All caps to the first letter of words following colons. If you subsequently edit the document and place your cursor to the right of a corrected letter and then begin typing, your characters will insert in all caps. To remove the all caps formatting, open the **Font** dialog box and remove the check mark at *All caps* or remove character formatting using **CTRL+Spacebar**. A variation of this macro can be found on the accompanying CD.

Create a Macro to Correct Missed Caps after a Digit

Similar to the macro described above, you can also create a macro to correct missed caps following a sentence that ends with a digit. Run this macro *after you have transcribed the document* to correct any missed caps. Begin a macro as described on page 466 and then continue with these steps:

1. Press **CTRL+H** (to open the **Find and Replace** dialog box).
2. In the *Find what* box, type ^#. ^$ (**Caret, Pound, Period, Spacebar, Caret, Dollar sign**). The caret+pound sign represents "any digit" and the

caret+dollar sign represents "any letter," so you are searching for the occurrence of a digit followed by a period, one space, then any letter. If you type with two spaces following a sentence, include two spaces between the period and the caret.

3. In the *Replace with* box, type ^& (**Caret, Ampersand**). This symbol represents the "find what text."

4. Select **Format** > Font.

5. Press **ALT+A** (to select *All caps*).

6. Press **Enter** to close the **Font** dialog box.

7. Click **Replace All**.

8. Press **Esc** to close the dialog box.

9. Stop the macro recorder.

Note: This macro adds the format All caps to the first letter of sentences that follow a sentence ending in a digit. If you subsequently edit the document and place your cursor to the right of a corrected letter and then begin typing, your characters will insert in all caps. To remove the all caps formatting, open the **Font** dialog box and remove the check mark at *All caps* or remove character formatting using **CTRL+Spacebar**. A variation of this macro can be found on the accompanying CD.

Create a Macro to Cap Words in a List

The macro described below will capitalize the first word of a numbered list. This will not work on an automatically numbered list—only a manually numbered list. Run this macro *after you have transcribed the document* to correct any missed caps. Start with the Seven Steps to Start a Macro on page 466 and then continue:

1. Press **CTRL+H** (to open the **Find and Replace** dialog box).

2. In the *Find what* box, type ^#.^t^$ (**Caret, Pound, Period, Caret, t, Caret, Dollar sign**). The caret+pound sign represents "any digit," the caret+t represents a tab character, and the caret+dollar sign represents "any letter," so you are searching for the occurrence of any digit followed by a tab then any letter. If you transcribe with spaces after the number instead of a tab character, replace ^t with spaces.

3. In the *Replace with* box, type ^& (**Caret, Ampersand**). This symbol represents the "find what text."

4. Select **Format** > Font.

5. Press **ALT+A** (to select *All caps*).

6. Press **Enter** (to close the **Font** dialog box).

7. Click **Replace All**.

8. Press **Esc** (to close the dialog box).

9. Stop the macro recorder.

Note: This macro adds the format All caps to the first letter of sentences that follow a sentence ending in a digit. If you subsequently edit the document and place your cursor to the right of a corrected letter and then begin typing, your characters will insert in all caps. To remove the All caps formatting, open the **Font** dialog box and remove the check mark at *All caps* or remove character formatting using **CTRL+Spacebar**. A variation of this macro can be found on the accompanying CD.

Create a Macro to Insert a Next-Page Section Break

Section breaks are important for managing headers and footers. If you will be adding section breaks to your document, you will appreciate having a shortcut key for this task. There is not a specific command for adding a Next Page section break. The built-in Word commands will only open the **Break** dialog box (where you have to choose the type of break), so this is a good application of the macro feature. Start with the Seven Steps to Start a Macro on page 466 and then continue:

1. To access the **Break** dialog box, do this:

    a. Press **ALT, I, B** (either version).

    b. In Word 2003, go to Insert > Break.

    c. In Word 2007, go to `Page Layout` > Page Setup > `Breaks`.

2. Choose Next page (or other type of section break needed).

3. Press **Enter** to close the dialog.

4. Stop the recorder.

Create a Macro to Copy Pre-Op Diagnosis to Post-Op

In the vast majority of cases, the preoperative diagnosis and the postoperative diagnosis are the same. Create a macro that will copy the preoperative diagnosis and paste the text into the postoperative diagnosis heading.

1. In the standard text for your operative note, type the preoperative diagnosis heading and format the section appropriately. Place an asterisk in the middle of the heading immediately in front of the word diagnosis (PREOPERATIVE *DIAGNOSIS).

2. Place another asterisk at the end of the preoperative diagnosis section. These asterisks will mark the beginning and end of the preop text to be copied.

3. For the postoperative diagnosis, type and format the word POSTOPERATIVE (only) and follow it with a single space and an empty field (**CTRL+F9**). Do not apply paragraph formatting to this paragraph—the paragraph formatting will be supplied when the preoperative text is pasted.

4. Begin a macro using the Seven Steps to Start a Macro (page 466). Record the remainder of these steps as your macro.

5. Press **CTRL+Home** (moves to the beginning of the document).

6. Press **CTRL+F** (opens the **Find** dialog box).

7. In the *Find what* box, type an **Asterisk** (*).

8. In the *Search* box, choose *Down*.

9. Click `Find Next`.

10. Press **Esc** (to close the **Find** dialog box).

11. Press **Delete** (to remove the asterisk).
12. Press **F8** followed by the **Asterisk** (this will select the text from the insertion point to the asterisk that marks the end of the preoperative section).
13. Press **Right** (to pick up the paragraph mark for the last paragraph in the preoperative diagnosis section).
14. Press **CTRL+C** (to copy the preop text).
15. Press **Right** (to remove the selection).
16. Press **Left** and then **Backspace** (to remove the asterisk at the end of the preop diagnosis).
17. Press **F11** (to place the insertion point at the postop section).
18. Press **CTRL+V** (to paste the text).
19. Press **Left** to move to the end of the postoperative section.
20. Press **Backspace** to remove the asterisk.
21. Press **F11** (or the arrow keys) to move the insertion point to the next position to begin transcribing.
22. Turn off the macro recorder.

To use this macro, type the preoperative section as dictated. Edit the preoperative heading to diagnoses (plural) if necessary. Run the macro. Two versions of this macro can be found on the accompanying CD.

Document Management

The following projects are designed to help you better manage your documents and document formatting.

Insert "Continued" in the Footer

When working with documents that exceed one page, you may want to include the word "Continued" at the bottom of each page. The following describes how to create a field that can be placed in the footer that will insert the word "Continued" at the bottom of each page but the last. Follow these steps:

1. Create a template for your report.
2. Make sure formatting marks are displayed (**CTRL+Shift+8**).
3. Open the footer space (**ALT, V, H**) and place the insertion point where you would like the word "Continued" to appear.
4. Press **CTRL+F9** to insert a field. Type the word `if` followed by a single space.
5. Insert a second empty field (inside the first).
6. Move the insertion point inside the second field between the two spaces and type `numpages`.
7. Move outside the second field and type one space followed by a greater-than sign and another space.
8. Insert another empty field.
9. Inside the second empty field type `page`.

(Continued)

10. Move outside the brackets of the second empty field and type "Continued" (including the quotation marks).

11. Your field should appear like the screen shot shown here (this screen shot shows the fields with field shading enabled):

{ if { numpages } > { page } "Continued" }

12. Be sure to include a space before and after each word and before and after the greater-than sign. You must insert the brackets as a field using **CTRL+F9**; you cannot simply type the brackets.

13. Once you create and test your field, select the entire field and save as an AutoText entry so you can insert it easily whenever you need it. This field works perfectly when placed in the footer of a document, as it will only appear when the document exceeds one page and will not appear on the last page. If you have selected *Different first page*, you will need to insert the field in both the first- and second-page footer.

Create a Macro to Open a New Document Based On a Template

Templates are a great way to streamline your work on a daily basis. Opening documents based on templates takes several steps, so this is the perfect application of a macro. Be sure to save these macros in the Normal.dot so they are always available.

For Word 2003, start with the Seven Steps to Start a Macro on page 466 and then continue:

1. Select File > New.

2. In the **New Document** task pane, click *On my computer*. This will open the **Templates** dialog box.

3. Select the template icon for the template file you need and click **OK**.

4. When the new document opens, use the arrow keys or press **F11** to navigate to the first position/field in the document where you will begin transcribing.

5. Click the **Stop** button on the Record Macro toolbar.

For Word 2007, start with the Seven Steps to Start a Macro on page 466 and then continue:

1. Go to **Office** > New.

2. In the **New Document** dialog box, click *My templates*. This will open the **New** dialog box.

3. Select the template icon for the template file you need and click **OK**.

4. When the new document opens, use the arrow keys or press **F11** to navigate to the first position/field in the document where you will begin typing.

5. Click the **Stop** button on the record toolbar.

Format Reports to Use Word's Line Count

One of the dilemmas many MTs face using MS Word is how to use Word's line count feature without counting blank lines. Word will count any line with a paragraph mark, so pressing **Enter** to create space between paragraphs creates a new line and thereby increases the line count. Some clients specifically will not pay for lines that do not contain text.

To work around this, format paragraphs using the Space before command. This will create spaces between paragraphs without inserting a paragraph mark. The shortcut key **CTRL+0** (**Zero** located above the **P**) corresponds to *Space before* located on the **Paragraph** dialog box and adds or removes (toggles) 12 points of space above the current paragraph.

This method works well if you completely format a template file and use empty fields to move the insertion point. Just remember that pressing **Enter** to exit a paragraph that has been formatted with the space-before attribute will carry the command with it. Remove this attribute for address lines and other areas of the document that should be single-spaced. It is easy enough to toggle **CTRL+0** to add or remove the space.

Display formatting marks (**CTRL+Shift+8**) so you can check for paragraph marks and then take a line count using Word's line count utility (**ALT, T, W** or in Word 2003, go to *Tools > Word Count*; in Word 2007, click the Word Count button on the <u>Status Bar</u>). You can also use the Document Property field to insert the line count directly into the document. Use this information to add to your log sheet and then delete before delivering to the client. See Special Project on page 465.

Create a Second-Page Header in a Template File

This project will show you how to set up a second-page header in a template file. This header will automatically appear when the report carries over to the second page.

1. Create your template file and place all standard text.

2. If the standard text does not extend to a second page, insert a page break (**CTRL+Enter**) to (temporarily) create page 2.

3. Open the header space (**ALT, V, H**).

4. To designate a different first-page header, do this:

    a. In Word 2003, go to *File > Page Setup* and select **Layout** > *Different first page*.

    b. In Word 2007, go to **Design** > <u>Options</u> and select *Different First Page*.

5. Type the standard text that should appear in the header area of the second page (see also the next project). Insert a page-number field (**ALT+Shift+P**) to insert the page number.

(Continued)

6.   Close the header space and delete the page break (if applicable).

7.   Save and close the template file.

Even though the template itself is only one page long, Word will "remember" the second-page header when an actual report based on the template exceeds one page.

Automatically Update Second-Page Headers with Patient Demographics

When patient reports exceed one page, the second page typically contains the patient's name, medical record number, date, page number, and/or other identifying information. You can create bookmarks and then create cross-references to the bookmarks that will automatically insert the information from the first page of the document into the second page. This technique uses bookmarks to "tag" the text on the first page and cross-references to "copy" the tagged text to the designated location. This method works very well, but you must follow these directions carefully.

1.   Create a template file with standard text.

2.   Begin by bookmarking an empty field. To do this, insert an empty field (**CTRL+F9**) at the point where you will transcribe the patient's name. Insert other fields for other information that will be needed on the second page (eg, date seen, MRN).

3.   Select the patient-name field (ie, the field brackets). Be sure not to include the paragraph mark or any leading or trailing spaces.

4.   With the empty field selected, open the **Bookmark** dialog box:

     a.   Press **ALT, I, K** (either version).

     b.   In Word 2003, go to Insert > Bookmark.

     c.   In Word 2007, go to Insert > Links > Bookmark .

5.   Type a name for the bookmark such as PatientName (no spaces or punctuation).

6.   Repeat steps 3 and 4 to bookmark the text for each type of information that will be needed on the second page (eg, DateSeen, PatientMRN).

7.   Now, create the cross-references for the bookmarked fields. To do this, go to the second page and open the header (**ALT, V, H**).

8.   Set the insertion point where the patient name (or other information) should appear.

9.   Open the **Field** dialog box:

     a.   Press **ALT, I, F** (either version).

     b.   In Word 2003, go to Insert > Field.

     c.   In Word 2007, go to Insert > Text > Quick Parts > Field.

10. Under Categories, choose Links and References. Under Field names, choose Ref. At Bookmark name, choose the bookmark name (eg, PatientName) that contains the text you want to insert at this position in the document.

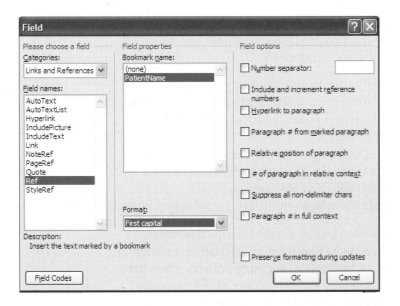

10. In the *Format* box, select the format to be applied to the text that will be inserted on the second page (uppercase, lowercase, Title case). For example, reports may have the name in all caps on the first page but title case on the second page. Word is capable of changing the capitalization on the second page while retaining the capitalization on the first page.

11. Click **OK** to close the **Field** dialog box.

12. Repeat steps 7–12 for each cross-reference to be placed on the second page.

13. Display bookmarks (faint gray brackets) to help you remember where bookmarks have been placed.

    a. In Word 2003, go to Tools > Options > View and place a check mark at *Bookmarks*.

    b. In Word 2007, go to **Office** > **Word Options** > **Advanced** > **Show document content** and place a check mark at *Bookmarks*.

When you are ready to transcribe a report, press **F11** to move the insertion point into the empty field that is tagged as a bookmark and type the appropriate information. If bookmarks are displayed, the gray brackets are right next to each other and will look like a capital letter I, but as you type text into the bookmarked field, the brackets will separate. *You must use the* **F11** *key to move the insertion point into the bookmarked field*. Typing in front of or after the field will not insert the text between the bookmark's brackets.

Note: For this method to work, you must transcribe your reports with field codes hidden (toggle **ALT+F9**). If field codes are displayed, pressing **F11** selects the field and typing into the field deletes the field. If the field is deleted, the bookmark is also deleted and the cross-reference field will not have a bookmark to cross-reference. At the point of your cross-reference, you will see a message "**Error: Bookmark not defined.**"

If you place these reference fields in a header, they will update when you close and then open the document. You can also force them to update using Update (F9). Open the header, press CTRL+A (select all) then F9.

It is also possible to create an AutoText entry to save your cross-references instead of inserting them into the header space of the template. To insert the cross-reference fields whenever and wherever you need them, create the bookmarks and cross-references as described above. Select the cross-reference fields and save as an AutoText entry. (Delete the cross-reference fields from the document after creating the AutoText entry if you don't need them in your template.) When transcribing a report, type the AutoText name and press F3. The information will automatically update when you insert the AutoText entry.

Cross-references are specific for the bookmark assigned to them. To create second-page headers that update correctly in files with more than one patient, you must create separate bookmarks and references for each patient. Place the standard text in the template file and include enough copies of the report to complete a typical day's dictation. Assign each field a unique bookmark name (eg, PatientName1, date1, medrec1, PatientName2, date2, medrec2) and create cross-references accordingly.

Automatically Insert Patient Demographics Throughout a Document

(Refer to the project above using bookmarks and cross-references.) If there is information that is used more than once in your document, you can create bookmarks and cross-references to quickly insert subsequent uses of that same information. For example, you can use bookmarks and cross-references to insert the patient's name in other areas of the document whenever needed. You can place the cross-reference in the standard text of your template if the information always appears in the same location (as described in the project above). If the placement of the information varies, save the cross-reference as an AutoText entry and insert that entry when needed. One advantage to this is approach is you can easily correct all occurrences of the information by correcting the bookmarked text (ie, the original entry). Once the bookmarked text is changed, the cross-reference fields will update to reflect the correction.

Insert Sections with Different Margins

To apply different page margin settings within a single document, you must divide the document into sections. Here is a quick way to insert section breaks with different page margins:

1. Type and select the text that will have different page margins.
2. With the text selected, open the **Page Setup** dialog box:
   a. In Word 2003, go to File > Page Setup (**ALT, F, U**).
   b. In Word 2007, go to **Page Layout** > Page Setup > **Margins** > Custom Margins.
3. Choose the **Layout** tab.
4. Set the appropriate page margins and choose *Apply to: Selected text*.

Create a Document that Includes the Envelope

If you create single-report documents or letters requiring an envelope, you can automatically insert an envelope at the beginning of the document to print at the same time as the document itself. Follow these steps:

1. Type the letter, highlight the address, and select:
   a. **ALT, T, E, E** (either version).
   b. In Word 2003, go to Tools > Letters and Mailings > Envelopes and Labels.
   c. In Word 2007, go to `Mailings` > Create > `Envelopes`.
2. On the `Envelope` tab, select `Add to document`.

This will create a new section at the top of your document with a formatted envelope. When you print the document, Word will prompt you to insert the envelope first. You can only create one envelope per file using this method. See the alternative method below for creating documents with more than one envelope.

Create an Envelope Document

This project creates a template where each "page" is actually an envelope. This approach works well if you have a lot of envelopes to print. To use this template on a daily basis, open the template and keep it open as you transcribe your letters and notes. Address an envelope to correspond with each letter you transcribe. When you are finished transcribing, load the envelopes into the printer and print them all at once. To create the envelope template, follow these steps:

1. Open Word and start a new document.
2. Press **F12** and name the template `EnvelopeDoc`. Save the template in the template folder (see page 236).
3. Open the **Page Setup** dialog box:
   a. In Word 2003, go to File > Page Setup (**ALT, F, U**).
   b. In Word 2007, go to `Page Layout` > Page Setup > `Margins` > Custom Margins.
4. Choose the `Paper` tab and set the Paper Size to #10 Envelope.
5. Choose the `Margin` tab and set to Landscape orientation.
6. On the `Margin` tab, set Top at 0.5 and Left at 0.5.
7. Close the **Page Setup** dialog box.
8. If you are using plain envelopes, type the return address in the left upper corner using 10-point font. If you create envelopes with more than one return address, create a separate template for each return address. Create the first template then create new templates based on the first template, changing only the return address. In this way, you only have to set up the envelope size and margins one time.
9. To set the address field, place the insertion point at approximately 2 inches ("At 2.0" on the Status Bar) and set a left indent at 4 inches. Place an empty field (**CTRL+F9**).
10. Insert a page break (**CTRL+Enter**).

(Continued)

11. Select all (CTRL+A) and save a copy of the envelope as an AutoText entry (ALT+F3).

12. Using your AutoText entry, insert enough "envelope pages" to accommodate a typical day of work.

13. Press CTRL+S to save your work and close the template.

To use, open a document based on the template, press F11 and insert an address. Press F11 to place the insertion point in the next address field. If you placed ten envelopes in your template file and only use eight envelopes, delete the extra envelopes before printing. Insert additional copies of the envelope when needed using the AutoText entry.

Alphabetize Patient Reports

If you transcribe multiple reports in a single file, Word can alphabetize the reports for you. For example, you transcribe 20–30 SOAP notes in a single document and the client would like the patient reports organized alphabetically—but of course the doctor dictates the reports randomly. Cutting and pasting the reports in alphabetical order is tedious, time-consuming, and prone to errors. Use the Outline feature in MS Word to alphabetize your reports. For this method to work, the patient's name must be on the first line of each report and the name must be formatted as last name, first name. Follow these steps:

1. Create a template file (as in Chapter 8). Place multiple copies of the SOAP note format (or whatever format is needed) one right after the other in the template file. Place enough copies of the format to accommodate a typical day of dictation.

2. For each copy of the SOAP note, apply the Heading 1 style (CTRL+ALT+1) to the line containing the patient's name. (The Outline feature uses the heading styles to create the Outline view of your document).

3. Save and close your template file.

To use your template, follow these steps.

1. Open a document based on the template file you created above and transcribe the reports as you normally do.

2. After you have transcribed all of the reports, save the file using CTRL+S one last time before stepping through the alphabetizing routine.

3. Change the document view to Outline (ALT, V, O).

4. While in Outline view, press ALT+Shift+1 to collapse the Outline so that only text with the Heading 1 style is displayed (ie, only the patient names).

5. To sort the names alphabetically, do this:

   a. Press ALT, A, S (either version).

   b. In Word 2003, go to Table > Sort.

   c. In Word 2007, go to Home > Paragraph > Sort (button marked with AZ).

6. Sort by Paragraphs, Text, Ascending Order. This will alphabetize the patient names; any text below the patient name will remain associated with the name.

7. Change the view back to Print Layout (**CLT+ALT+P**) and the reports will be in alphabetical order.

8. Open the **Find and Replace** dialog box (**CTRL+H**).

9. Set the insertion point in the *Find what* box and then click **More** > **Format** > *Style* > *Heading 1*. This will search for occurrences of the Heading 1 style.

10. In the *Replace with* box, choose the Normal style (**Format** > *Style* > *Normal*).

11. Click **Replace All**. This will replace all occurrences of the Heading 1 style with the Normal style, so your patient names will be formatted as regular text.

Be sure to save the file before changing to Outline view in case there is an error in the sort routine. If a problem arises while in Outline view, close the file without saving changes and re-open the file.

If you need to format the patient name in a format other than the Normal style, create a new style that corresponds to the style needed and use the **Find and Replace** dialog to replace the Heading 1 style with your new style.

Tip: The above steps starting with step 4 can be recorded as a macro to make this even faster.

Automating Log Sheets

Sometimes creating log sheets can be as time-consuming as transcribing your documents. You can use macros to copy information from the document and paste the data to a log sheet. A macro can include the following steps: copy needed information and add to a log sheet, save changes to the transcribed document, close the document, open a new document, and place the insertion point to begin typing. Typical data for a log sheet might include dictation file number, the number of characters with spaces, patient name, date of visit, and report type.

Since the information needed to build a log entry is typically scattered throughout a document, you can use styles to identify the information within the document to be copied to a log sheet. Create a template with standard text as explained in Chapter 8. Insert Document Property fields to display the final character count (**ALT, I, F** > *Document Information* > *DocProperty* > *CharactersWithSpaces* > **OK**). You can delete the field before returning the file to the client. Choose any other fields that contain information you need about the document (see Chapter 11).

Create a new style with the same attributes that you will use to transcribe the document. The style itself will be the "marker" that Word uses to identify the text within the document that needs to be a part of your log sheet. To create a new style, open the **Styles** task pane (**ALT, O, S**) and click **New Style** (button located at the top of the task pane in Word 2003 and at the bottom of the task pane in Word 2007). In the **New Style** dialog box, type a name for your style (any name you choose). Select *Paragraph* style and base your style on the *Normal* style. Set any other attributes for the style as needed.

Now, go through your template file and select each area of the document that contains information you need for your log sheet and apply your new log style. The dictation file number and the character-count fields can be inserted into the document long enough to be recorded and then deleted. Be sure you use empty fields to navigate through your standard text so you don't accidentally hit the Enter key and carry your "log style" forward to a new paragraph. You only want the specific text that is part of your log sheet to carry the log-sheet style.

After transcribing the document, follow these steps to gather the information for the log sheet:

1. Lock any fields that are based on specific information within the current document (eg, the character-count field, document-name field, etc). If you copy/paste the fields to a new document (without locking or converting to text first), they will update based on information in the *log* sheet and your data will be incorrect.

2. Open the **Find** dialog box (CTRL+F).

3. Click More > Format > Styles.

4. Select your log style name.

5. In the **Find** dialog box, place a check mark at Highlight all items found in, Main document.

6. Click Find All.

7. Press Esc to close the **Find** dialog box.

8. All text within the document formatted in the designated style (ie, log style) will be selected. Press CTRL+C to copy all selected information.

9. Open a new document that will be your log sheet and paste (CTRL+V) the results.

10. Continue to paste the information from each transcribed document into the log sheet document.

11. Select the text in the log file and open the **Convert Text to Table** dialog box:

    a. Press ALT, A, V, X (either version).

    b. In Word 2003, go to Table > Convert > Text to Table.

    c. In Word 2007, go to Insert > Tables > Table > Convert Text to Table.

Choose the appropriate number of columns (eg, three columns if gathering patient name, date, and MRN) and Separate text at Paragraph marks. This will create a nice, neat table with data in columns.

Managing Macros

The following projects will help you manage and share your macros.

Seven Steps to Start a Macro

When recording a macro, start with these seven steps and continue with the steps in the specific project as described.

For Word 2003, follow these steps:

1. Open a document based on the template that you want to use to store the new macro. Open any document if you want to store the macro in the Normal.dot.

2. Turn on the Macro recorder (double-click REC on the Status Bar or select Tools > Macros > Record New Macro).

3. Name your macro (no spaces and no punctuation).

4. Type a description in the lower box (optional).

5. Open the *Store macro in* drop-down box and select a template to store the macro. The macro will be stored in the Normal.dot by default, so you only have to designate a template if you want to store it in the current document template (ie, not the Normal template).

6. Click **Keyboard** to assign a shortcut key or **Toolbar** to add an icon to a toolbar. Assign the shortcut key or toolbar button and then click **Close** on the **Customize** dialog box.

7. Proceed to record your macro.

 For Word 2007, follow these steps:

1. Open a document based on the template that you want to use to store the new macro. Open any document if you want to store the macro in the Normal.dot.

2. Turn on the Macro recorder:

   a. Click the Macro icon on the Status Bar (if the icon is not displayed, right-click the Status Bar and place a check mark next to Macro Recording) OR

   b. Go to **View** > Macros > **Macros** > Record Macro.

3. Name your macro (no spaces and no punctuation).

4. Type a description in the lower box (optional).

5. Open the *Store macro in* drop-down box and select a template to store the macro. The macro will be stored in the Normal.dotm by default, so you only have to designate a template if you want to store it in the current document template (ie, not the Normal template).

6. Click **Keyboard** to assign a shortcut key or **Button** to add an icon to the Quick Access toolbar. Assign the shortcut key or button and then click **Close** on the **Customize** dialog box.

7. Proceed to record your macro.

Copying Macros to Another Computer

You have several options for copying macros to another computer.

- If you are moving to a new computer and want to transfer all your shortcuts, macros, AutoText entries, and customizations, then copy the Normal.dot/Normal.dotm file to the new computer (see more about moving to another computer on page 476).

(Continued)

- If you want to share a single macro with another user, you will need to copy the actual code for that *one* macro from the Visual Basic Editor and paste that macro's code into the editor on the other computer (see instructions on page 470).
- The other option for sharing macros is to copy the entire module containing the macros to a template file on the destination computer using the **Organizer**.

To use the **Organizer** to copy an entire module of macros, follow these steps:

1. Place a copy of the template (`*.dot` in Word 2003 or `*.dotm` in Word 2007) that contains the macros onto removable media such as a USB thumb drive.
2. Place the removable media containing the template file in the appropriate drive of the destination computer.
3. Open the **Macro** dialog box (**ALT+F8**) and click Organizer.
4. Click Macro Project Items. Word displays the modules in the active document in the pane on the left and the modules in the Normal template in the pane on the right.
5. On the left side, click Close File, which will toggle to Open File. Click Open File (the same button). Browse to the removable media and locate the template file. Select the template file and click Open.
6. The right-hand pane will display the contents of the Normal.dot on the local computer. Now that you have both the source and the destination templates appearing in the **Organizer** panes, check to see if both modules have the same name (most likely both will be called NewMacros). Select NewMacros on the removable media and click Rename. Type a new name for the module to be copied (eg, NewMacros1). You have to rename the module to be copied because you cannot have two modules with the same name in the same template.
7. Select *NewMacros1* in the left-hand pane and click Copy. All the macros from the other computer will now be in their own module stored within the Normal template on the destination computer.
8. Close the **Organizer** dialog box and open the **Macros** dialog box (**ALT+F8**) to see a list of all macros, including those just copied.
9. If the module you just copied contains macros you do not need, simply delete them using the **Macros** dialog.

Any key assignments or toolbar buttons associated with the macros just copied will *not* copy to the new template. Use the **Customize** dialog box to assign shortcut keys or toolbar buttons to the macros just copied.

Use Macros, Styles, and AutoText Entries from Other Templates

You may find it helpful to temporarily attach a template file to a document in order to access macros, AutoText entries, or other items stored in that template file. This is an easy way to share any of these items with another user or to make items available when you are working in another template. Follow these steps:

1. Open the **Templates and Add-Ins** dialog box:

   a. Press **ALT, T, I** (either version).

   b. In Word 2003, go to Tools > Templates and Add-Ins.

   c. In Word 2007, go to **Developer** > Templates > **Document Template** . If the **Developer** tab is not displayed, go to **Office** > **Word Options** > **Popular** > *Show Developer tab in the ribbon*.

2. Click **Attach** .

3. In the **Open** dialog box, browse the file list to locate the template file containing the items you want to use.

4. Select the template file and click **Open** .

5. On the **Templates and Add-Ins** dialog box, click **OK** .

6. If you would like to use the styles that are stored in the template that is being attached, click *Automatically update document styles*. See page 244 (Word 2003) and page 256 (Word 2007) for an explanation and warning.

7. If you will use this template often, record these steps as a macro and assign a shortcut key.

8. To remove the template, open the **Templates and Add-ins** dialog box and delete the file and path name in the *Document template* box.

Note: Place the template in the **Templates** folder and macros will automatically be enabled. If you store a template outside the **Templates** folder, you will have to either manually enable macros each time you use the template or change your macro security settings. See page 71 for the location of the **Templates** folder. See page 143 (Word 2003) and 166 (Word 2007) for more explanation of the macro security feature.

Attaching a template *does* make styles available and can *potentially* affect formatting of the current document. *Adding* a template as a global template (see next project) has *no effect* on styles or formatting.

Use a Global Template to Share Macros and AutoText Entries

Some power users prefer to store macros and other items in a global template other than the Normal.dot/Normal.dotm and add the global template when they want access to items stored in this template. You can also use this method to easily share macros, custom toolbars, and menus with other users without affecting their Normal.dot/Normal.dotm file. Follow these steps:

1. Create a template file with macros and other customizations that you would like to either have available at all times or easily made available when you need them. Save the template in your **Templates** folder.

2. Open the **Templates and Add-Ins** dialog box:

   a. Press **ALT, T, I** (either version).

   b. In Word 2003, go to Tools > Templates and Add-Ins.

(Continued)

    c. In Word 2007, go to [Developer] > <u>Templates</u> > [Document Template]. If the [Developer] tab is not displayed, go to [Office] > [Word Options] > [Popular] > *Show Developer tab in the ribbon*.

3. Click [Add].

4. Select the template from the **Templates** folder.

5. The template name will appear in the list of *Global Templates and Add-ins*.

The template name will remain on the list of add-ins (even if you switch to another document or close and re-open Word) but you can remove and then replace the check mark as needed to make the template's contents available. The template will attach to all documents as long as the template is checked. *Adding* a template as a global template has *no effect* on styles or formatting. *Attaching* a template *does* make styles available and can *potentially* affect formatting (see project above).

Editing Macros and Inserting Code

If someone shares a macro with you by giving you the actual code (eg, the code is pasted into a Word document or listed on a website), you need to copy the code into the Visual Basic Editor. Follow the steps outlined below to create a new macro and insert the code.

1. Copy the text of the macro that has been shared with you *excluding* the line that contains the macro's name. The macro name always starts with the word Sub and ends with two parentheses like this: `Sub MacroName()`

2. Open the **Macros** dialog box (**ALT+F8**).

3. In the *Name* box, type a name for the macro (no spaces or punctuation).

4. Click [Create]. The Visual Basic Editor will open. Do not move the insertion point when the Editor opens. It should be located on a line just above the words `End Sub`.

```
Sub CreateNewMacro()
'
' CreateNewMacro Macro
' Macro created 7/17/2009 by Laura Bryan
'

End Sub
```

5. Immediately paste the code at the location of the insertion point.

6. Go to the File menu and choose Close and return to Word.

7. Using the **Customize** dialog box, assign a shortcut key or toolbar icon to the macro that you just added.

Notes: In the Visual Basic Editor, an apostrophe at the beginning of a line of code will cause the text that immediately follows the apostrophe to be ignored. In other words, the line will not be considered a part of the macro to be executed. Programmers call these lines comments. Comments will appear in green type.

All macros begin with the macro name that is formatted as `Sub MacroName()`. If you copy/paste a macro that contains this first line of code directly into the Editor, the Editor will automatically create a new macro using the name as indicated. Be sure that you don't paste the line of code containing the macro name into the middle of another macro in the VB editor.

All macros must end with the line `End Sub`, so be sure you insert code above that command line and be careful not to repeat the command line within a single macro.

If the macro that has been shared with you includes the macro name as the first line of the code, and you would like to use that same name, you do not have to create a new macro using the **Macros** dialog box (as described in steps 4 and 5 above). Simply open the Visual Basic Editor, press **CTRL+End** to set the insertion point at the end of the other macros, and paste the entire macro code into the Visual Basic Editor. Close the Editor and the macro will appear on your list in the **Macros** dialog box. (To open the Editor, select any macro name from the **Macros** dialog box and click **Edit**.)

Run Macros Using the Macro's Name

There are many ways to run a macro in Word. You can assign shortcut keys, toolbar buttons, or use the **Macros** dialog box. As explained here, you can write a macro that allows you to use the actual macro name to run the macro. In other words, this is a macro that allows you to run macros by typing the name of the macro you want to use. This can be helpful if you have a series of macros that have simple names but would "gobble up" a significant number of shortcut keys if you were to assign a shortcut key to each one. To create the macro, follow these steps:

1. Open the **Macros** dialog box (**ALT+F8**).
2. In the *Name* box, type a name for the macro (eg, MacroInserter).
3. Click **Create**. The Visual Basic Editor will open. Do not move the insertion point when the Editor opens. It should be located on a line just above the words `End Sub`.

```
Sub MacroInserter()
'
' MacroInserter Macro
' Macro created 7/17/2009 by Laura Bryan
'

End Sub
```

4. Insert the following code on the line just above `End Sub`. You can either type the code as it appears below, or you can copy the macro code from the Macros section on the accompanying CD. *You must type the code exactly as it appears with the spacing between words exactly as displayed here.* You do not have to worry about capitalization; the Editor will format capitalization when you end the line with the **Enter** key.

(Continued)

```
Dim·mySelection·As·String
On·Error·GoTo·ErrorOut
Selection.MoveLeft·Unit:=wdWord,·Count:=1,·Extend:=wdExtend
mySelection·=·Selection
Selection.Cut
Application.Run·MacroName:=mySelection
Exit·Sub
ErrorOut:
MsgBox·"Incorrect·Name"
```

5. Go to the File menu and choose Close and return to Word.

6. Using the **Customize** dialog box, assign a shortcut key to the macro inserter that you just created. Choose an easy-to-use shortcut key such as one of the F keys that you are not already using.

To run any macro by name, type the actual name of the macro (as it appears in the **Macros** dialog box) and press the shortcut key that you assigned to the "macro inserter" macro. For utmost efficiency, use short names for macros that you intend to run using the macro inserter.

Utilities

The following ideas and projects will help with printing, troubleshooting problems, and backing up your files.

Use Print Screen to Troubleshoot Problems

A handy feature in Windows is Print Screen. The **Print Screen** key, located in the upper-right corner of the keyboard, will take a "picture" of your monitor's display and place that image on the Windows Clipboard.

When you want to capture what is on the display, simply click **Print Screen**. It will not appear that anything has happened—the screen will not change and you won't hear a sound. After capturing the display, paste (**CTRL+V**) the image in a Word document or any other program that will accept graphics. To capture only the active window instead of the entire screen, press **ALT+Print Screen**.

Use this technique to make a record of options and settings in dialog boxes before making changes so you can return to previous settings if you do not like the results. After making choices, repeat the process to keep a permanent record of your settings in case you have to reload your computer.

Another handy way to use this feature is to capture an error message. If you are having technical problems, click **Print Screen** to capture the message box and then save and/or print. Make notes on the page about the circumstances, the date, resolution, etc. Keep these printouts in a notebook. You can also attach this document to email or fax directly to tech support. Also, you can often use the error number or other information contained in the message box to search for a solution. Type the information into the Google search box and see what you can learn.

Two-for-One Printers

If you find yourself switching print preferences, you can save yourself some time by creating "virtual" printers. Even though you only use one printer, you can install the printer twice (or three times) and each time assign a different name to the printer based on the task you would like it to perform. For example, name your "printers" Letterhead, Plain paper, Sticky paper, Labels, etc. The virtual printer is really just another printer icon that displays on the list of printers in the **Print** dialog box.

Follow these steps for Windows XP:

1. Go to Start > Settings > Printers and Faxes and click the Add a Printer icon. Step through the installation a second time but use a different name for the printer so that the name indicates its purpose (eg, HP for Letterhead).
2. After installing, return to the **Printers and Faxes** folder.
3. Select the new printer icon. Right-click and choose Printer Preferences.
4. Set the preferences that correspond to the printer icon's purpose. Click OK.
5. When printing, choose this printer icon's name in the **Print** dialog box when you want to print with the selected preferences.
6. Be sure to designate the printer with the settings that you use most often as the Default Printer. To do this, right-click the printer's icon in **Printers and Faxes** and choose Set as Default Printer.

You can also create a shortcut on your desktop for each printer. Right-click the printer icon under **Printers and Faxes** and choose Send to > Desktop (create shortcut). Open a document folder, select the documents to print, drag and drop the selected files' icons on top of the appropriate printer icon.

Follow these steps for Windows Vista:

1. Go to Start > Control Panel > Classic View > Printers > Add Printer and step through the installation a second time but change the name of the printer to a name that clearly indicates its purpose (eg, Epson for Letterhead).
2. After installing, return to the Control Panel and select the printer's new icon.
3. Right-click and choose Printer Preferences from the right-click menu.
4. Set the preferences that correspond to the printer icon's purpose. Click OK.
5. When printing, choose this printer icon's name in the **Print** dialog box when you want to print with the selected preferences.

(Continued)

6. Be sure to designate the printer with the settings you use most often as the Default Printer (right-click and choose Set as Default Printer).

You can also create a shortcut on your desktop for each printer. Right-click the printer icon under **Printers and Faxes** and choose Send to > Desktop (create shortcut). Open a document folder, select the documents to print, then drag and drop the selected files' icons on top of the appropriate printer icon.

Use the AutoCorrect Utility

Microsoft provides an AutoCorrect utility which creates a document listing all AutoCorrect entries. This document can be used to back up, view, edit, move, and restore the AutoCorrect list. This approach is different than backing up the Normal template and the AutoCorrect list, as this method creates an actual document with all entries listed in a table. This method also backs up *only* the AutoCorrect list. This may be the best approach to make extensive changes to your AutoCorrect list. Just be very careful when editing the document. The entries are listed in a table, so the safest way to remove entries is to delete the entire table row that contains the entry. You may also be able to use this document to convert AutoCorrect entries to a different format to import into a third-party text expander. Follow these steps to use this utility:

1. Locate the Support.dot file on your computer (or copy the file from the accompanying CD onto your hard drive). The path for the Support file for Word 2003 is C:\Program Files\Microsoft Office\Office11\Macros. Word 2007 does not include the Support.dot but you can still use the AutoCorrect utility from the Support.dot supplied with Word 2003. *Only use the AutoCorrect Utility in Word 2007; do not use the other two utilities included in the Word 2003 Support.dot.*

2. Open the folder containing the Support.dot and double-click the file to open. When asked, choose Enable macros. If you place this file in the **Templates** folder, the macros will automatically be enabled.

3. On the face of the document, click AutoCorrect Backup.

4. In the message box, click Backup.

5. In the **Save As** dialog box, name the file and choose a folder to store the document. You can choose any folder to store this document.

6. Click Cancel on the message box and close the document that was opened based on the Support.dot. Be sure to click Cancel, as Word will not perform any other actions with this message box open. You may have to switch back to the support document to close the message box—it may not be the top window.

7. Open the folder that you chose to store the backup document and open the document to view your list of AutoCorrect entries. The entries will be formatted as a table. Entries with the word "False" in the third column are unformatted entries.

To restore your AutoCorrect list using the backup document, follow these steps.

1. Open the Support template (as in steps 1 and 2 above).

2. On the face of the document, click AutoCorrect Backup.

3. In the message box, click [Restore].

4. In the **Open** dialog box, browse to the folder containing the backup document that you created (as above) and select the document. Click [Open].

5. The utility will begin restoring the entries, so wait until a message box appears indicating the process is complete.

6. Click [Cancel] on the message box and close the document that was opened based on the Support.dot. Be sure to click [Cancel], as Word will not perform any other actions with this message box open. You may have to switch back to the support document—it may not be the top window.

Automatically Back Up Critical Files

You can create a simple backup routine for the Normal.dot/Normal.dotm, Custom.dic, the AutoCorrect file, document templates, Building Blocks.dotx (Word 2007) and any other important file. To create a backup routine, follow these steps:

1. Open Notepad, a text editor program supplied by Windows, (**Logo+R**, Notepad, **Enter**) and type the commands into the Notepad file as explained below.

2. Follow the pattern shown below where *file name* is actually the complete path name of the file you want to back up. You can back up more than one file at a time—just give each file a separate line in the code. Each path name must be in quotation marks. Replace A with the actual drive letter (on your computer) that will contain the backup media (eg, a USB thumb drive). Note: In the image below, the dots represent a space. There should be one space following the word copy, one space before the drive letter, and one space between the back and forward slashes. See additional sample text below. You may also choose to use the text provided in the Backup document located on the accompanying CD.

```
@echo
cd\
copy·"file·name"·A:\·/y
copy·"file·name"·A:\·/y
rem·finished·copying·files
;end
```

3. Select File > Save As and change the *Save as type* to *All files* *.*. In the *Name* box, type Backup.bat (be sure to use the file extension .bat). In the *Save in* box, choose *Desktop*.

4. Close Notepad.

To run this routine, place the backup media in the appropriate drive and double-click the Backup.bat icon on your Desktop. It's that easy!

(Continued)

To back up to a different drive (for example, a backup folder on a server), replace `A:\ /y` with `H:\Backup\ /y` (where *Backup* is the name of a folder on a server, and *H* is the disk name on the server). Be sure to place a single space between the back and forward slashes.

The following is an example of the text as it might appear if you are using Word 2003 on Windows XP and backing up to a USB thumb drive designated drive E. This example will back up the Normal.dot, the Custom dictionary, and the AutoCorrect list. Remember, path names vary depending on the operating system and the version of Word. For specific information on file locations, see page 71. More sample text for automatically backing up files can be found on the accompanying CD.

```
@echo
cd\
copy "C:\Documents and Settings\Laura\Application Data\Microsoft\Proof\Custom.dic" E:\ /y
copy "C:\Documents and Settings\Laura\Application Data\Microsoft\Templates\Normal.dot" E:\ /y
copy "C:\Documents and Settings\Laura\Application Data\Microsoft\Office\MSO1033.acl" E:\ /y
rem finished copying files
;end
```

Tip: An easy way to place the file names without making a typo is to use the *Target* path in the **Shortcut Properties** dialog box. To do this, locate and/or create a shortcut icon for the files you wish to back up (see page 103). Right-click the shortcut icon and choose Properties. Select the path listed in the *Target* box and copy (CTRL+C). Paste (CTRL+V) this path name in the code as above. The *Target* path name will already include quotation marks.

Move to Another Computer

If you need to move to a new or different computer (or your hard drive has been reformatted or replaced on the same computer), you will want to reestablish your copy of Word as before. Files associated with MS Word that you will want to copy to the new computer/hard drive, referred to as the destination computer, include:

- Normal.dot/Normal.dotm
- Any document template files that you have created
- AutoCorrect list (MSO1033.acl)
- Custom dictionary (Custom.dic)
- Building Blocks.dotx (if you use Word 2007 and store AutoText entries in this file)

Be sure to close Word before copying these files. Locate the above files on your current computer and copy them to removable media. File locations for each version of Word and Windows can be found on page 71.

On the destination computer, paste these files into the appropriate folder based on the version of Word and Windows that are installed on the destination computer. If the versions of Word and Windows are not the same, use the folders that correspond *to the version that will be using the files*—not the version that originated the files. Be sure to reinstall your electronic medical spell checker also.

If you are upgrading from Word 2003 to Word 2007, see instructions below.

Moving from Word 2003 to Word 2007

If you have *upgraded* from Word 2003 to Word 2007 on the same computer, follow this first set of instructions. If you are moving your data files from Word 2003 to a new computer running Word 2007, follow the second procedure described below.

Refer to page 71 for the complete path names and instructions for locating the files and folders described here.

Upgrading to Word 2007

The following describes how Word handles your files when you upgrade to Word 2007 on a computer already running a previous version of Word:

- Normal template (Normal.dot): This file is renamed Normal11.dot (the 11 refers to Word 11, another name for Word 2003). It is stored in the **Templates** folder.
- Document templates: Any templates that you created that were stored in the **Templates** folder remain in the **Templates** folder.
- Custom dictionary (Custom.dic): A copy of this file is moved from the usual **Proof** folder to the **UProof** folder. Word 2007 uses the Custom.dic file located in the **UProof** folder.
- AutoCorrect list (MSO1033.acl) remains in the **Office** folder.

To migrate the Normal.dot file so you can access your AutoText entries, formatted AutoCorrect entries, macros, custom shortcut menus, shortcut key assignments, and other customizations, follow these steps:

1. Make sure Word is closed.
2. Open the **Templates** folder.
3. Locate the Normal.dotm and rename the file Normal.old. (The Normal.dotm file will not exist until you have opened Word 2007 and made some changes). If you cannot locate a Normal.dotm file in the **Templates** folder, proceed to the next step.
4. In the same **Templates** folder, locate the Normal11.dot file. Rename this file Normal.dot.
5. Double-click this Normal.dot file. Word will open and Compatibility Mode will be displayed in the Title bar.
6. Now close Word. If asked to save changes to the Normal template, answer **Yes**. Opening and closing Word will convert the Normal.dot to Normal.dotm. Your AutoText entries, formatted AutoCorrect entries, macros, and other customizations will be available.

(Continued)

To migrate your document templates, follow these steps:

1. Locate the **Templates** folder.

2. Right-click on a template file name and choose Open.

3. Press **F12** (Save As).

4. In the **Save As** dialog box, open the *Save as type* drop-down list and choose *Word Macro-Enabled Template (*.dotm)*.

5. Close the template file.

6. Repeat steps 2-5 for each document template.

7. The original template file (with the extension dot) will still be in the **Templates** folder. Move this file to a different folder or delete it from the **Templates** folder to avoid possible confusion from having two versions of the same template file in the same folder.

Note: Macro-enabled templates (*.dotm) are marked with a yellow exclamation mark superimposed on the template's icon.

You will want to decide how you would like to handle your AutoText entries. Word 2007 has incorporated AutoText entries into the Building Blocks feature. Building Blocks have their own storage file (Building Blocks.dotx). The AutoText entries that were contained in your previous Normal.dot file (that you converted above) are fully functional and available at all times, so you don't really have to make any decision about your entries. But if you would like to store your AutoText entries in the Building Blocks.dotx file, use the **Organizer** to move each AutoText entry from the Normal template to the Building Blocks template. See page 294 for instructions.

Moving to Word 2007

If you are moving files from a computer that was using Word 2003 (or previous version) to a computer using Word 2007, you will need to first move the necessary files to the appropriate folder and then convert the files to Word 2007's format. Copy the following files from the computer running the previous version to removable media (eg, CD, USB thumb drive):

- Normal template (Normal.dot)

- Document templates that you have created

- The Custom dictionary (Custom.dic)

- The AutoCorrect list (MSO1033.acl)

Place a copy of the MSO1033.acl file in the **Office** folder and place a copy of the Custom.dic in the **UProof** folder. These two files are compatible across all versions of Word and do not require a conversion step.

To migrate the Normal.dot file so you can access your AutoText entries, formatted AutoCorrect entries, macros, custom shortcut menus, shortcut key assignments, and other customizations, follow these steps:

1. Make sure Word is closed.

2. Open the **Templates** folder.

3. Locate the Normal.dotm and rename the file Normal.old. The Normal.dotm file will not exist until you have opened Word 2007 and made some changes. If you cannot locate a Normal.dotm file in the **Templates** folder, proceed to the next step.

4. Place a copy of your Normal.dot in the **Templates** folder.

5. Double-click the Normal.dot file. Word will open and Compatibility mode will be displayed in the T̲i̲t̲l̲e̲ bar.

6. Now close Word. If asked to save changes to the Normal template, answer `Yes`. Opening and closing Word will convert the Normal.dot to Normal.dotm. Your AutoText entries, formatted AutoCorrect entries, macros, and other customizations will now be available.

To migrate your document templates, follow these steps:

1. Place a copy of your document templates in the **Templates** folder.

2. Right-click on a template file name and choose Open.

3. Press **F12** (Save As).

4. In the **Save As** dialog box, open the *Save as type* drop-down list and choose *Word Macro-Enabled Template (*.dotm)*.

5. Close the template file.

6. Repeat steps 2–5 for each document template.

7. The original template file (with the extension dot) will still be in the **Templates** folder. Move this file to a different folder or delete it from the **Templates** folder to avoid possible confusion from having two versions of the same template file in the same folder.

Note: Macro-enabled templates (*.dotm) are marked with a yellow exclamation mark superimposed on the template's icon.

You will want to decide how you would like to handle your AutoText entries. Word 2007 has incorporated AutoText entries into the Building Blocks feature. Building Blocks have their own storage file (Building Blocks.dotx). The AutoText entries that were contained in your previous Normal.dot file (that you converted above) are fully functional and available at all times, so you don't have to make any decision about your entries. But if you would like to store your AutoText entries in the Building Blocks.dotx file, use the **Organizer** to move each AutoText entry from the Normal template to the Building Blocks template. See page 294 for instructions.

Frequently Asked Questions

AutoCorrect

Where are AutoCorrect entries stored? p. 273

How do I choose between AutoText and AutoCorrect? p. 278

Why did inserting an AutoCorrect entry insert a hard return? p. 266

Can I prevent AutoCorrect from expanding/correcting? p. 270

Can I print my AutoCorrect list? p. 474

Can I edit my AutoCorrect list? I need to add/delete a lot of entries. p. 474

How can I add "-year-old" to my AutoCorrect list? p. 267

I added an AutoCorrect entry but it does not insert with the correct formatting. p. 266

AutoText

How do I back up AutoText entries? p. 285, 296

Can I share AutoText entries? p. 285, 296

How do I choose between AutoText and AutoCorrect? p. 278

Can I print my AutoText entries? p. 285, 296 (see also Macro Sample Code on the accompanying CD)

Why does the font change when I insert an AutoText entry? Word 2003, p. 281; Word 2007, page 291.

I created an AutoText entry but I don't get the suggestion box to insert it. Word 2003, p. 286; Word 2007, page 290.

Yesterday, I created several AutoText entries, but today they are gone. p. 246 (Word 2003), 257 (Word 2007)

Backing Up

How do I back up important files? p. 71-74

Which files should I keep backed up? p. 71-72

File Management

I work in Word 2003 but my colleagues use Word 2007. What do I do when they send me files in Word 2007 format? p. 70

I work in Word 2007 but my colleagues still use Word 2003. How can I send them documents that they can use? p. 70

What is the best way to save my documents? p. 75

Where should I store my reports? p. 33 (Windows XP), 49 (Windows Vista), 150 (Word 2003), 164 (Word 2007)

Why is there an exclamation point on the template icons in Word 2007? p. 316

Formatting

How do I change the formatting of documents created in Word 2007? p. 202

How do I get rid of the extra space after the paragraphs in documents created in Word 2007? p. 202, 212

Why does my font revert back to Times New Roman? p. 205

Why does my font change in the middle of the document or at the last line of the document? p. 205

OOPS! What did I just do and how do I undo it? p. 372

How do I create a hanging indent? p. 218

I deleted some text and now my formatting has completely changed. How do I fix it? p. 222

How do I keep Word from changing "cc" to "Cc"? p. 267

How can I reveal codes? p. 127, 222

How do I get a tab stop to "stick?" p. 213

How can I set the date at the right margin? p. 215

Can I tell Word to automatically cap after a colon? p. 454

The Automatic Capitalization feature does not always work. p. 272

Word will not automatically capitalize words following a sentence ending in a digit. p. 454

Why does Word convert some fractions to single-space fractions but not all (eg, 1/4 to ¼)? p. 206

How do I format terms like H_2O and mg/mm^2? p. 206

How do I keep words from separating across a line like titles and surnames and numbers and units of measure? (nonbreaking spaces and nonbreaking hyphens). p. 208

I opened a document and the font appears huge (or too small). p. 126

There's no "white space" or "paper edges" between pages, just a line separating one page from the next. p. 127

Headers and Footers

I'm not seeing headers or footers but I know they should be there. p. 123 and 224

How do I change the header or footer on the second page of my document? p. 225 (Word 2003), 227 (Word 2007)

All of my headers and footers look the same; I need them to be different. p. 225 (Word 2003), 227 (Word 2007)

The font in the header and footer is different than the rest of the document. p. 199 (styles), 205 (default font)

Macros

How do I create a "stop" in a macro like I did in WordPerfect? p. 299

How do I back up macros? p. 71-72

Can I share macros with another person? p. 324

How do I copy macros? p. 321

Where are macros stored? p. 321

Word will not allow me to copy a macro using the Organizer. p. 468

My macro shortcut key doesn't work. p. 396

Locking Up

Word locked up and I had to shut down. Can I get my documents back? p. 75

Word locked up. What do I do now? p. 68

Why does Word ask me to save changes to the Normal template (Normal.dot) and what do I do? p. 247 (Word 2003), 257 (Word 2007)

Why do I get this error: "File in use by another user"? p. 246

Word shut down and now I have recovered documents. What do I do with the recovered documents? p. 75

Miscellaneous

OOOPS! What did I just do and how do I undo it? p. 372

Can I add numbered lines to my document? p. 210

When I try to draw a line for the doctor's signature, Word creates a line across the page. p. 157 (Word 2003), 179, 157 (Word 2007)

How can I use Word's line count without counting blank lines? p. 459

I work in Word 2007 and am sending documents to a person using Word 2003. What do I do? p. 70

Every time I press a key, more text is selected. p. 365

I have shaded boxes appearing in my document. p. 305

Suddenly I have red lines, blue text, and/or red text appearing in my document. p. 376

I will be getting a new computer. What files do I need to copy to the new computer? p. 476

Suddenly typing replaces text already typed instead of adding to the document. p. 138 (Word 2003), 169 (Word 2007)

My Page Up and Page Down keys work differently now. p. 301

Can I turn off the dots, arrows, and paragraph marks? p. 127, 222

Will others see the dots, arrows, and paragraph marks in the document? Will they print? p. 127-128

What's the best way to shortcut "-year-old"? p. 267

I'm seeing codes and "gibberish" between brackets in my documents. p. 305

Normal.dot/Normal.dotm

What is the Normal.dot/Normal.dotm? p. 235

Word asks me if I want to save changes to the Normal.dot/Normal.dotm. How do I answer? p. 247 (Word 2003), 257 (Word 2007)

Numbered Lists

When I try to type an indented numbered list, pressing the Tab key causes the text to indent further. p. 217, 219

Word automatically indents a numbered list. How do I get it back to the left margin? p. 330

How can I create a numbered list where the text lines up under text? p. 218

How do I create a sublist? p. 331

The numbered list did not start with number 1; how do I fix that? p. 333

The numbered list is not numbered correctly but I can't edit the numbers. p. 333

Shortcut Keys

How do I print a list of shortcut keys? p. 183

I pressed a shortcut key but nothing happened. p. 84

How do I remove a shortcut key assignment? p. 394 (Word 2003), 403 (Word 2007)

How do I change a shortcut key assignment? p. 394 (Word 2003), 403 (Word 2007)

Spelling and Grammar

How do I turn off spelling and grammar (ie, get rid of the red and green sawtooth lines)? p. 142 (Word 2003), 162 (Word 2007)

Word does not mark words in ALL CAPS that are misspelled. p. 142 (Word 2003), 162 (Word 2007)

What's the fastest way to check spelling? p. 354

Why does Word change the language used when spell checking? p. 359

Templates

Where are templates stored? p. 71

Can I use templates from earlier versions of Word? p. 248 (Word 2003), 258 (Word 2007)

What's the difference between a template and boilerplate? p. 128-129

Toolbars and Menus

I don't like the way the menus and toolbars are constantly changing in Word 2003. Can I change that? p. 152

Can I change the ribbon in Word 2007? p. 399

access key	A specific key that executes a command. Access keys are displayed next to the command in a small box called a KeyTip. To display access keys, press ALT.
active window	The actual part of the screen that will respond to keyboard commands. The active window is indicated by a colored Title bar.
alpha character	The first character of a file, folder, shortcut name, or item listed in a drop-down box that serves as the hot key for accessing the item.
AppData	A folder found under each user's profile in Windows Vista that stores the user's preferences, settings, and options for a variety of applications. The Office suite of applications makes extensive use of the AppData folder.
Application Data	A folder found under each user's profile in Windows XP that stores the user's preferences, settings, and options for a variety of applications. The Office suite of applications makes extensive use of the Application Data folder.
AutoCorrect	A feature in Word designed to automatically correct typographical errors and common spelling errors. Its use has been extended to changing formatting and expanding text.
AutoFormat As You Type	A feature in Word that applies formatting as you type based on contextual clues.
automatic numbered list format	A defined format that includes the list number (as a number field), an indent, and a hanging indent. It is called "automatic" because the numbering is controlled by the formatting commands and each new list number will insert automatically.
AutoText	A productivity feature built into Word for quickly inserting words, phrases, boilerplate text, graphics, and other document elements.
boilerplate	A boilerplate is a block of text that is used repeatedly.
browsing	Moving from one folder to another folder or from one website to another.
Building Blocks	A feature in Word 2007 for storing elements of a document such as boilerplate text, headers, footers, graphics, cover pages, and more.
Clipboard	A temporary "container" for information that has been copied or cut. The Clipboard is controlled by Windows.
Comments	A tool built into Word for providing feedback or for flagging text with questions.
Custom dictionary	A reference list created by the user to augment the Main dictionary. Words added to the Custom dictionary are not marked as misspelled during spell check.
Customize dialog box	A dialog box used to make changes to keyboard assignments, toolbars, and menus. Opening the dialog box also puts Word in customize mode.
Customize Keyboard dialog box	A dialog box in Word that is used to make changes to keyboard assignments.
customize mode	A state in which Word allows changes to be made to the keyboard assignments, toolbars, and menus. Opening the Customize dialog box puts Word in customize mode, which changes the way Word responds to the keyboard and mouse.
data field	A set of instructions placed at a specific point within a document that automatically carries out a specific action or function. The results of the action are positioned in the document at the point of the field.
default	Refers to setting or action that results if the user does not take an action or does not supply a preferred value.
default font	The font used by Word in all new documents unless otherwise specified. The default font is part of the Normal (paragraph) style definition.

default tab stop	A preset interval that determines how far the insertion point moves when the tab key is pressed. The initial default tab stop in Word is ½ inch.
demote	To indent a list or create a sublist. This is often used in reference to an outlined list where some items are subordinated or demoted.
Desktop	The main screen that appears after a full startup of your computer
dialog box	An element of the Windows interface that is used to give and get information. Dialog boxes use tabs, buttons, check boxes, radio buttons, lists, slide bars, text input boxes, and a variety of other methods for specifying options and settings
direct formatting	Formatting attributes applied to a paragraph that are not part of the paragraph's style definition.
Document properties	A document's metadata (data that describes data). Document properties include the document's file name, the author, the title, subject matter, statistical information, and many other types of information that describe the file.
document template	A file that is used as the basis of a new document for a given document type or report type.
document view	A way of displaying the contents of a document. The document view changes how a document appears on the screen but does not affect the way a document will print.
Documents	One of the user's personal folders created under each profile in Windows Vista. The Documents folder is the default working folder for the Office suite of applications. See also My Documents for Windows XP.
Draft view	A document view in Word 2007 that hides headers, footers, graphics (except those placed in-line with text), and other non-text elements. This view also does not show white space, page margins, or page boundaries.
electronic dictionary	A dictionary formatted electronically as opposed to being printed and bound in a book. Like a traditional dictionary, electronic dictionaries provide spelling, pronunciation, etymology, and definitions.
electronic drug reference	A drug reference stored electronically as opposed to a printed and bound book.
electronic reference	A reference (dictionary, word list, drug list, etc) that is stored electronically as opposed to printed and bound as a traditional book.
electronic spell checker	An electronic reference list to aid in spell checking a document. Spell checkers are typically sold as specialty lists such as medical and pharmaceutical terms or legal terms.
empty field	A field that does not contain field codes. Empty fields can be used to create jump points for navigating boilerplate text.
Extend mode	A feature in Word that is used to select text. Extend mode essentially "locks" the keyboard in select mode so you can use the keyboard to quickly and precisely select any amount of text.
extension	A three- or four-letter suffix that is used by Windows to identify the file type and to associate the file with a particular program.
field code	The instructions contained within a field.
field results	The information obtained based on the field instructions.
Find	A tool in MS Word for finding words, phrases, symbols, formatting marks, and styles contained within the current document.
Find and Replace	A tool in MS Word for replacing or deleting words, phrases, symbols, formatting marks, and styles.
Font dialog box	A dialog box in Word that contains formatting attributes that can be applied to characters.
formatting marks	Symbols (representing paragraphs, spaces, tabs, line and page breaks) that are displayed in the document space that aid in formatting, editing, and troubleshooting formatting problems. These marks are displayed on the screen but do not print.

Formatting toolbar	One of two main toolbars in Word 2003 that contains a collection of commonly used commands for formatting text and paragraphs.
function keys	The keys located across the top of the keyboard labeled F1 through F12.
global template	A template file with the extension dot, dotx, or dotm that stores AutoText entries, Building Blocks (Word 2007), macros, and customizations to be used across many document types. A Global template makes information available to all documents as long as it is active.
Grammar Settings dialog box	A dialog box in Word that is used to adjust the grammar checking feature. This dialog allows the user to select the grammar issues to mark and those to ignore.
Graphical User Interface (GUI)	A standardized set of graphical elements that creates a consistent, predictable, and easy-to-use working environment. The graphic elements are capable of acting as computer commands.
gridlines	Faint gray lines that display on the screen to represent the borders of tables. Gridlines can be used to manage a table when the borders themselves are hidden.
hanging indent	A format in which the first line of a paragraph is closer to the left margin compared to the second and subsequent lines of the paragraph.
header and footer	The space at the upper and lower edges of a document that typically contains the letterhead, page number, and patient demographic information. The header and footer spaces are separated from the body of the document so the text within the body of the report can be edited without affecting the placement of the text contained within the header and footer.
horizontal alignment	The setting that determines the orientation and appearance of the left and right edges of a paragraph. Alignment commands include Left, Right, Centered, and Justified.
Horizontal Ruler	A ruler that is displayed across the top of a Word document that contains formatting markers to indicate tabs, indents, and margins.
hot key	A specific key which executes a command. Virtually every command, whether listed on a menu bar, drop-down menu, submenu, shortcut menu, or dialog box, has a hot key which invokes that command when the menu or dialog box is active.
indent	(noun) The space between the margin and the edge of the text. (verb) To move text away from the right or left margin.
KeyTip	A small box displayed next to a command that gives the access key associated with the command.
line spacing	The setting that determines the amount of vertical space between lines of text within a paragraph.
Lock	A command that prevents a field from updating.
Logo key	One of the modifier keys. This key may also be referred to as the Windows key. The Logo key is marked with the Microsoft "waving" window logo; When pressed alone, the Logo key will open the Start menu; when pressed with another key, it executes a specific command.
Look Up (Research)	A feature in Office that includes a dictionary and a thesaurus as well as other resources.
macro	A feature in Word that bundles a series of commands into a single executable.
Macro Recorder	A tool in MS Word that is used to create macros.
Macros dialog box	A dialog box used to manage macros.
Main dictionary	The reference list used by the spelling and grammar feature that installs with Office. Words contained in the reference list are recognized as correctly spelled.
menu	An element of the Windows interface that contains a list of commands that are grouped by category or specific types of tasks.
modifier keys	Keys that are used to change the normal function of a key (eg, inserting the letter A versus the command Select all using CTRL+A). Modifier keys are either pressed

	simultaneously with the key they modify or they are pressed sequentially. The modifier keys include CTRL, Shift, ALT, and the Logo key.
module	A unit of storage for saving macros in MS Word. Individual macros are stored in modules, and modules are stored in templates and documents.
My Documents	A personal folder in Windows XP that is used as the default working folder for the Microsoft Office suite of programs as well as many other applications (see also Documents for Windows Vista).
navigation keys	The keyboard keys that are used to move the cursor and insertion point. Navigation keys include the arrow keys (Up, Down, Left, Right), Page up, Page down, Home, and End.
Normal style	The default paragraph style used by Word.
Normal template (Normal.dot, Normal.dotm)	The main template used by MS Word. The Normal.dot file stores the default font setting, the default paragraph style (Normal style), the default page margin settings, customized toolbars and shortcut keys, and many other preferences.
Normal view	A document view in Word 2003 that hides headers, footers, graphics (except those placed in-line with text), and other non-text elements. This view also does not show white space, page margins, or page boundaries.
object	Any distinct item on the display such as an icon, image (graphic), text, a window, or part of a window.
Office Button	The icon in the left upper corner of the Word 2007 interface that opens the main Program menu.
Office Clipboard	A "container" for temporarily storing information. The Office Clipboard works in addition to the Windows Clipboard. The Office Clipboard is managed by the Office applications (not Windows) and is capable of storing up to 24 separate items that have been copied or cut.
Options dialog box	A dialog box in Word 2003 that brings together 11 different dialog boxes covering a variety of categories. These dialog boxes contain commands for changing settings and preferences.
Organizer	A tool in MS Word for managing items stored in template files.
Paragraph dialog box	A dialog box in Word that contains commands for formatting paragraphs. Commands found in the Paragraph dialog box are associated with the paragraph mark.
paragraph mark	A formatting mark, created by pressing Enter, that represents the end of a paragraph.
path	A description of a file's location using the disk, folder, and subfolders that contain the file. Windows locates and identifies each file or folder by its unique path, also referred to as an address.
pointer	The on-screen indicator controlled by the mouse. The pointer is used to select items anywhere on the display. The pointer not only points to objects on the screen, it also gives feedback to the user to indicate the computer's mode. The mode is indicated by the shape of the pointer or by another icon attached to the pointer.
Print Layout view	A document view in Word that shows text, graphics, headers and footers, and other elements as they will appear on the printed page. Print Layout also displays white space and page boundaries.
Print Preview	A document view in Word that gives the best representation of the document as it will actually print. Use this view as a final check for margins, headers, footers, page breaks, and overall layout.
promote	To decrease the indent or to elevate the level of a sublist. Often used in reference to an outlined list.
Properties	Refers to a file's attributes or the way an object appears or behaves. See also Document Properties.
query	A word or phrase that best describes the information you are searching for.

Quick Access toolbar	A toolbar that sits alongside the ribbon in Office 2007. Initially, the toolbar only contains icons for Save, Undo, and Redo, but you can add other commands that you use often.
Quick Launch bar	Part of the Taskbar that sits between the Start button and the Taskbar buttons. The Quick Launch bar contains icons that respond to a single click so you can use this area to access frequently-used items.
RAM (random access memory)	A form of memory that stores information while it is in use. When you open a file, Windows retrieves information about the file and the program used to work with the file and moves a copy of the information to RAM. As long as you are working on the file (ie, the file is open), you are actually working on the data that has been copied to RAM.
read-only	A file attribute that prevents a file from being changed. A read-only file can be opened, but it cannot be edited (ie, you can open the file but you cannot save any changes to the file).
Redo	A command that reverses the Undo command.
Replace text	The text that is typed into the Replace text box in the Find and Replace dialog box.
Reveal Formatting task pane	A task pane in Word that displays formatting information based on the current location of the insertion point.
Run	The command for "playing back" a macro.
Save	A Windows command that causes information to be written to the hard drive for storage and safekeeping. When a file is first created, the Save command opens the Save As dialog box, which allows you to name the file and designate a place to store the file.
Save As	A command in Windows that allows you to save a copy of the file that is currently open using a different file name or a different file location.
Search	A Windows feature that searches your computer for files and folders based on whatever information you can provide.
search mode	An approach to searching an electronic reference. Search modes typically include Browse Index and Search Index (also called Search on Headword or Search on Entry).
section break	The point at which one section ends and another section begins within a Word document. Sections divide documents into parts that can be managed individually. Sections can have their own margins, headers, footers, page sizes, and orientations.
select	To distinguish the object on the screen from everything around it in order to perform an action on that particular item.
Send To	A submenu that is available when you right-click a file or folder. This particular menu can be used to move or copy a file, attach a file to an email message, or to create a shortcut icon.
set tab	A specific tab setting that stabilizes column formatting and also guides the indent commands. Paragraphs with set tabs will have tab indicators displayed on the Horizontal Ruler.
short form	An abbreviation that expands into a word, phrase, paragraph, or boilerplate.
shortcut icon	An icon that takes you directly to the item it represents, called the target. Since shortcut icons are links (not the actual file), you can create as many as you like, rename them as you please, and place them wherever you want.
shortcut key	A key sequence that executes a command and functions as if you clicked an icon or menu command using the mouse.
shortcut menu	A menu containing helpful commands that displays when you right-click an object. Every object displayed in the Windows interface—icons, shortcut icons, files, folders, toolbars, text, graphics, tables, disks, drives, and printers—has a shortcut menu associated with it.
source	The information referenced by a field.

Spelling and Grammar dialog box	A dialog box in Word for spell checking a document and correcting grammar errors.
Spelling and Grammar shortcut menu	A shortcut menu in Word for correcting spelling and grammar errors.
standard text	Text that appears in most, if not all, documents of a given report type.
Standard toolbar	One of two main toolbars in Word 2003.
Start menu	The main menu in the Windows operating system and the gateway to the files and programs installed on your computer.
Status Bar	The bar that creates the lower border of a Word window. The Status Bar displays information related to the page count, cursor location, and the current mode. In addition to giving information, all areas of the Status Bar are active and will respond to mouse clicks.
style	A defined set of formatting commands that simplify formatting tasks by bundling formatting attributes into a single definition, allowing you to apply several formatting commands to a paragraph or a word in one step.
sublist	A list within a list.
task pane	An element of the Windows interface that combines features of drop-down menus and dialog boxes. Task panes remain open while you continue to work within the window or document.
Taskbar	The bar that sits along the bottom edge of the Desktop. The Taskbar acts as the command and control center for the activities on your computer.
template	A file type used by Word to store settings, standard text, macros, shortcut key assignments, and other customizations. A template is used to create new documents, and information stored in the template determines how new documents based on the template appear. Templates have the extension dot (dotx and dotm in Word 2007).
Templates folder	The folder that stores the Normal.dot/Normal.dotm and other template files.
text expander	A utility that allows you to type a short form that inserts text into the document. See also third-party text expander.
third-party text expander	A separate software program that runs in conjunction with your word processor. These programs store short forms that insert the corresponding word or phrase directly into the document when the short form is typed.
toggle key	A type of command that either alternates between "on" and "off" (think of a light switch), or cycles through a series of related commands or a collection of buttons.
Undo	A command for reversing the previous action(s). The command works in Windows and in Office and includes actions taken deliberately by the user or any of the automatic actions by Word (eg, changes made by the AutoFormat As You Type feature).
universal keys	Shortcut keys assigned by Windows that work in most, if not all, circumstances.
unlinking	To sever the relationship between a field and its source. A field result will become regular text when it is unlinked from the source and cannot be updated.
Update	A command that causes a field to refer back to the source of the information and make necessary changes to the results.
view	The way you see information. The view can be changed to hide or display information or rearrange information without deleting or losing information.
Visual Basic for Applications (VBA)	The programming code (programming language) used by Word to record and execute macros.
white space	The space on the page between the first and last line of text and the top and bottom edge of the page. The white space is always hidden in Normal/Draft view, but is optional in Print Layout view.

Windows Explorer	An application provided by Windows that is used to see the hierarchy of folders on your computer and to manage your file system. Use Windows Explorer to copy, delete, move, rename, and create files and folders.
With text	The text that is typed into the With text box in the AutoCorrect dialog box.
Word Options	A set of dialog boxes in Word 2007 for setting preferences and options.
zoom	A feature in Windows and many other applications that causes the document to appear larger or smaller on the display but does not affect the way the document prints.